The Herbal Apprentice: Plant Medicine and The Human Being.

Abrah Arneson Cht RH

What is life?
It is a flash of a firefly.in the night. It is the breath of a buffalo in the winter time. It is the little shadow which runs across the grass and loses itself in the Sunset.
- Blackfoot 1890 on his deathbed.

CONTENTS

Dear Reader;

The Herbal Apprentice: Plant Medicine and The Human Being will help you think like a herbalist.

There was a time when a herbalist planted a garden and wandered her local woods and meadows to pick her medicine. Her apothecary, based on her knowledge of local herbs, contained anywhere between 50 to 150 plants. Each plant she knew intimately from stories passed on by her mentors. She was introduced to the plant's character and habits by observing their growth in her garden and the wild. Birds, wild animals and her familiars taught her about the healing plants as she watched the animals heal themselves with berries, grasses, barks and roots. She knew the scent a healing plant left on her hands after grinding it and the texture each plant created in her mouth as she slowly chewed on a leaf to determine if it was time to pick its medicine. She knew her plants from the way they interacted with vinegar, brandy or milk. Her knowledge of medicinal plants arrived each time she used them to help others in their birthing, dying and all of life's bumps and knocks in between.

In the modern world, it is impossible for a herbalist to know everything about her plants. To begin, it is difficult for many people to find hands on training with the plants that grow in backyards or local woods. Training in plant medicine is academic and the person offering advice on the use of the plant often does not know the plant only flowers in moon light, or that the flowers leave behind a red stain on finger tips when the medicine is ready to harvest. How could the herbalist know when the plants she uses are grown on other continents, far from home and arrive encapsulated ready to use?

Today some herbalists explain plant medicine using clinical studies and pharmacology. Others attempt to know a plant's medicine by connecting with the plant's spirit. There are books of folk tales offering advise on the use of plants for healing, scientific journals reporting the effects of plants on rats or descriptions of what happens when phytochemicals interact with liver cells in petri dishes. Herbalists study ancient treatises on plant medicine from China, India, and Europe in hopes of uncovering some new/old methods of applying plant medicine to disease. And a journey beyond the intellect to a spiritual knowing of plant medicine by imbuing hallucinogens from the Amazon or a fungus growing on old growth forest floors can also reveal previously unknown uses for plant medicine. Herbalists have been known to undertake such adventures. The simplicity of wandering in the woods and collecting a basket of leaves to steep in a jar with brandy is almost a lost art in this insanely complex world of plant medicine.

At times being a herbalist means you are barraged with conflicting information, opinions and ideas about plant medicine. Everyone from the local shaman to the university researcher to your client that tells you she has been miraculously cured by yarrow has some idea about plant medicine without ever seeing the living plant!

Sometimes it is even difficult to know what to call medicine made from plants. Those of a scientific bend prefer phytotherapy, others who sell pre-packaged plant medicine use the term botanicals, some call it herbology, while other describe their remedies as plant medicine.

In my practice I have learned that everyone is right and everyone is wrong when it comes to plant medicine and its effect on the human body. (Or, should I say, the human body's effect on plant medicine.) It is my experience that to be skilled in plant medicine is not based on what you know (although this important) but how you think. To practice herbal medicine successfully, you need to think like a herbalist.

A good herbalist understands that the body/mind is as much part of nature as the plant medicines she uses. This knowledge is the foundation of the practice of herbal medicine. When the bedrock of herbalist's appreciation of plant medicine is based on the interdependence of life on this planet, all the conflicting views and methods of using plant medicine in the modern world are either easily incorporated into her practice or dismissed for their lack of deeper understanding, such as a plant's effect on a rat's liver.

Herbalists, or those who think like a herbalist, are in the unique position to help humanity to bridge the gap between a seemingly isolated singular existence and the dynamic weaving of life. The foundation of herbal medicine is the authentic understanding of the interdependence of life. With feet firmly planted in the awareness of interdependence, herbalists offer life-affirming medicine. *The Herbal Apprentice: Plant Medicine and The Human Being* unearths the alliance between the plant world and the human body. It is my wish that this book will be a healing balm for all of you who have lost faith in a reductionist understanding of both plant medicine and the human being, and seek knowledge of medicine based on a complex, dancing web of life.

Plant medicine is based on the profoundly dynamic ancient relationship between plants and the human being. Plant medicine is more than understanding the chemistry of a plant, just as the kidney is more than a filtration system. The study of plant medicine is vast and complex, and yet simple and heartfelt. The practice of plant medicine is for the intellectually curious, those guided by sudden intuitive illuminations and the careful of heart.

In this time of strident restrictions on the making of plant medicine, the herbalists' art of preparing medicine from local plants is being tossed aside for standardized patent medicine manufactured in industrialized settings. It is not just the knowledge of plants and simple methods of extracting their medicine that is being lost, but even more important, we are losing the ability to think like herbalists. Academic training encourages memorization of abstract chemical diagrams, ignoring the traditional gift of reading a plant's medicine with the senses and teaching trust in an intuitive analysis of a plant while discovering her heartfelt, healthful connect to nature.

Over twenty years ago I was sitting in a Buddhist Temple listening to my teacher talk about the future. He said that when people begin to commit suicide in the streets, we would have reached the point of no return in the destruction of the life-sustaining environment this planet offers to an approximate 8,700,000 species (not including bacteria and viruses). In 1996 the first suicide bomber exploded in a café, and by 2001 there were 81 individuals who strapped bombs to their bodies and blew themselves up in a public setting. In 2005 there were 460. It seems each year since that time there have been more tsunamis, hurricanes, tornadoes, and earthquakes, each one more destructive than its predecessors. This past weekend there was even an earthquake that woke people in their beds about a 45-minute drive from my home. I live in a place where the last earthquake occurred beyond memory.

Twenty years ago my teacher asked his students, "What are you going to do to help sustain life through the impending dramatic changes that are going to take place?" I decided to become a herbalist who could walk through the woods and discover plant medicine. Once I had a basic understanding of plant medicine I would share what I learned to the best of my ability.

There are many herbalists who are much more skilled than I am. I encourage anyone interested in becoming a herbalist to seek out many teachers--both well renowned and the not so well known. *The Herbal Apprentice* is the knowledge I have gathered about plant medicine to this point. I offer it to support individuals who want to help others and this beautiful planet during this intense time of transformation.

Like a child, a book is not grown in isolation. My heart is filled with gratitude to my two teachers, who have since both passed on, Namgyal Rinpoche and Cecilie Kwiat. They shook me awake from a self-destructive hedonistic dream and insisted I do more with my life than write bad poetry and get high. This book is dedicated to these two inspiring, unruly, wise, brave, and compassionate souls.

All of my clients and those who have joined me on the journey of discovering the rich world of plant medicine are part of this book. Without them I would not have the courage to ask hard questions or the discipline required to learn and write.

I want to thank my friends Aly Seymour and Dionne Jennings who encouraged me to continue writing while offering valuable critical analysis of *The Herbal Apprentice*.

To my husband, Mark Arneson: well, let's just say, a man is either born to be a herbalist's husband or he isn't. I thank you for your tenderness, sweet kindness and wisdom. It is rather convenient that you are also a photographer who enjoys making pictures of plants. Thank you for your photographs.

And to herbalist and photographer Rosalee de la Forêt, your photographs have inspired me since the first day I saw them. Thank you for bringing your eye for beauty to *The Herbal Apprentice*.

Finally, I must not forget the plants. I am always inspired by the patience of the plant world. It seems no matter how much stumble, I am always caught by Earth's Blanket, the green plants. I thank the green ones for their friendship and their generous teaching.

May the plant world's green blessings shine, Abrah

It's All About the Environment

From Earth with Love

I remember walking across a vast meadow between two small mountains in the Yukon. The month is June. The meadow welcomed the midnight sun with an ecstatic dance of wild rose, fireweed, flax and the pungent scent of sage. Bird song from groves of stunted poplars gladdened the morning while gophers whistled and ran for cover. Overhead, hawks circled. For all its beauty, life seemed chancier in the wilderness.

During my first days in the immense landscapes of the Yukon, I was frightened. There are no fences in the Yukon dividing the land into yours and mine. I was raised on land tamed by the straight lines of sidewalks where I did not walk on another's lawn or through a flowerbed. The Yukon, with few people and even fewer highways, is fiercely wild and its lack of predictability made me edgy.

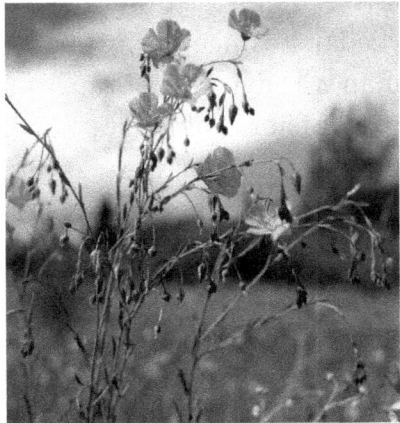

Flax   Mark Arneson

1

One afternoon, lying in on my back, amongst the blue of flax flowers competing with the blue of sky for brilliance, I let go. The warmth of the earth held me.

My bones are made with minerals harvested from Earth by green plants. My blood runs with water drawn from deep underground rivers. My cells float in an ocean contained by skin. The wind, causing me to pull the collar of my coat closer, is my breath. When the sun rises I wake from sleep. At night I dream under the moon. Every day I am renewed with blueberries, apples and sun-kissed oranges.

For years, I sought the place where I felt I belonged. I remember an elderly German woman, who ran from the bombing of Berlin and the shame of the holocaust telling me, "Eventually I stopped long enough to discover I am a citizen of the Earth. I belong everywhere."

Now, after I have laid amongst the flax flowers in that Yukon meadow, played in the cold waves on the far west coast of Canada, lived in a tree house among the green giants of Sumatra, thirsted in the desert, and held smooth river stones in my hand, I understand I belong here. I am Earth.

I was thinking the other day about a woman I cared for when I worked in hospice caring for the dying. The I was thinking of woman was dying of a brain tumour. The tumour pressed in on the part of her brain that controlled her appetite. Her brain continually told her she was hungry. All day and night she ate: watermelon, lemon tarts, hamburgers, and olives, anything she could get her hands on. The food she loved the most was popcorn, lightly tossed with butter. She devoured it by the fistful.

Her best friend was angry. With a bitter voice, she complained, "She used to take such good care of herself. She read all those alternative health books and took all those vitamins and herbs. She followed her diet (prescribed by a nation-wide weight loss program) religiously. A half-cup of popcorn without butter once a week was all she ever ate. She looked fabulous. She is too young to be here and eating through her last days."

At the time I was in herb school. The friend's lament made me consider deeply my studies in herbal medicine. Surfing the internet it is not hard to find miraculous claims about plant medicine. So what is the truth?

Perhaps the truth was found lying on my back while the flax flowers danced.

We are earth; we are not separate from her. All we have comes from the earth. This includes bulldozers, skyscrapers, nuclear bombs, and cell phones, pharmaceutical and herbal medicine. Nothing is separate in this vast matrix of life called earth. Every living being belongs here. Knowing this is enough. Being here is enough. This understanding brings contentment. Contentment creates health.

When some inner belief tells us we have to be more, we deny the rich heritage of belonging to this great planet. Trying to do more, be more, have more, we lose our ground. When we grasping for answers that to make everything right, herbs that to fix imperfections, and affirmations to change who we are, we lose connection to what is right, what does not need to be fixed and the marvellous miracle of who we are. We lose sight of the incredible beauty and power of life on this planet that cannot be separated from the very essence of our being.

The woman I cared for at the hospice loved popcorn lightly tossed with butter. Long before the tumour formed, some inner voice inside did not allow her the simple pleasure of a full bowl of popcorn. Some belief told her she had to be as thin as she was when she was 18, before her babies, if she was to have the right to be loved. I do not mean loved by others, but by herself. She took her herbs and vitamins and ate all the "right" foods, not because she loved life, but because she did not feel right in her life. Somewhere along the way, she had lost sight of her connection to earth and her right to be here now.

A wise person once told me, "Everything you put in your mouth is made by sunlight and sparkling waters. It comes from tender seeds waking in rich soil under the caress of moonlight. Every mouthful of food is a testament to the nurturing provided by generations of mothers and fathers, farmers, and any person who has ever loved another enough to offer a carefully prepared meal." This person went on to say, "Food, medicine, clothing, housing; everything is created from love's generous nature. This planet Earth is love."

So what is the truth of herbs and their ability to create miraculous cures? I know this is cliché but "every day is a miracle." Live it. If you are ill use the best medicine you can find. That medicine may be a walk in a forest, sleep, water, a good talk, plants, or a pill, or perhaps a little bit of everything. Do not grasp medicine with fear; accept it because medicine comes by way of love.

The Foundation of Herbal Medicine (Besides Plants)

The greatest challenge in developing a well-established foundation for the practice of herbal medicine is arriving at the understanding that herbal medicine does not treat illness. Traditional practices of herbal medicine seek to shift the environment of the body/mind to create a terrain where disease cannot thrive.

The body/mind matrix continually seeks balance. Physiologists call this lively body/mind activity homeostasis. Holistic practitioners define homeostasis as the body's intrinsic ability to seek balance. Homeostasis is healing from within. As the body/mind regains balance, illness has only one option to cease its activity.

The journey to balance is one of hills and valleys. Rarely is healing a one-time event. Commonly the process of healing is compared to an onion. Each layer of the onion represents a layer of ill health, whether it is of the mind, body or both. A skilled herbalist assists the person in peeling back one layer at a time, all the while encouraging trust in the intrinsic wisdom of the mind/body. When a steady confidence in the mind/body's healing ability has developed, balance can truly be restored.

In this chapter we will begin to explore how to read a body's state of balance using the language of traditional herbalists. We will start this journey with a look at the how we arrived at the current condition of the orthodox medical system. We will cross-oceans to explore the language of herbalists in China and India. From there we will voyage back in time to the roots of western medicine and explore the healing methodology of the ancient Greeks.

How We Arrived At This Point

I will never forget a piece of wisdom I received in 1967; on the first day I learned to clone stem cells in graduate school. It took me decades to realize how profound this seemingly simple piece of wisdom was for my work and life. My professor, mentor and consummate scientist, Irv Konigsberg was one of the first cell biologists to master the art of cloning stem cells. He told me that when the cultured cells you are studying are ailing, you look first to the cell's environment, not to the cell itself for the cause....cell biologists would have done well to post, "It's the environment stupid," over our desks... - The Biology of Belief- Bruce Lipton.

Orthodox western medicine does not support the body as it realigns itself in each moment of seeking health. Western medicine uses reductionist methods, either to treat disease or the symptoms of disease. It is important to note that many of the healing processes the body uses to regain balance, such as fever and inflammation, are treated as diseases in western medicine.

Medical doctors have been hung up on reductionist medicine for approximately 150 years, since Louis Pasteur proposed The Germ Theory.

In the 1870's an epidemic among silk worms threatened to destroy France's thriving silk industry. Louis Pasteur, a chemist and microbiologist, saved the day when he discovered the silk worms fell prey to the mysterious disease only in overcrowded conditions. Healthy silk worms were separated from sick ones and the spread of disease stopped.

When in 1879 an anthrax epidemic swept through France killing many sheep, the French government asked Louis Pasteur to rescue the sheep industry.

Pasteur discovered that *Anthrax bacillus* was present in the dead sheep, and concluded that it was the anthrax killing the sheep. Pasteur went on to develop a vaccine against the anthrax and inoculated a number of sheep. The vaccinated sheep lived even when exposed to infected animals. From this research, Pasteur was a proponent of the Germ Theory/credited with proving and promoting the Germ Theory : the belief that infectious disease is caused by micro-organisms within the body, and to this day the short term economics of the Germ Theory are preferred by those of limited vision: killing the pathogen is cheaper than providing healthy living environments.

During Pasteur's time medical professionals were losing a desperate battle against infectious disease. Over-crowded cities and poor sanitation were killing thousands across Europe. Doctors overwhelmed by infectious disease grasped at The

Germ Theory as the absolute truth. This led to significant shifts in the medical profession's treatment of disease and the layperson's understanding of illness and their body. Two examples are:

1. The conviction that poisoning a pathogen results in a cure. This belief has led to the development of pesticides, antibiotics and numerous vaccines. In the past two decades we have seen bacteria and viruses mutate, defending themselves against these poisons. The use of pesticides has led to massive factory farms for both plant and animal foods. Chemical farming practices have resulted in dead soil and nutrient deficient food. With the introduction of so many chemical poisons into the environment rates of cancer, autoimmune diseases and allergies are on the rise. There are now serious challenges to the belief that poison creates health with the rise of antibiotic resistant bacteria, water replete with synthetic hormones, degraded soil, and etc.

2. Over the last century, diagnosis and treatment of disease has become completely reliant on reductionist principals. No longer is the whole body considered when assessing health or illness. The belief that microorganisms are the cause of disease has led to the manipulation of minute biochemical processes within the body. It is commonly believed that hormones lead to health challenges in women and men, renegade cells cause cancer, chemical messengers triggering an immune response are responsible for autoimmune diseases, and an imbalance in neurotransmitters are responsible for a person's unhappiness. Rarely is the environment, whether within or outside the individual, assessed. The body's ability to heal itself is dismissed.

The Germ Theory and the rise of reductionist medicine have led to the superstitious belief that the body's response to illness is illness itself. Many now believe that the body is the cause of the illness.

In the late 1800s not everyone was convinced that Pasteur's Germ Theory was the ultimate truth. Florence Nightingale, while nursing fallen soldiers in over-crowded hospital wards wrote:

"The specific disease doctrine is a grand refuge of weak, uncultured, unstable minds, such as now rule the medical profession. There are no specific diseases; there are specific disease conditions."

Charles Bernard, a contemporary and foe of Pasteur, vigorously challenged The Germ Theory. He said repeatedly that it was an acidic environment within the body that supported the growth of bacteria and viruses. He believed an alkaline environment within the body was the key to preventing disease.

Even Pasteur questions his own trademark theory that brought him fame and wealth. On his death bed, Pasteur recanted his theory when he exclaimed, "Bernard is right. The pathogen is nothing. The terrain is everything."

Herbal medicine treats the terrain.

The Terrain: a tract of country considered with regards to its natural features.

Alkalizing herbs:
Many tonic herbs are known for their alkalizing nature. A simple tea made with one or a combination of these herbs will help alkalize your body. This is a great place to start any herbal treatment. These herbs include:
Nettles (Uticaria dioica)
Alfalfa (Medicago sativa)
Chickweed (Stellaria medica)
Rosehips (Rosa acicularis)
Dandelion leaf (Taraxacum officinalis folia)
Raspberry leaf (Rubus idaeus)
This is list is far from comprehensive.

Having understood that the herbalist treats the environment of the body (not only the disease or symptoms of disease) it is necessary to consider what the terrain is and learn a language to navigate it.

The Language of Traditional Healing Systems

There was a time when a healer, no matter their tradition, prepared herbal medicine based on the firm understanding that the body/mind is not separate from the earth. The language of the ancient healing systems from China, India, the Middle East, Europe and North America reflect the intimate relationship between the Earth and the health of the body/mind. This is the language of the elements.

Around the world healers talk about hot or cold (fire), dry or wet (water), vibration (air/wind) and solid (earth) in terms of illness, plant remedies and health. Different traditions have variations of the elements, some combine them, and others have added other substances the earth produces, but the basic language of healing returns to the earth and her elements.

The Elements and Healing Traditions from around the World

Ayurvedic Medicine

The essence of all beings is Earth. The essence of the Earth is Water. The essence of Water is plants. The essence of plants is the human being.   *Chandogya Upanishad I.12*

Approximately 6,000 years ago the teachings of ancient healers living in what we now call India was recorded in a philosophical text called The Rig Veda. Over time, these teaching became known as Ayurvedic medicine. The word Ayurvedic comes from the ancient Sanskrit language: "ayu" meaning life, and "vedic" meaning knowledge.

During ancient times, before technology gripped the imagination of healers, Ayurvedic herbalists sought understanding of health and illness directly from nature and her many faces. Ayurvedic medicine is founded on nature's eternal dance of balance: day becoming night, night becoming day, the moon following the sun, plants flowering after rain, and withering during the dry season.

The Ayurvedic practioner offers herbs with the intention of creating harmony between the individual and nature. As nature continually seeks balance, once the individual is aligned with nature's harmony, health of body/mind will follow as naturally as spring follows winter. The steps of nature's dance are the flow of the elements. In Ayurvedic medicine there are five elements.

The Five Elements of Ayurvedic Medicine:

The first element, ether, arises from the consciousness that pervades all life, animals, plant and mineral. This cosmic consciousness presents as clarity and manifests in matter as ether. Ether can be defined as the subtle essence of life. In a plant, ether is dominant in the fruit.

The second element, fire, arises from energy. It is measured as the degree of warmth that pervades life and manifests in matter as radiant energy. In plants, it is dominate in the flower. A plant's temperature is a measure of the fire element's presence and will determine how the herbalist uses it.

The third element, earth, arises from inertia. In matter, the earth element manifests as solidity. For example, a diamond contains higher levels of earth than a feather. In plants, the earth element is dominant in its roots. Herbalists often describe the taste of roots as earthy.

The fourth element, air, arises from the mingling of clarity of consciousness and energy called ether. It manifests in matter as gas. In plants the air element is associated with leaves that tremble and sway in the slightest breeze.

The fifth element, water, arises from energy trapped in inertia. In matter it reveals itself as liquid. The plant's stem, the tube where sap flows to nourish parts of the plant, is associated with the water element. Considering the body's relationship to moisture is essential in understanding the overall health of the body. The water element carries all nutrients to the body's cells while removing waste.

Ayurvedic medicine combines the elements into three dosas: Vata, Pitta and Kapha. Each dosa describes the predominating flow of the elements within an individual's mind/body continuum. An individual's dosa can all be called his constitution. Ayurvedic herbalists assesses a client's constitution before offering herbs to be sure their medicine supports the natural balance of the body.

The Three Dosha

The Vata constitution is a mingling of the elements air and ether. These individuals tend to live with their heads in the clouds and their feet not so firmly planted in the earth. As the air dries up moisture lying stagnant on the earth, Vata types tend towards dryness. Lacking earth, they can be deficient in minerals, often suffering with osteoporosis as they age. Herbs offering nourishment, warmth and soothing moisture bring their constitution into balance with nature.

The Pitta constitution is dominant in the fire element with a dash of water element. These individuals are on the go. Movement is essential for their well being. Their fiery nature

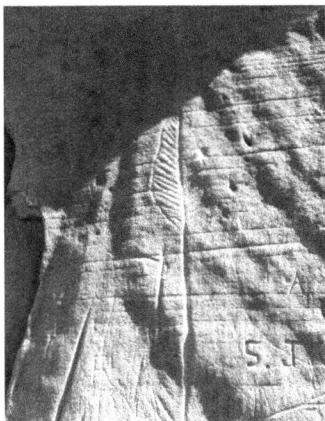

The Earth Element contains the records of this planet, if not the universe. Petroglyphs like the ones found at Writing On Stone Provincial Park, Alberta are only a hint of the many people and cultures who have been nourished by this planet. Meditations on the earth element reveals one's ancestors as well as the potential of your life.

loves adrenaline. Cooling, calming herbs are essential to their well being.

The Kapha constitution is a mix of the elements of water and earth. This individual's motto is: one must not be too hasty. They are the salt of the earth. When having fallen out of balance

Tonic Herbs for Each Dosha
Vata - Wild Oat Seed (Avena sativa)
A tincture made with fresh oat seeds is a perfect tonic for those with a Vata constitution. It soothes the nervous system and is strongly nourishing.
Pitta - Alfalfa (Medicago sativa)
Alfalfa's high mineral content supplies the extra nourishment the Pitta type needs, keeping their active body alkaline and clearing the extra metabolic waste created by adrenaline surges.
Kapha - Nettles
There is an old saying: nettles get the body moving. This is why it is part of a spring cleanse after a winter on the couch. Nettle has a warm and drying character that keeps the water flowing in sluggish Kapha.

their body/mind becomes cool and sluggish. An herbalist offers the Kapha spicy herbs to dry up the stagnant waters.

The following chart outlines the qualities of each dosa.

Feature	Vata (Air and Ether)	Pitta (Fire and Water)	Kapha (Earth and Water)
Frame	Thin	Medium	Thick
Appetite	Variable, low	Good, excessive	Slow but steady
Health challenges	Nervous disorders, pain	Heat, infection and inflammation	Excess water and mucous

Bowel movements	Dry, hard, constipated	Soft, oily, loose	Thick, slow, oily, heavy
Physical activity	Varies	Moderate	Lethargic
Mind activity	Restless, curious, active	Aggressive and intelligent	Calm, slow and receptive
Emotional challenges	Anxiety and fear	Aggressiveness and jealousy	Greedy and attached
Pulse	Thready, feeble, moves like a snake	Moderate, jumps like a frog	Broad and slow, moves like a swan
Memory	Short term good	Sharp	Slow but does not forget
Quality of herbs offered	Nourishing, warming, moist	Cooling and calming	Warming and drying

Traditional Chinese Medicine (TCM)

"Heaven has four seasons and five elements to allow cultivation, growth, harvesting and storing. It produces cold, heat, drought, humidity and wind. Man has five vital organs that transform the five influences to engender happiness, anger, vexation, sadness and fear." Yellow Emperor's Classic of Internal Medicine 4000 to 6000 years ago The Story of the Rainmaker

Dr. Carl Jung, an eclectic, groundbreaking psychiatrist who sought to understand the mind through the study of both science and the mystical arts practiced by cultures throughout the world, enjoyed telling this short story about balance. It very much underlines an herbalist's use of herbs within Traditional Chinese Medicine. It is a story to consider when harvesting plants, making medicine, listening to a client and creating their formula. This story comes from the Taoist tradition in China.

There was a great drought; for months there had not been a drop of rain and the situation became catastrophic. Finally some said: "We will fetch the rain maker." And from another province a dried up old man appeared. The only thing he asked for was a quiet little house somewhere, and there he locked himself in for three days. On the fourth day clouds gathered and there was a great snowstorm at a time of year when no snow was expected, an unusual amount, and the town was so full of rumours about the rain maker that my friend went to ask the man how he did it. In true European fashion he said, "They call you the rain maker, will you tell me how you made the snow?" And the little Chinaman said, "I did not make the snow, I am not responsible." "But what have you done for three days?" "Oh, I can explain that. I come from another country where things are in order. Here they are out of order, they are not as they should be by the ordnance of heaven. Therefore the whole country is not in Tao, and I am also not in the natural order of things because I am in a disordered country. So I had to wait three days until I was back in Tao, and then naturally the rain came."

From C.G. Jung on Nature, Technology and Modern Life.

Like herbalists in India, Chinese herbalists turn to nature for inspiration and guidance when seeking insight into the art of healing. They too have a profound understanding of the ever-flowing dance of nature. This flow, the laws of the dance, is called the Tao. The yin/yang symbol is used to elegantly convey the balance of opposites contained by life, the harmony within the Tao. This symbol defines health through the continually changing needs of an individual living in alignment with nature. A person who sleeps during the dark of night and is active during the light of day promotes health through living in harmony with nature's ever changing rhythms.

Again, like the Indian herbalists, Chinese herbalists observe nature's expression of the elements. The interactions between the elements are used as metaphors to describe the flow of day into night, winter into spring, childhood to old age, health into illness and the passage back to health. These observations have led Chinese healers to develop a set of elements specific to their understandings and sensibilities: wood, fire, earth, water and metal.

I was not trained in Traditional Chinese Medicine, so in some ways I feel like I am peering into mysteries of this ancient healing tradition from the outside. I do not particularly use the five element system for understanding plants and their medicine, but I certainly find it useful for some mind/body challenges my clients struggle with.

The first element is wood. When the wood is balanced in an individual, she is compared to a young sapling, open to possibility. She is creative in her activity and thoughts. Wood unbalanced is withered growth, stuck, frustrated, and lacking creativity.

Because wood breaks through earth, when earth is excessive, wood brings it balance. Keep this in mind when we explore the virtues of earth. On the other hand, metal controls the overgrowth of wood. Metal cuts wood. An individual who is unable to prune down his activities suffers with an overgrowth of wood. The metal axe cuts through dense and thick overgrowth like mental clarity can sort out a scrambled mind.

The second element is fire. Fire, as in Ayurvedic medicine, is the warmth of life. The sun, the source of the fire, brings life to our beautiful planet. In balance the fire element gives us the ability to use our life energy with skill and compassion. The fire element brings to life a joyful heart. It is easy for us to give and receive.

When the fire element is deficient one feels cold and alone in life. To replenish life's fire the wood element is nurtured. Remember the wood element brings creativity and new life. This relationship between a low fire remedied by the wood element is synonymous with the seasonal change of winter into spring. When the fire element is weak, creativity and newness is offered just as the first green leaves of spring gladdens the heart.

When the fire element burns out of control, it is easy to overindulge and a feeling of entitlement dominates restraint. Water extinguishes a raging fire. Water is likened to the cooling nature of compassion. A compassionate heart cannot place her own needs above another.

The third element is earth. A person with balanced earth is self-

Tibetan Medicine

Tibetan medicine is considered to be a blend of TCM and Ayurvedic medicine. Tibetan doctors have a unique way of classifying illness into four categories.

Passing illnesses. This category includes: colds and flus. They are treated with herbs and rest.

Lifestyle illness. These illnesses are associated with poor nutrition, lack of exercise, etc. They are treated with changes in lifestyle.

Karmic illness. These are inherited illnesses or illnesses that come from previous lives. They are difficult to treat, requiring herbs and spiritual practice.

Demonic possession. These illnesses could be considered mental illness. They are difficult to treat, requiring herbs and spiritual practices.

motivated, centred, grounded and able to digest life. When earth is deficient, he is easily overwhelmed by other people and events and continually seeks support for his emotional and physical needs. This is an individual who requires constant reassurance. To balance deficient earth, fire is needed. Fire ignites his heart's passion, and allows him to give and receive all that life has to offer.

The individual with excess of earth tires easily and complains. To break through stuck earth, call on the wood element. Recall the image of the sapling breaking through the earth. The excess earth individual stuck in the mud of life needs the sapling's thirst for light.

The fourth element is metal. Metal is the distilled spiritual essence in each of us. Spiritual essence is defined as a living awareness of the interdependence of life. It is the interactions of the other elements, earth, fire, water, wood that refines gold, the most precious metal.

The individual with balanced metal can remain centred while completely aware of the interdependence of life. She lives with passionate equanimity.

When the element of metal is lacking, she is tossed about by circumstances and has difficulty differentiating between self and others. The centeredness of the earth element steadies unstable metal.

An over-abundance of metal creates mental tension and rigidity in the body. I like the metaphor of a heart encased in a metal cage while the head tries to figure out, compile and create order from the apparent chaos of existence. The person with excess metal seeks a rarefied existence, free of the feelings associated with the physical world. To heal the erudite the passions of the heart need to be fired up. Fire melts thought's rigid cage around the heart and ignites feelings, offering the opportunity to engage intimately with the world.

The fifth element is water. Just as life on this planet emerged millions of years ago from water, the Chinese herbalist imagines the water element as the potential of all life. In TCM, water represents the spirit of one's ancestors, the resources one has inherited, strengths and weakness as well as one's physical constitution. Water also gives one the ability to flow from the past into the present and on to the future.

Excess water creates a leaky environment. This individual has porous boundaries and is unable to contain emotions and restrain physical impulses. She lacks willpower and needs to be shored up by the earth element. The earth fills the cracks in her foundation and helps build a supportive container for her sense of self.

Too much water creates stagnancy, almost like earth. However, in the case of excess water, the stagnancy is not caused by a lack of creativity as in earth, but by fear. Fear freezes activity, like the north winter chases everyone inside their home, on couches, under blankets, watching mind-numbing TV. The excess water individual is rigid with fear. The antidote to fear caused by excess water is the understanding of interdependence of life bestowed by metal. Developing an awareness of a sense of belonging in life cuts through fear.

European Herbal Medicine: Humourism

Orthodox western medicine is supposedly derived from the healing principals developed by Hippocrates who practiced herbal medicine in Greece between 460 to 370 BC, and is referred to as The Father of Western Medicine.

Hippocrates grew up in a culture that believed illness was caused by fickle gods. When a disease overpowered health, the first step back to wellness was to invoke a dream. The dream was then interrupted by a priest who performed the appropriate rituals to appease the gods. Hippocrates called this system of healing nonsense. He, along with others, advocated and developed for a more rational system of medicine called humourism.

Humourism focuses on the patient's lifestyle and their prognosis. For example, the severity of a patient's imbalance is assessed; the path to balance through lifestyle changes is advised. As opposed to curing a specific illness, humourism balances the four humours in the body: yellow bile, black bile, blood and phlegm. Humoural practitioners believe that a proportionate mixture of humours creates health while a disproportionate mixture creates ill health. Plant medicine is used to restore the balance of the humours.

In humoural medicine, herbs, like illnesses, are classed in terms of their qualities: hot and cold, dry and moist. Each quality is further divided into degrees from 1 to 4. Cayenne pepper, the fieriest herb in the apothecary, is considered to be hot in the first degree. Hops, a sedative, is consider to be cold in the third degree. Humourism applies herbs with the understanding that "contraries cure contraries". To generate the proper mixture of humours within the body, the herbalist offers herbs to counter balance the humour's quality. The herb's quality provides the body with the opposite effect of the humoural imbalance. This returns the body to equilibrium.

Essentially, western herbalists still practice "contraries cure contraries."

Like the elements in TCM and Ayurvedic medicine, each humour is associated with a season, an element, an organ or organs, quality and temperament. Quality is defined as the activity of the humour on the body. The humours are also the basis for four temperaments: choleric, melancholic, sanguine, and phlegmatic. Temperament defines a patient's character. Body/mind medicine is an essential component in humourism.

The Four Temperaments, Humours and Qualities

Yellow Bile - Fire

The choleric temperament has a disproportionate amount of yellow bile. Yellow bile manifests in the body as the quality of dry heat. When an individual is described as choleric, she knows how to use aggression to get things done. She is ambitious, and does not fear using anger to get her way. She focuses on her goals and is not concerned about what others think. Like anyone who burns brightly and rushes into action, for the choleric there is always the moment when doubt enters the mind. A tiny voice in the background suggests the possibility that the goal will not bring lasting reward. This voice, creates a pause in the choleric's activity. She broods. If the dark mood is not checked, she falls into depression.

In literary language the word bile is synonymous with anger, annoyance, irritation and rage. The quality of yellow bile in the body is hot and dry. The heat of anger dries out the body. Herbs with cooling and moistening qualities are used to soothe the inner burning and dampen down the fire. Chickweed (Stellaria medica) or Dandelion root (Taraxacum officinalis radix) are excellent tonic herbs to offer the choleric.

It is noteworthy to mention a condition the Chinese refer to as *liver heat*. This condition is also associated with anger and frustration.

Blood - Air

The sanguine's dominant humour is blood. The quality of blood is hot and damp. The sanguine personality could be described as a "red blooded American" (from a Canadian's point of view). The sanguine is confidant, proud, bold and extrovert. Like the choleric individual, he rushes into action. Unlike the power hungry choleric, the sanguine temperament is completely in it for the pleasure. It is difficult for the sanguine individual to accept the law of diminishing returns - the tendency for a continued application of effort or skill toward a particular project or goal to decline in effectiveness after a certain level of result has been achieved. In other words, he is great at starting new adventures but is not in it for the long run.

His life of over-indulgence in food, wine and women, leads to disease of excess. Cool, dry herbs are offered to balance a sanguine temperament. Two classes of herbs are specific for balancing blood: herbs high in flavonoids, and astringent herbs that dry up dampness. Two examples of astringent herbs are: raspberry leaf (Rubus idaeus) and agrimony (Agrimonia spp.). Herbs high in flavonoids provide the anti-oxidants necessary to counter the sanguines over-indulgent lifestyle. Hawthorn berry (Crateagus oxycantha) and rose hips (Rosa spp.) are examples of herbs high in flavonoids.

Phlegm - Water

The phlegmatic's dominant humour is phlegm and has the quality of cold and wet. The phlegmatic temperament is the pillar of tradition. She plans the Christmas dinner, using her grandmother's recipes. Dinner is served on her mother's china. Everyone at her table must sit in their assigned places. She uses nametags. She does not like change, and is always ready to offer a stabling influence. The phlegmatic leaves adventures to the choleric and sanguine types. If she does not like what you have to say you won't hear a word from her. She will offer you her cold shoulder. The phlegmatic freezes like a stone. The phlegmatic prefers a stationary lifestyle (remember she does not welcome change) and tends towards diseases of stagnation including the varied illnesses associated with obesity. To introduce some movement and spark to the phlegmatic's world, hot dry herbs are given. Ginger (Zingberis officinalis) is a great herb to warm up the phlegmatic.

Black Bile - Earth

The melancholic's dominant humour is black bile and has the quality of dry and cold. The melancholic carries the world on his shoulders. He writes poetry about the cruelty of love, reassures trees at the sound of chain saws and saves whales, kittens, and damsels. He philosophizes about relationships while forgetting to engage in the "real" rough and tumble of life. In this way his ideal world is never challenged. The melancholic can become lost in the romanticizing of death and darkness. The melancholic, unable to digest life, suffers with illnesses associated with malnourishment. Warm, moist herbs are offered to the melancholic to soften the sharp lines of his idealism and warm up his heart.

Wild oat seed (Avena sativa) is a nourishing nerve tonic suitable for the melancholic.

Herbal Medicine Today

Fast forward....!

I am in herb school. After spending ten years living on and off in a meditation retreat center, I decided I needed a "real" job. To do this, I think I need a "real" education. I decide to go to herb school to become an herbalist. Many people looked at me quite strangely when I told them my plans for my "real" job and "real" education. Fortunately I had been studying the nature of reality for some time, and knew that reality is fluid.

After studying a variety of programs available in Canada, I enrolled in the oldest North American school of herbal medicine, Dominion Herbal College.

During my time at the meditation center, I learned about the importance of tradition. If I was going to spend money and time on my education, I wanted to study herbal medicine with tradition supporting it.

While studying meditation, I learned it is essential in the spiritual life to acknowledge and study the words of the ones who have walked the path before you, broken ground, opened doors and seen the light. This is called honouring one's lineage. There are many reasons for understanding lineage, one of the greatest being to build confidence in the teachings and meditations offered. Lineage demonstrates that the teaching and meditation have for a very long time helped others who are not really very different from oneself. The meditation I practice has been used by human beings for over 2000 years to mend broken hearts and infuse confused minds with clarity. When going through a bumpy patch, one can look to those who have already made it to the other side and gain the confidence needed to take another step forward.

I could not find such a lineage in western herbal medicine. I asked my teachers who their teachers were and where they had learned herbal medicine. Many of them could not answer my question. They had their diplomas or degrees but I was looking for more detailed answers. Some spoke about Galen and Culpepper, but there was little relationship to what these historic herbalists taught and what I was learning.

So I looked to the east and found Traditional Chinese Medicine (TCM) and Ayurvedic Medicine. Both these traditions have lineage. These traditions use the same language and principals of healing as they were used thousands of years ago. Yet in the core of my being, (which I do occasionally listen to!), I knew that neither of these traditions was the one I would practice. I needed a form of herbal medicine that is from my culture.

I mulled this question over in my garden, forests, meadows and mountains. I went back and studied Culpeper and Galen some more. I discovered Samuel Thompson's teachings, watched grainy Doctor Christopher videos and still I was not satisfied. I studied a picture of the founder of the school I attended, a stout woman in a black dress standing in a garden back in the 1930s.

"Where did you learn your medicine from?" I asked her silent stare. I really, really wanted a lineage with names and dates; one I could recite. A lineage of herbalists who had performed amazing cures with plants, an honoured and respected lineage of healers. Healers I could supplicate in times of need.

Sitting under my thinking tree one sunny afternoon, my herbal lineage came to me in a flash. I realized that the plants do not care about traditions and lineage. These are human constructs. The plants themselves contain the knowledge of medicine and they pass it on. Humans create a consensual language to pass on information learnt from the plant themselves. Plants are the Gurus in herbal medicine and they transcend tradition.

There is an old expression: "Do not mistake the finger pointing to the moon for the moon." The finger is the books, seminars, workshops and other herbalists. The moon is the plant and its relationship to every other living thing on this planet.

(Note: Since that time I wrote this I have done considerable reading on the history of Western Herbal Medicine. There is a rich lineage but one has to dig deeper than in the traditions of the East. A good place to begin your study is with Matthew Wood's books, *Vitalism* and *Practices of Traditional Western Herbalism*)

Why consider the elements in today's herbal clinic?

In 2002, 3,226 users of herbal medicine took a survey on the ConsumerLab.com website. The survey asked why they took herbal supplements. The following are the results:

For general health 67%

Colds 53%

Energy enhancement 37%

Cholesterol lowering 29%

Cancer prevention 28%

Allergies   27%

For four or more conditions 54%

Another 2002 survey of 2,590 users of herbal medicine discovered the ten most common reasons people took herbal medicine:

Health, they are good for you 16%

Arthritis   7%

Memory improvement 6%

Energy   5%

Immune booster 5%

Joints 4%

Supplement the diet 45%

Sleep aid 3%

No reason specified 25%

All others including weight loss, menopause, etc. 45%

Note that not one person took herbal medicine to ease dryness resulting in constipation, or used plants to moisten a dry cough. No one was taking herbal medicine to reduce liver fire, or calm wind. No one was interested in taking herbs to reduce blood, for bad blood or to encourage yellow bile. Yet in both surveys, consumers of herbal supplements rated high levels of satisfaction.

If herbal medicine can be used like pharmaceutical drugs, to reduce symptoms of an underlying lifestyle challenge, why bother with archaic healing principals? In a society where most people do not even feel a connection to the earth, the sun, the wind, and prefer soft drinks over water can the traditional language and practices of herbalist be relevant?

If, as a herbalist, you are interested in helping people achieve the greatest level of health with the least amount of effort, the traditional modes of herbal medicine need to be considered in your herbal clinic. When a herbalist understands the overall imbalance occurring in the body and offers herbs to correct that imbalance, cures are the result, not just symptom control.

Developing a visceral understanding of the elements in the human body and in plants takes the practice of herbal medicine to a whole new level of healing. Far beyond feverfew (Tanacetum parthenium) for migraine headaches, milk thistle (Silybum marianum) for cirrhosis of the liver and St. John's Wort (Hypericum perforatum) for depression. Standing on the shoulders of the great healing traditions of the past, you can benefit many.

For instance, let's consider peppermint (Mentha piperita). Many herbals state that peppermint is contra-indicted in heartburn. When a plant is contra-indicated, it aggravates the condition. In my clinical practice, I have successfully used

The Races and the Medicine Wheel

First Nations peoples use the medicine wheel for many purposes. The Hopi people use the medicine wheel as a template to describe the history of human beings and the role each race of people have in caring for the earth.

Hopi elders tell of a time when all races were one. The Great Spirit divided humans into four groups and sent each group into one of the four directions telling them they would one day become the colour of that direction.

The group sent north was given the task of caring for fire. White is the colour of north, and these people became white Europeans. The group sent east was responsible for air. Yellow is the colour of the eastern direction, and these people became Asians.

To the south the group responsible for earth was sent. South is red in colour, and these people became Native Americans.

To the west the group responsible for water journeyed. Black is the western colour and these people are Africans.

It is interesting to note that western herbalists are focused on controlling the fire in the stomach. As the race responsible for fire, perhaps the whites need to temper their use of fire. This certainly is true with the white obsession with fiery weaponry.

peppermint to cure heartburn. If digestion is damp and sluggish, dominated by earth and water, heartburn results from a slow emptying of the stomach. Frequently bloating and a sense of fullness precede this type of heartburn. Often the individual suffers with constipation. If this condition continues, eventually heartburn is added to this person's list of digestive complaints.

A traditional herbalist assesses this individual as having inadequate digestive fire. The digestive fire has been extinguished by excess water and earth. Peppermint is a dry, warming herb. It has a fiery nature. The dry, warming quality of the herb counters the damp stagnation in the gut, improving overall digestion and easing any heartburn.

If the digestive system is burning too hot, as when anxiety accompanies heartburn, and the body is acidic, peppermint's heat will only increase the burn. In this case, the moist, cooling action of chamomile (Matricaria recutita) will calm the fire of both heartburn and anxiety and peppermint is contra-indicated.

A word about phytotherapy and molecular biology: The reductionist approach to healing

As a herbalist it is essential one does not become entrenched in the dogma of the day. Today the best herbalists are comfortable with one foot in the world of the reductionist methods scientists use in researching plants and their complex chemistries, while their other foot is firmly planted in the intuitive approach used since beyond memory to understand the relationship between the body and plants. Do not be fooled by language, viewpoints or others' ideas about how plant medicine should be practiced. There are many ways to approach the body and plant medicine. Both the human being and plants carry the vast intelligence of this planet called Earth.

Beginning at the Beginning: Sensing

They suggested that matter, at its most fundamental, could not be divided into independently existing units and indeed could not be fully described. Things had no meaning in isolation; they had meaning only in a web of dynamic interrelationships.
Lynn McTaggart, author of The Intention Experiment on describing the findings of quantum physicists Niels Bohr and Werner Heisenberg

The study of physiology opens a window on the dynamic dance called the human body. There are the many actions our body makes responding to our wishes: climbing mountains, making love, sprawling on the couch, or dancing to the music in our hearts. Then there are the actions our bodies perform on our behalf, without us thinking about it: sweating, blinking, sleeping, ovulating, sensing. Our bodies are activity. It is a misnomer to refer to the human body as a noun. There is nothing stagnant about the human body. Even after death, the body is in the continual process of decomposition. Perhaps we are consciousness (formless) woven into motion called form and commonly referred to as a human being. Being is a verb.

My personal quest for wholeness - physical, emotional, mental and spiritual - began when I heard the following statement: In this fathom long body, subject as it is to illness, old age and death, I show you the coming in to being and the passing away of a universe – Shakyamuni Buddha.

With this single statement, huge questions shook me to the very core of my being. What is this body? This thing I dress, adorn and take to work, conferences, parties, coffee dates, etc.? Am I this breathing, eating, excreting, flesh and bones that brings me so much pleasure and so much pain or am I simply a guest within it? How is it I am a living universe? The most important question to me is: how can I hear the pulsation of stars in my body? These questions have inspired many adventures over the years leading to glimpses of possible responses.

Adventure's adversary is an answer. Answers in my life have led me to dead-ends and rigid uncompromising beliefs. Luckily my karma always runs over my dogma, and sends me on an adventure again, renewing the BIG questions in my life. How can I hear the universe in my body? It is this question that shapes my understanding of my body, the universe and my place within this complex matrix called life; not a diagram in a textbook or Latin names for body parts and plants.

A glimpse into the complex workings of your body empowers you to listen more deeply to the body's needs. Understanding the body allows you to develop confidence in your ability to heal. This is the foundation of one's personal health and guides your to help others enhance their well-being.

Let's begin by exploring the physiology of learning: sensing.

Three Sensing Stories
Story One

I live on a stretch of land that bridges the foothills of the Rocky Mountains and the flat lands of the prairie. This area, treed by the hardy poplar, is known for its unpredictable weather. The North wind can bring snow in July. The West wind carries temperatures of 15C over the mountains in January. Today began as a sun kissed May morning. My mood and my body as felt light as spring breeze: optimism ruled the day.

By 2 o'clock this afternoon, my body was beginning to feel heavy. My shoulders slouched. My mind became dull. All I could think of was napping. By 3:30 thick grey clouds hung low in the sky and the wind picked up. I asked the clouds to release their rain and lift the weight the low air pressure was exerting on my body/mind. At 4:00 the clouds burst. By 5:00 the storm had past, the sun shone and my body and mind lightened. My body had sensed the storm hours before it arrived.

Story Two

Every summer students of Tibetan medicine hike the vast Himalayan valleys, dramatic plateaus and treacherous cliffs sniffing, tasting and observing plants to finely tune their senses to the medicine found in plants. By learning to read the plant with their senses the future Tibetan doctors learn how to harvest medicine with respect for

Green Tara is a healing meditation from Tibet, although the roots of this practice reach much deeper into history. She is a called a protector and one asks for her protection when undertaking difficult tasks like scaling the Himalayan mountains seeking out wild plant medicine. An important part of healing is offering protection under difficult circumstances.

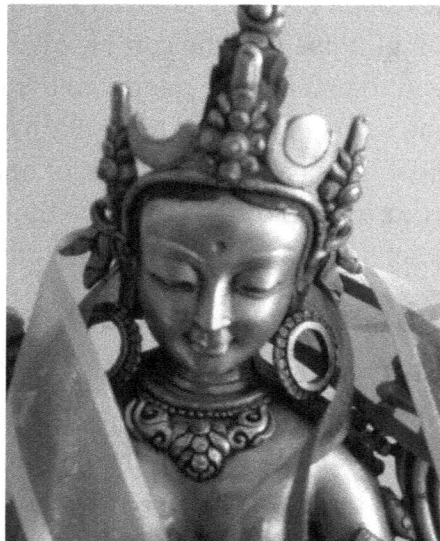

the fragile ecology of the highest mountains on our planet.

At the end of seven years of study, students of Tibetan Medicine use blindfolds to prepare for their final exams. Without the use of sight, the students practice identifying plants solely through taste and smell for their final exam on materia medica. If successful in identifying the medicine in plants simply through his sense of taste and smell, the student will pass on to become a Doctor of Tibetan Medicine.

Story Three

Several years ago I was living in a meditation retreat house. My role was head cook and bottle washer. One day a man dropped by who had heard we offered meditation classes. He sat at the kitchen table and I offered him tea. Another woman staying in the house joined us. The man told us about himself, in particular his journeys as a shaman. His stories were fantastically wild with multidimensional visions of alternate realities. When we finished the pot of tea the man left. Then my friend turned to me and told me the man was schizophrenic. I asked her how she knew. She told me she had been married to a schizophrenic and this man had the same odour that her husband had. The man did have a very distinctive and unpleasant odour.

Since that day I have known three other people who had the same odour. Each of them was completely preoccupied with "out of body experiences."

The Senses

When it comes to learning you have no greater tool than your senses. It is with impressions gathered by the senses that we evaluate, analyze and develop a deeper understanding of ourselves and the world we live in. For an herbalist to do well in her trade, acute sensing is essential. Herbal medicine is not learned from books, although study does help. It is learned through tasting and smelling the medicine in plants. To understand clients' needs, herbalists must clearly see, smell, hear and touch them.

The Four Functions

For a moment let's consider Carl Jung's, a Swiss psychiatrist with a deeply mystical nature, map of consciousness to guide our understanding of the relationship between sensing and learning. He called this map of consciousness "The Four Functions".

The four functions of consciousness are:

Intuition

Feeling   Thinking

Sensing

Jung theorized that each individual has one function that is stronger than the rest and is her comfortable way of interacting in the world. Each individual also has a secondary function that she is comfortable using but it is not how she gets through the day. Then we all have an awkward relationship with a third function and the fourth function is our Achilles' heel.

It is important to know which function is your strength and which is your weakness. This gives you the opportunity to develop the function you find most inaccessible while playing up your strength.

Let's explore each function:

Intuition is "gut feelings". It is an immediate experience, one that does not require thought. It just happens. Intuition creates a big picture instantly from random bits and pieces of data. It is an internal, non-analytical process. Intuition is the "aha!" moment when suddenly everything falls into place. The clearest example of the intuitive function is when working on a puzzle. For a while it is difficult to find pieces that fit together. Then suddenly several pieces fall into place without any effort. This is the intuitive at work, slowly gathering information and then bursting into understanding.

Sensing is perception of the physical world through the senses. It is the direct experience of touch, sight, hearing, smell and taste. Sensing is deeply in tune with our heart experience of the world. Beauty is discovered through our senses. The experience of beauty nourishes our hearts.

The sensing and intuitive functions are both receptive in nature. These functions are open to the moment, not action based.

Feeling has an analytical quality to it; only it is not analysis with the mind (as thinking is), its analysis with the heart. Feeling function is aware of the meaning of relationships and seeks to create harmony between opposing forces. For example: a dog is very sick, and will not live for long. The person who is dominant in feeling function wraps the dog in its favourite blanket.

Thinking also has an analytical quality. It is analysis using the mind. These individuals focus on facts over relationships. Those strong in thinking function see many sides of the same issue and choose the favoured course according to the facts of the situation. For example, the thinking function sees the dog is dying and decides the kindest action is to put the dog down. She does not think about a blanket.

Great herbalists are able to shift between each function with ease. However, collection of data through the senses is essential in understanding the health challenges of clients and the plant medicine to be dispensed. Without a meaningful sensual relationship with both clients and plants, the herbalist's medicine is as dry as an aspirin. To be sensitive to the input from your senses offers you more information to objectively think through the challenges faced by clients and assess scientific data of plants without falling into bias. Flowing between the sensing and thinking functions strengthens your ability to communicate without judgment to your clients and dialogue with those who have a reductionist attitude towards life. When a herbalist has finely tuned senses, lightning flashes of intuition strike and she clearly knows both a plant's medicine and her clients in the most intimate manner: from the heart. When she masters the feeling function her medicine is offered with kindness and warmth.

Who is sensing?

The senses are portals to the world outside our body. Through your senses, information flows into your being. The senses do not interpret information and create meaning. The brain does that. Details of the outer world reach your senses via wavelengths, light waves and molecules. The brain categorizes these bits of data and endows them with meaning overlaid with emotions based on your past experiences. Because all information is assessed through the lens of experience, seeking new experiences enriches your ability to expand life's meaning.

The Art of Seeing

It's not what you look at that matters, it's what you see. – Henry David Thoreau

The saying "beauty is in the eye of the beholder," begs the question, who is doing the seeing? It certainly is not the eye.

The retina on the back of your eye captures flickers of light, transforming them into nerve impulses. The nerve impulses speed along approximately 1.2 million optic nerve ganglions to the occipital lobe at the back of your brain.

Upon arriving at the occipital lobe, the light is categorized and painted with your previous experiences, preferences and emotions. It is in the brain where your visual idea of the world is created. In the blink of an eye, the play of light on the retina takes on a reality that can overwhelm you with beauty, cause you to run with terror or pull out your wallet and purchase the treat you deserve. The person walking down the street transforms into the man one woman loves, while another woman sees him as a stranger to be feared. A herbalist seeing St John's Wort (Hypericum perforatum) presses the plant's yellow flowers between the tips of her finger to see if the medicine is ready, while a farmer goes to his shed to find a pesticide to kill the noxious weed in his monoculture field. Beauty is not in the eye of the beholder, it is in the individual's previous experiences.

Be aware, no matter how extraordinary the brain's ability to give meaning to the light that shines on the back of the retina, this complex physiology is as beguiling as a magician's hand or as fluid as a dream. It is easy to be fooled by the play of light and shadows. On a long hot car trip the heat waves on the highway appear as water. A coiled rope strikes the fear of a venomous snake in the heart. It's easy to believe the shiny new car will make you happy. A friend of mine, who is liberally minded, once confessed to sitting on a bus and thinking a young man was a drug dealer because of the colour of his skin. She was horrified that she had passed judgment on an individual who she knew nothing about.

As a herbalist, it is important to become aware of how your previous experiences and preferences taint your perceptions, forming your personal version of reality.

Case Study of Seeing

The other day, in my clinic, a woman arrived early, in a bluster about parking. She sat down before I offered a chair and exhaled with a huff. Before I sat down she began to tell me about her troubles with other people. Her lips were tight with tension and the tendons in her neck were taut. She avoided making eye contact and sat on the edge of her chair ready to spring into action. Her skin, although tanned, lacked luster. She wanted nothing to do with my questions and offered me vague answers. She was intent on reciting the trials others were putting her through. I put down my paper and pen and observed her dispassionately while she ranted. After about ten minutes the tension in her lips softened and she sat back in the chair. Half an hour later her skin began to take on a healthy glow. Once her skin changed I asked her if she was feeling better. She paused for a moment, looked me in the eye for the first time and said, "Yes". I then began to ask my questions and she answered them with thoughtfulness.

She had to tell her side of the story. When I saw the subtle change in her skin, I knew she had said enough and had relaxed to the point where she could take in new information. If I had become caught up in her story and followed her down the path of discontent, I would have never seen the shift in the colour of her skin Without observing the changes in her physical appearance, together we would of continued to through fuel on her unhappiness. This would of been in direct conflict with my story for being there in the same room as her which was to soothe and ease her unhappiness.t is only through patiently seeing that I have learned to assess when to let someone go on with their story and when to take charge of the interview and move forward with my needs for a proper assessment.

A Final Note on Sight

It is impressive to consider the complex mirages neurons puzzle together in the

Iridology

Iridology is an assessment tool many herbalists use. By studying the patterns and markings on the iris, an iridologist discovers an individual's constitutional strengths, inherited weaknesses and health of organs. An iridologist can understand a client's digestion and level of inflammation in their body. Most importantly, an iridologist can read their client's eyes when he has shifted from chronic illness to healing.

back of our brains. It challenges our intrinsic sense of reality to consider that the world we see out there is created inside our brains. There is, however, one more fact that requires deep consideration. Our senses develop over time according to the environment we find ourselves in. Fish swimming in the depth of the ocean are as blind as earthworms. If it were not for the sun, there would be no eyes. Eyes, the crow's, salamander's, elephant's, trout's, have all appeared as a response to the light cast off by the heat from our fiery star, the sun. If there were no sun shining its beautiful warm light down onto our lovely, ever changing planet, there would be no eyes. Eyes and the joy of seeing are a response to a world with light. Eyes have not developed in isolation.

The Art of Hearing

Ancient dissectionists spoke of the auditory nerve being divided into three or more pathways deep in the brain. They surmised that the ear was meant, therefore to hear at three different levels. One pathway was said to hear the mundane conversations of the world. A second pathway apprehended learning and art. And the third pathway existed so the soul itself might hear guidance and gain knowledge while here on earth. – Women Who Run with the Wolves by Clarissa Pinkola Estes, Phd

Hearing and the feelings of the heart have a profound relationship. A ballad sung by Emmy Lou Harris can make a hardened heart weep. A child's cry stirs a silent longing in a barren woman's heart. Screaming heavy metal triggers aggression behind the wheel. An ambulance's siren brings us to alert attention. The shaman's drum guides seekers on visionary quests to alternate landscapes where the mysteries of the universe are unlocked. Sound touches the most vulnerable places of our being. Moments after conception, to the rhythm of our mother's heart, our cells begin to divide. Bathed in the thrumming drum of a loving heart, our brain, heart, liver, arms and legs develop. By the fourth month of life our ears are tuned into the meaning behind the heart's many rhythms.

Listening to a client with your heart is a rare healing offered in these days of diagnostic technology. My friend, Robert Rogers, a skilled clinical herbalist who over many years has earned the gift of plant wisdom through listening deeply to both people and plants, tells this story:

Robert had travelled to the rocky shores of Newfoundland. There he met a retired medical doctor who referred to himself as "old fashioned". In other words, he made house calls! Robert and the doctor stayed up late one night sharing a bottle of scotch and swapping stories of practicing medicine. Sometime after midnight, the good doctor leaned over towards Robert and whispered, "If you listen long enough to a patient, they will tell you what is wrong with them."

Hearing your client's story with your heart open creates an environment in which the most profound healing can occur: healing at heart level. Without even having offered any herbal medicine, your client will leave your office feeling better. You may never see the client again. But if you listened with warmth and integrity during their time with you, you can be assured you helped them in some way.

Case Study in Hearing

One day a woman in her early 60s came to see me. She had the presence of a woman comfortable with herself, yet seemed unsettled, uncertain. When I asked her why she had come to see me, she told me she could not stop crying. Through her tears, she told me her story.

She had recently moved with her husband from another part of the country to care for her mother who had fallen ill with Alzheimers. It was important to her that her mother's final years were spent in her own home. Several Kleenexes later, she told me how trapped she felt in the house. "I can't even go to the toilet without my mother following me," she said and blew her nose into another Kleenex.

The woman woke at night and found her mother staring at her. At the same time, she had to maintain a constant surveillance on her mother as she would turn on all the burners of the stove and walk away, make random phone calls to strangers, and walk out the front door with only her underpants on. The daughter was exhausted and felt terribly alone.

At one point in the story, the tears stopped and we paused for a moment sipping our tea. Suddenly, she looked up at me and smiled, "I know what is wrong with me," she said, "I miss my friends from back home."

After speaking with her husband about her insight, she decided to regularly visit her friends across country, leaving her mom in respite care. That was the end of the tears-- no herbs needed.

The Element of Hearing

Without the air element, we would not hear the flutter of leaves, the caw of the crow or a child's laughter in a pool on a summer's day. Sound hums across space, vibrating one air molecule at a time, like dominoes tumbling one after another. The pulsating molecules, called sound waves, flow through space like flocks of birds in the autumn sky.

Some people, particularly those with a well-trained ear, experience sound waves as colours. Imagine for a moment a rainbow of sound entering your ear and tapping out a rhythm on your eardrum. Red is the frenetic dance of fire; yellow's pulse is as uplifting as sunlight, and sky blue has a soft, spacious rhythm while midnight blue has a deep, long, penetrating beat.

The colours swirl through the ear canal and shimmer across the eardrum. Passing through the eardrum into the middle ear, the colours ripple their distinct pattern over the malleus. The malleus passes the vibration onto another bone, the incus, and finally onto the third in the series, the stapes. The tinkling stapes triggers a fluid wave within the inner ear. This wave spirals through the cochlea flowing over delicate nerve endings; imagine infinitesimal hairs, tossing to and fro, like seaweed swaying in the ocean tide. The hair-like nerves register the fluid's movement and relay the rhythms to the temporal area of the brain.

Leaving the cochlea, sound travels down two separate neural pathways. Most sound heard by the right ear is carried on a wide pathway into the left temporal brain, while sound caught by the left ear travels to the right temporal brain.

Tinnitus and Gingko biloba

Tinnitus is ringing, roaring, clicking or hissing in the ear. It maybe intermittent or constant, mild or cause hearing loss and/or insomnia. Causes of tinnitus include: side effects from medication, exposure to loud noises, allergies, high or low blood pressure, tumours, jaw and neck tension, or heart disease. In a multi-center double blind drug vs. placebo study, Gingko biloba showed effectiveness in reducing tinnitus resulting from a variety of causes in all 103 participants of the study. Gingko does this by improving blood flow to the delicate blood vessels of the brain and the ears.

Each hemisphere of the brain interprets different aspects of sound.

The right side of the brain, receiving most of its sound impulses from the left ear, names and classifies sound waves based on previous experiences. The left side of the brain, open to transmissions from the right ear, hears rhythm and melody, the intangible meanings in the sound.

In Traditional Chinese Medicine (TCM) these two different ways of hearing are used in a diagnostic system called The Five Elements. The Five Elements is a framework to assess a client's constitution, state of health and possible cause of illness. This meaningful analysis of human health and causative factors of disease requires the development of the herbalist's sensing and intuitive functions. The herbalist needs to be as skilled in tuning into the rhythm and melody of the client's voice with the left side of her brain as she is in grasping the meaning of client's word with the right side of her brain.

The five elements system of analysis explores the balance of elements within the body/mind complex through listening to the client's voice. Using the five elements, the herbalist listens not only to the client's symptoms, but also to the quality of his voice. Understanding how the music of the voice relates to the client's health does not depend on the naming or analytical function of the right brain. Rather interpreting the flow and tone of the voice is dependent on the left-brain. The herbalist needs to rest in the place of not knowing, and just listen, to truly apply this ancient system of assessment.

A loud or shouting voice, even when there is nothing to shout about, suggests an imbalance in the wood element. A sing song voice, like the lilt at the end of a sentence so many women have when trying to convince you of a truth, represents the need to develop more earth element. Excessive laughter, or the complete lack of it, indicates fire imbalance. Disturbances in the water element manifest in a groaning quality to the voice, and include many sighs and moans, signalling deep fatigue. An imbalance of metal creates sounds like crying and sobbing.

The Art of Smell

You can always trust Nature to be economical. When something works she sticks with it. Nature does not reinvent the wheel: she leaves that to humans. Nature is particularly efficient in her use of shapes.

Spirals are an intricate design aspect of the ear, eye, nose and finger tips.

The Journey of Scent

Every in breath you take spirals through your nose in a swirling motion created by a series of circular canals called turbinates. Turbinates lengthen the breath's journey through the nose. As the breath enters your nostrils eddies of air linger over the moist membranes lining your nose. This extended time in the outer nose serves two purposes. First: the air reaches body temperature before flowing deeper into the body, and secondly, the fine dust particles and other irritants are trapped in the fine hairs and mucous membrane lining the nose.

Energetic Sense Organs

Within human beings there is an energetic body that can be seen through the mind's eye and felt with sensitive hands. Sensing organs within the energetic body are called chakras. There are seven primary chakras and many, many more secondary ones throughout the energy body. Just as the outer physical senses use the spiral to carry information into the body, so do the chakras. Chakras spin in either a clockwise or counter clockwise spiral, depending on how they are sensing and transmitting information. A clockwise spinning chakra is opening up to the flow of energy in the environment. Spinning counter clockwise, the chakras close off to the energies in the environment. Both the opening and closing movements of the chakras are important for balance and well-being in life.

This reduces the chances of the offending particles penetrating deeper into the respiratory system and causing infection or damage to tender tissue.

On the roof of your nose, a small patch of nerve tissues called olfactory receptors allows you to smell your way through life.

The olfactory receptors take the shape of minuscule hairs called cilia, similar to the hairs in the cochlea. As the air churns over the hairs passing scent molecules are trapped. Once the fine hairs sniff the molecules out, the scent information is transmitted to both the limbic system of the brain (considered the primitive brain) and temporal regions (part of the cerebral cortex, or the higher brain).

The Act of Smelling

Walking with my lab, Bubbaloo, her intense need to sniff every tree, mailbox, or stop sign, pulls me this way and that. Her unrelenting need to smell conflicts with my need to walk in a straight line. Once off leash, I am astounded at her quick about turns and sudden dashes across the meadow as she catches a whiff of something that is a complete mystery to me. All I smell is perhaps snow or wild roses, depending on the season. What is even more amazing to me is how attracted she is to a dead animal! She loves the stench of death so much; she can't help but roll on the rotting carcass, covering her shining black coat in slimy, retching stink.

Bubbaloo uses smell to mark her territory, and she knows who has passed through. I suspect the dead animal perfume she loves to wear has some kind of mating significance which, in her domesticity, has long since lost its meaning to her.

I was surprised when I read the following passage in a physiology textbook for nurses:

The sense of smell in human beings is generally less acute than in other animals. Many animals are known to secrete odorous chemicals called pheromones that play an important part in chemical communication in, for example, territorial behaviour, mating and the bonding of mothers and their newborn offspring. The role of pheromones in human communication is unknown. --Anatomy and Physiology by Anne Waugh and Allison Grant.

My sense of smell may not be as refined as Bubbaloo's, but I too use pheromones to mark my territory, mate and bond with those I love. When my husband has been away, and we embrace at the airport for the first time in weeks, I deeply inhale his unique scent and immediately feel the comfortable familiarity we share settle over my body/mind. Women,

Sniffing Out Disease

Traditional herbalists smelled their patient's urine, armpits, stools, wounds and even the webbed gap between toes to assess how deeply the disease had penetrated into the body and to determine the prognosis of the illness. Some suspect that the invention of the stethoscope was driven by a physician's desire to distant themselves from the multitude of odours ill bodies omit.

Smelling and the Mind

Schizophrenics, manic-depressives, low weight anorexics, Alzheimer sufferers and those who experience frequent migraines have a deficiency in their smelling abilities. It is suggested that an olfactory exam should be used in diagnosis of some mental illness. Supplementation with zinc can improve some smelling deficiencies.

after the pain of labour, gently sniff their new born, welcoming the sweet baby scent into every cell of their being. The new born, if not drugged from the birth, uses her sense of smell to find her mother's nipple. There are many studies that suggest the subconscious scent of estrogens attracts a man to a woman. Upon entering a hotel room you are greeted by a mix of cleaning agents and stale air smell. It's a distinct "non-lived in" smell. You immediately know the hotel room is a temporary dwelling. A healer I have known for years refuses to do telephone consultations with clients. He says he can't counsel people if he can't smell them. Humans, no matter how sophisticated and perfumed, continue to rely on scent to help them meet their most basic needs.

Scent molecules are decoded deep inside the limbic brain where many of our unconscious or primordial responses to life are governed. It is estimated that our five to six million olfactory nerves are capable of distinguishing 10,000 different odours. Few of these scents register consciously. Most leave behind a vague feeling that is difficult to put into words. In the limbic brain there is no language - only instinctual knowing.

Most plants create a series of chemicals called volatile oils to imbue themselves with a unique scent. The rose blends over 400 separate volatile oils to create its scent of seduction. Over a hundred volatile oils are mingled in the peppermint plant to produce its spirited scent.

Like animal pheromones, a plant's volatile oils mark their territory and attract pollinators. The chemical nature of volatile oils interferes with the replication of bacteria, fungi and viruses that attack plants. The sun's warmth excites the plant's volatile oils stimulating their release into the air. Dancing on breezes, the volatile oils' scent entices pollinating insects to the plant's sweet nectar.

In the human body, these scented chemicals generally have both a calming and stimulating effect on the nervous system while offering anti-microbial action. The stronger the plant's scent, the stronger the medicine.

Sniffing Herbs

When you are picking, making or buying herbal medicine it is important to smell it. If the yarrow in the garden does not carry the strong musky odour of yarrow in the meadow, harvest the yarrow in the meadow. If you cannot smell the herb above the smell of the alcohol in a tincture, the tincture is probably weak. If the powdered herb in the teabag carries no scent, it should not be used as medicine. When sniffing a salve, if you cannot smell the beeswax, it is probably made with a petroleum product.

Herbalist/chemist Lisa Ganora recommends sniffing herbs like a wolf. Place your nose close to the plant and gently sniff. Cautiously approach the herbs taking deeper sniffs; finally stuff your nose right into the herbs, grunt and sniff with vigour. The plant's scent invades your olfactory bulb and diffuses into your limbic brain. Rest for a moment. Feel your body/mind and its response. Consider the following questions:

Is the scent repulsive or are you craving another sniff? Does it evoke a memory or a feeling tone in your body? Where do you feel your body respond to the scent?

What emotion does the smell trigger?

Would you describe the scent as a high note, low note or middle note? Hint: Scents with a high note dissipate quickly while a scent described as a low note lingers. For example: peppermint has high notes, woody scents are low notes, and lavender has a middle note.

Does the scent have a colour?

Sniffing plants in this manner trains your nose to recognize a specific plant, its quality of medicine and quite possibly learn ways to use it that are not recorded in books, but in the genetic history of human kind. Or in other words, your ancestral memories stored away in the limbic system.

To enhance your sniffing of herbs have a small canister of ground coffee handy. Sniffing the coffee between each herb will clear your olfactory receptors, preparing them to receive a new scent.

When picking plants either in the garden or the wild for medicine, if the volatile oils have been dissipated in the warmth of the sun leaving the plant with no scent, it is best to wait for another day to gather medicine.

It is not just leaves and flowers that are high in volatile oils; many roots are rich with scent. When first digging roots, smell them, as many have a distinct odour. If the roots have had their thirst quenched, their scent will be diffuse. If they are thirsty, their scent will be odorous and their medicine strong. Thirsty plants always make better medicine.

The Element of Scent

Although the odorous molecules travel on the air into our nasal passages to trigger the experience of scent, it is the water element that is essential for an acute sense of smell. A dry nose has a poor sense of smell. The olfactory nerves enjoy bathing in the moist mucosa of the upper nose. Mucus allows the odorous molecules to linger over the olfactory receptors helping us catch their scent.

When people who have smoked for years quit, they often note how much more of the world they smell. The cigarette smoke's heat dries out mucous membranes of the nose. Olfactory receptors have a difficult time transmitting scent in hot, dry environments.

The Art of Tasting

This morning I nibbled on a leaf of wild mint. Its sharp bite startled me. The taste sparked a flame in my mouth, waking up all my senses, brightening my mind. From one taste I understood a lot about the wild mint's medicine and I knew it was time to harvest it.

A herbalist tastes herbs like a sommelier savours wine. After deeply inhaling the fragrance of the herb, place a piece of the plant in your mouth. Chew it slowly. Let the plant mingle with the saliva in your mouth. Become aware of the environment the plant is creating in your mouth. The tannins in astringent herbs make your mouth dry. Demulcent herbs moisten your mouth with their mucilaginous substances. Open yourself to the evolving play of the plant's flavour on your taste buds. Chamomile begins sweet and tender and finishes bitter. Raspberry initially leaves a floral imprint on the tongue that quickly transmutes to a dry, minerally blunt, earthy taste.

The sensations and evolving flavour each plant leaves on your tongue reveals its medicine. Chamomile's sweet nature soothes, while its bitterness supports digestion, calms the nerves and grounds the flighty mind. The dry

Chickweed (*Stellaria medica*) is cooling and moist in the mouth. On a hot summers day, find a patch of chickweed and touch the soil under her green leaves. Her cooling moist nature will be revealed. Photo credit: Rosalee de la Forêt.

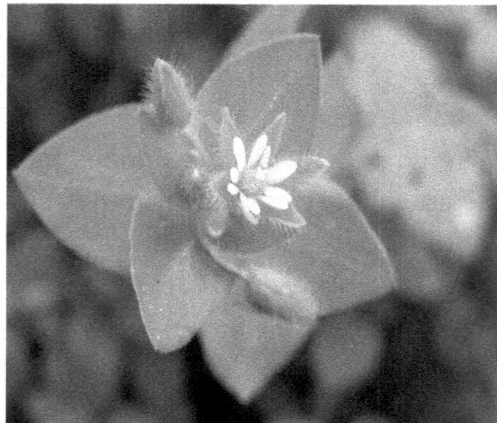

Chickweed   Rosalee de la Forêt

texture of raspberry alerts the herbalist to raspberry's astringent nature. Raspberry's blunt meatiness is a signature for the plants high mineral content.

To Taste is To Smell

To smell is to taste. There is an urban myth that goes like this: if someone blindfolded you, plugged your nose and fed you a piece of raw onion you would not be able to discriminate it from a strawberry. As food is macerated between your teeth, scent molecules are released and waft up the pharynx to tickle the olfactory receptors at the top of the nose. Without smell, we only sense.

Because taste appears to be so insensitive on the surface, it is the least understood of the senses. Research to enhance our understanding of the relationship between taste, the tongue, the nose and the brain, has not been well funded. The epidemic of obesity is changing this. A New York Times article

Spit Medicine

Aboriginal peoples around the world prepare plant medicine by chewing on the leaves, roots or seeds. In the Polynesian Islands, the lovely, peaceful kava plant was prepared by first cutting up the root into bite size pieces and then intensively chewed by virgins until it was mush. The mush was then spat into a bowl and shared by the community. It is recorded that the Polynesians believed the virgins' purity was necessary for good medicine. But I suspect that keeping those just entering puberty mellow with kava and occupied was useful to the community. As Aristotle concluded more than 2,300 years ago, "the young are heated by Nature as drunken men by wine." In herbal first aid, saliva is a useful solvent for the extraction of plant medicine. It is a blend of digestive enzymes: amylase and lipase prepare the fat and carbohydrate portions of medicine for absorption. Salvia supports the defense of the body with a bacteria-killing enzyme called lysozyme and immunoglobin A. Saliva dissolves a plant's water-soluble medicine.

printed on August 4, 1994 sums up the state of taste research today:

To modify people's "taste appetites" to aid weight control, make dull, nutritious food taste better, improve taste perception and appetites of the elderly, produce tastier substitutes for sugar and salts and develop drugs to counter taste disorders.

Since 1994, the sense of taste has been rediscovered. First, throw out the taste map of the tongue that was charted in 1901: the one with bitter on the root of the tongue, sweet on the tip and sour and salty on the sides. That is not how taste works. The old map did not even include the fifth taste (which a good cook always knew was there)--umami. Umami is a meaty or savoury taste believed to be triggered by amino acids.

Today's map of the tasting tongue records clusters of taste buds (papillae) dotting the sides, tip and root of the tongue, the roof of the mouth and on the back of the throat or pharynx. The papillae on the pharynx are particularly sensitized to strong bitter flavours and will trigger the gag reflect. Each cluster is made up of approximately 50 to 100 taste buds. Each taste bud contains 50 to 150 taste receptor nerves. It is uncertain whether taste receptor nerves can sample all five tastes but have a preference for one, or whether each taste bud contains nerves with different tasting abilities. At the base of each bud are nerves that are sensitive to pain, pressure and temperature. The whole package - the five essential tastes, texture, temperature and aroma, is called the flavour factor. The flavour factor is what the herbalist assesses to know a plant's medicine.

The tongue is the servant to three cranial nerves that feed directly into the brain stem. The brain stem is the most primitive area of the brain. We have no conscious awareness of the comings and goings of messages within the brain stem. This means most of the information gained through tasting remains completely unconscious. For example, when a herbalist offers a strongly bitter medicine, the patient may complain of gagging. It is not because the patient strongly dislikes the taste of the medicine (which they probably do) but because the medicine stimulates the bitter taste receptors on the pharynx triggering the automatic gag reflex. The response to the medicine is beyond conscious control. The innate intelligence of the body uses the gag reflex to protect itself from poison.

Within plants is a diverse group of chemicals called alkaloids. Generally alkaloids are bitter and in large doses can be poisonous. The gag reflex stops the ingestion of these dangerous plant constituents. Herbalists do frequently use plants with alkaloids, but in smaller doses. (For more on alkaloids: see medicine making.)

The tongue is a complex weaving of different types of tissue. As the cells divide in a woman's womb, growing a new human being, the tongue develops from two different types of tissues. It begins as ectoderm tissue. This is the tissue that covers the growing fetus and becomes both the nervous system and skin. The presence of temperature and pressure sensing nerves on taste buds offers a glimpse of the shared origin between the skin and tongue. These specially designed sensing cells are also found on the skin.

Within the layer created by the ectoderm, the endoderm tissue grows. This tissue is found throughout the lining of the digestive, respiratory and urinary systems as wells as many organs. This is the tissue that holds us together. Endoderm tissue also creates pores for fluids to flow through the body. For example, within the endoderm of the digestive tract are goblet cells which secrete mucousthat keep the lining of the esophagus, stomach and intestines moist and slippery. Because the tongue is made of both endoderm and ectoderm tissue, it has a close affinity for both the digestive organs and the nervous system.

Taste and the Immune System

The root of the tongue is covered in lymphatic tissue called lingual tonsils. The lingual tonsils monitor everything we put in our mouth for pathogens. When you taste something with an "off" flavour natural killer cells within the tissue of the lingual tonsils and throughout the respiratory tract have been mobilized.

A strong tincture of Echinacea (Echinacea angustifolia) should leave your mouth tingling like fireflies sparkling in a meadow on Midsummer Eve. A class of plant constituents called alkamides causes this tingling effect. In Echinacea the specific alkamides are referred to as isobutylamides.

Herbalists suspect that the tingling in the mouth is created by isobutylamides triggering an immune response. Echinacea's tingle could easily be interpreted as the unpleasant sensation left in the mouth after taking a bite of potato salad left out in the sun a little too long at the family reunion. The tongue knows something has just come into the mouth that is not quite right and should be spat out immediately.

The physiological effects of the isobutylamides are significant:

- Modulating the activity of macrophages. Macrophages are literally large mouthed white blood cells that gobble up everything in the body that does not belong there.
- Temper the activity of cytokines. Cytokines are messenger proteins that tell immune cells where to go and what to look for.
- These combined activities ease inflammation while creating a more effective immune system.

Remember Echinacea's activity begins with a tingle.

The Bitter Taste

When a patient has you stumped, and you do not know what to do recall herbal medicine's golden rule: keep it simple. This fundamental principal of plant medicine has been recited to me by a Cheyenne medicine man, a Ukrainian dermatologist/herbalist, and a grey haired, hunched back woman infused with wild plant medicine knowledge. Offering bitter tasting herbs supports this basic principal in herbal medicine.

Simply by offering a tea brewed with mildly bitter herbs, or a strongly bitter tincture, the client's senses are woken up, his appetite enhanced, digestion stimulated and depression eased. In my practice I have offered a mildly bitter tea before bed to cure chronic insomnia.

The Bitter Taste and the Vagus Nerve

When the tongue senses a bitter taste the vagus nerve in the brain stem is stimulated. The vagus nerve turns on the parasympathetic nervous system (PNS). If you want to recall the activity of the PNS think of "rest and digestion".

The vagus nerve, also called the wanderer, begins in the brainstem and reaches deep into the body, calming the heart muscle and stimulating digestive secretions from the stomach, gall bladder, bile duct and pancreas.

A bitter taste on the tongue turns on the vagus nerve's activity and prompts the release of bile

Gentian *(Gentiana lutea)* is the most bitter herb in the apothecary besides wormwood (*Artemsia absinthium*). Both wormwood and gentian have the ability to ground flighty, scattered minds and help the restless to sit for a meal and relax. A couple of drops of gentian taken in a 1/2 glass of warm water 15 minutes before a meal will guarantee less bloating and ease of digestion as well as absorption of nutrients. Gentian is frequently added to formulas to improve uptake of iron in cases of chronic anemia.

from the liver, gastric secretion from the stomach, and digestive enzymes and bicarbonate from the pancreas. Bitter herbs are the solution for many who struggle with a sluggish, uninterested digestive system.

Many people who endure depression and insomnia have a slow moving digestive process. One could say during sleep the mind digests the day. Enhancing the appetite and improving overall absorption of nutrients in the digestive tract helps those with tense minds that have difficulty giving way to sleep.

A caution: too much of a bitter taste will cause a hardening in the body just as too much bitterness in life hardens the heart. The remedy for a bitter heart is sweetness.

The Sweet Taste

The sweetness of mother's milk is the first taste of life. The newborn's sense of smell guides him to the breast. Tiny glands on the underside of the mother's breast release minute amounts of hormone that carries a scent similar to amniotic fluid. The infant, recognizing the womb's perfume, is drawn to the breast, roots out the nipple and an ancient inner knowing recalls suckling. The sweet taste stirs deep memories of that first moment of nourishment, loving embrace and complete satisfaction. Sweetness is the pleasure that releases the dramatic tension and uncertainty of birth.

Herbalists prepare sweet tasting medicine to rebuild the body after chronic stress, severe disease, starvation and depletion of physical and mental resources. Just as mothers provide new borns with sweet milk to grow and become strong, Mother Nature offers an array of sweet herbs to replenish our health after bitter times have left us floundering with low immunity, no libido and generalized malaise.

Sweet medicine is offered in a similar manner as bitter medicine-- a little bit at a time. Too much sweetness is not always in the best interest of health and balance.

The Dark History of Sweet Pleasure

The human history of sweet tastes is one of greed, slavery and now chronic illness. Sweetness was at one time found in an apple or pear. The sweetness of maple syrup or honey was a very special treat, and saved for times of famine. White sugar was so precious it was at one time called White Gold, and used as a spice such as cinnamon is today. Before the discovery of the Americas making sugar from sugarcane was both labour intensive and expensive. Most could not afford the sweetness of sugar.

The slave trade erupted when Christopher Columbus, trained in the import and export of the sugar trade, led the way to colonization of the West Indies. The hot moist climate of the tropical islands was perfect for growing sugar cane. Land was expropriated from the indigenous people, Africans kidnapped from their homelands, and sugar plantations were established. Stolen land and stolen people made sugar's pleasure affordable to everyone.

Industrial farming techniques make it possible for the average North American to consume an average of 5 pounds of sugar a month. That is a lot of sweetness. Addiction to the sweet flavour is evident in rising obesity among children, diabetes, and even cancer rates. Cancer is unchecked growth. Recall that the sweet taste creates growth.

Today sweet tastes have become a necessity of life for many people. Check out the breakfast cereal aisle in grocery stores. It is not unusual to see a child crying because her mother has refused to buy the latest sugary taste advertised during Saturday morning cartoons. This is the challenge of sugar. Sweetness becomes an addiction. Something in sugar's refined taste evokes the belief of entitlement. If we do not get our sugar, something feels out of place, wrong, our needs are not being met. Many clients say, "I feel like I am missing something, then I eat the bag of cookies."

The sweet taste in herbal medicine is not the sickly sweetness of cane sugar poured into soda pops, boxed breakfast cereals, candy or donuts. In my practice I am always suspicious when a client refuses to take a bitter tasting herb. "I can't stand the taste," they'll say with head turned, nose pointing to the sky.

It is my experience that individuals who only allow the sweet taste into their mouths act like children when life throws them a

Clinical Skills

A swollen tongue with teeth marks suggests a damp gut. In this case ask the client how much sugar is eaten in a day and recommend a reduction in sugar intake. Don't forget to ask about fruit and fruit juices.

challenge. They have a temper tantrum and threaten to take their toys home. They blame others for their misfortune and are unwilling to look into their own hearts. These individuals are the most difficult clients as they are unwilling to taste any part of life that is not sweet. At times I have almost advised these clients to go to the medical doctor and take her sugar coated pills.

One could say that those who crave and consume large amounts of sweetness have lost the connection to the sweetness in their hearts. They have lost their confidence in the ability to meet and overcome challenges. The sweet addiction turns life into a sickly sweet niceness. She can no longer stand her ground and face unpleasant truths. Instead, she hides in a dark kitchen eating fistful of chocolate chips, trying to fill the emptiness left behind by too many sweet smiles when a furrowed brow would be more to the point.

That being said, for those going through another round of chemotherapy, or having lost significant weight after the death of a loved one, or the teenage girl who carries the sufferings of the world on her shoulders and can no longer eat, these individuals need sweet medicine to counteract the sharp corners of life that has left them bruised to the bone. Sweet herbs will rebuild their bony frames and wrap them in warm flesh.

Wild oat seed (Avena sativa) is a sweet herb offered to those with frayed nerves and no buffer against life's many twists and turns. The oat's seed is swaddled in a fine green husk that protects it from the elements until it is ready to germinate. The husk's shape is reminiscent of the myelin sheaths found along nerves in the body. Deterioration of the myelin sheath results in a chaotic nerve transmission commonly referred to as frayed nerves. Herbalists recommend oat seed tea or tincture to sooth and restore frayed nerves.

The sweet taste of oat seed is favoured for those who have depleted their resources with extreme living: too much sex, drinking and drugs. It is invaluable when a crack habit has left an individual dried out, stressed out and frizzled out. Wild oat seed soothes and restores.

Wild oat seed is a friend to those who struggle with infertility. It calms the heartache of a barren woman and comforts her soul. Oat seed replenishes both partners' resources, when trying for a child has sucked the life and passion from their partnership.

Some of wild oat seed's regenerative power can be attributed to its high mineral content that includes magnesium, calcium, silica and chromium.

The Pungent Taste

Imagine biting into a hot chili pepper. The burning heat left behind on your tongue by the pepper makes your eyes water, your face flush and your nose run. The pungent taste is not really a taste. It's a mild (and sometimes not so mild) pain experience. Pungency, or heat, in food and herbs interacts with pain receptors at the base of the taste buds. Recall that the tongue is partially derived from the same embryonic tissue as the skin and rich in pain receptors.

The tingling or burning sensation on the tongue created by a pungent herb is interpreted in the brain as a threat to the body. Your brain turns the burning sensation on your tongue into a real burn. Remember the brain interprets the input from sense without regard for the reality of the moment.

Responding to the pungent taste, the brain orders up an immune response to clear away the debris of dead cells and intercept possible bacteria attempting to penetrate the area of the burn. In other words, a mild inflammatory response is initiated.

Herbalists use the pungent taste to get the fluids of the body moving, enhance the distribution of medicine contained in other herbs, and to stimulate the mind and fight infection.

Pungency takes advantage of the following law of nature: heat flows to cool. Consider the cooling effect of stretching out on cool grass in the shade of a poplar tree on a hot day. The heat drains from your body into the cool grass. Using this basic principal, herbalists offer pungent herbs to move stagnant interior heat towards the cool periphery of the body. This regulates the temperature of the body and enhances circulations. The pungent taste lifts the mind, increases blood flow throughout the body, and breaks up both energetic and physical blocks in the body.

The hypothalamus, located just above the brain stem, secretes neurohormones that control many metabolic functions in the body including temperature. The hypothalamus interprets the pungent taste as a burn and in order to reduce heat sends messages to the blood vessels near the surface of the body to dilate. Warmth from the body's core is carried in the blood to the cooler surface of the body. Sweat glands open up to further release heat. The cooling system used by the hypothalamus to reduce internal heat whether caused by hot yoga, a fever or a summer's day, can be activated by the pungent taste on the tongue.

In the classic herbal *Bartram's Encyclopedia of Herbal Medicine*, the following case is used to demonstrate the stimulating action of herbal medicine's most pungent herb: cayenne (Capsicum minimum).

"I was called in haste to a lady who was dying. I found her gasping for breath with no wrist pulse and very cold. Seven specialists had treated her and were positive nothing could be done. I gave her tincture of Capsicum in one-drop doses, often and persistently. The specials made all kinds of fun of me. The patient became well and strong at 80 years. I suggest that if Cayenne pepper had been given in all cases where whiskey had been taken for relief, many of those who are now dead would be alive." (C.S. Dyer, MD)

If the good Doctor Dryer had been practicing Traditional Chinese Medicine, he would have said, "The heat in the cayenne pepper stimulated the old woman's Qi".

Pungency and the Vital Force

In the physiology of TCM, Qi (pronounced chi) is the energy of life or the activating force in the body. The existence of Qi is the pivotal healing force encouraged by herbalists around the world. In traditional European medicine Qi is called the vital force. In India, Qi is referred to as prana. Japanese herbalists named it Ki and Hawaiians call it mana.

Most cultures believe the vital force rides the breath through the body, mind and spirit, nourishing and replenishing depleted energies while removing the causes of disease and obstruction. It is felt that the vital force pervades all life on this planet: humans, animals and plants.

A foundational belief for many traditional healers is that the vital force found in plants is no different from the vital force that animates the human body. Traditional herbalists offer plant medicine knowing the vital force that maintains the beauty and life of the plant will interact with the human body in the same way. Plant medicine nourishes the vital force in the human being. For this reason, traditional herbalists pick medicinal plants with prayers and take care that their mind and heart is in a state of love when drying and preparing plant medicine. It is not unusual for herbalists to carry on a lively conversation with the plants to encourage the exchange of vital forces between humans and plants.

Pungent herbs have a special affinity with the vital force. Life is warm. To be full of life is to be vibrant, have a sparkle in the eye and a passionate heart. These are metaphors for the fire element, the heat of life. To call a man or woman "hot" means they stimulate one's sexual appetite. It is the sexual appetite that creates life. To burn with creative fire is to produce meaningful (even if only to yourself) works of art.

When I cared for the dying it always surprised me how quickly the body became cold after

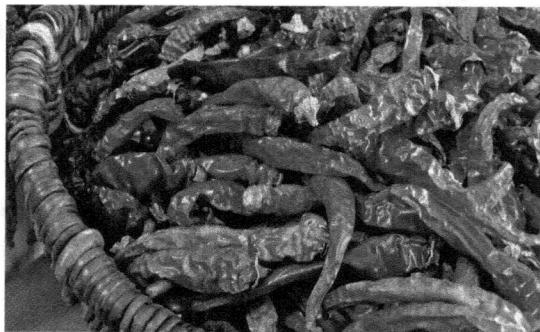

Cayenne Peppers   Rosalee de la Forêt.

life fled with the final breath. When the body went cold it reminded me of dead wood. The person, the heat that animated the flesh, was no longer present.

Warmth conveys the ability to feel. A cold heart refuses to be touched by life. It prefers morose isolation. Coldness walls us off from life. Just as frostbite leaves extremities numb and without feeling, when we call a person cold we are saying they lack feeling. They are numb to the heat of life.

To offer pungent herbs is to encourage life. As with the old woman treated by Dr. Dryer, pungent medicine wakes up the body's vital force, stimulates blood flow and removes cold obstructions.

Pungent herbs force a response by irritating the body. The pungent taste can be used to initiate a cough or sweating. They increase digestive powers and encourage the heart to beat with force. Pungent herbs fire up the body and the mind.

Offering pungent medicine requires care. One uses pungent herbs in the same way as one builds a fire. I am reminded of watching herbalist Rosalee de la Forêt gently blow on a nest of bark filled with downy tinder. Nestled in the nest was a small red coal. As if she was breathing life into a tiny bird, Rosalee sent her breath over the coal, encouraging its heat to mingle with the tinder. Like magic riding Rosalee's breath, a flame leapt from the nest.

When igniting the inner fire, one must use similar care. Gently offer pungent herbs to encourage the body to create its own warmth. There is an old Blackfoot saying:

"If you blow on a fire too hard, strong winds will burn the prairie grasses." This is true for the herbalist as well. Always handle pungent herbs with care.

Plants with a bitter pungent taste

Everything in nature is made up of all the elements. One or two elements will be more dominant than the others in any given season, time of day, plant, body, illness, geographic region, or even belief systems. Tastes, like the elements, have many basic qualities as well. Herbs have a primary taste and then many secondary and tertiary tastes.

Many plants, particularly their roots, have a bitter and pungent taste. Plants with this taste combination are effective in reducing pain. I use these herbs to ease the pain of migraine headaches and its accompanying digestive distress.

Western medicine considers one cause of migraine headaches to be the rapid constriction of arteries surrounding the brain followed by their sudden dilation. The sudden change in blood flow triggers a flurry of chemical activity around the blood vessels. Those chemicals ignite inflammation and can cause excruciating pain.

Many people who suffer with migraine headaches know that the very first sign of a headache is felt in the stomach. It is an uneasy feeling that progresses to nausea and vomiting. For this reason, traditional herbalists believe migraine's pain arises from the digestive organs and advise a bitter pungent herb be taken at the first turning of the stomach. In this way, the migraine may be averted, or at the very least the pain mitigated. There are a number of pungent bitter herbs that can be used. I have had success with both sweet flag (Acorus calamus) and lovage (Levisticum officinale).

Chewing a piece of the root of either plant ignites the pungent effect on the tongue, opening up blood vessels and moving the obstructed Qi. The body relaxes deeply, releasing the tension of migraine pain.

The root's bitter flavour lingers on the tongue and mingles with saliva while stimulating the vagus nerve, hence relaxing the digestive system. Digestive upset eases as the bile released by the liver stimulates peristalsis and the bowels move. The tightening grip of the migraine is loosened and one feels the light of life return.

The Salty Taste

"You must not lose faith in humanity. Humanity is like an ocean; if a few drops of the ocean are dirty, the ocean does not become dirty." — Mahatma Gandhi

In my mid-twenties I spent 8 weeks in a Singapore hospital breathing through a machine. When the plane landed in Vancouver I weighed 85 pounds. My bony body ached with each breath, step and thought. It was late May.

A profound melancholy often follows a serious illness. Perhaps it is the body's way of keeping our life quiet while wounds heal. Perhaps it is the sudden awakening to life's vulnerability, or maybe we need the melancholy to search for meaning after illness while asking life's deeper questions. Possibly it is the reorganization of priorities that follows the

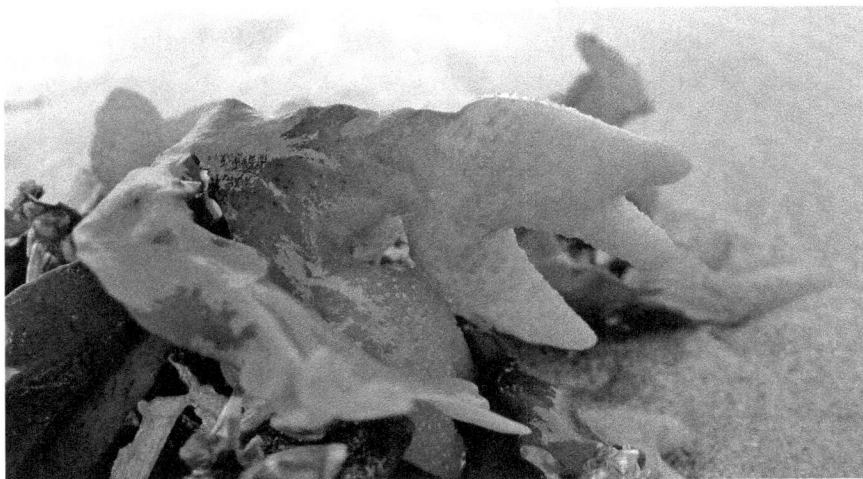

Fucus spp.   Rosalee de la Forêt.

remorse felt after reckless, casual decisions resulting in consequences that threaten life. In any case, weak and exhausted by illness and living in a strange city where nothing evoked memories of whom I had been before journeying to Asia, I took to the beach.

Each morning I hobbled down the hill to the beach with my journal. Wrapped in a wool blanket, as my body had not yet recovered its warmth, I counted waves or simply gazed at the restless ocean. Day after day I practiced expanding my lungs hardened by trauma and scar tissue, breathing in the ocean's salty air.

The ocean's steady pulse beating on the sandy shore gently relaxed muscles that were rigid with pain, untangled the tight knots trauma had tied in my mind and eased the fear from my heart. The ocean was my healer in those first days of recovery.

In Traditional Chinese Medicine it is believed that salt weaves the body/mind together and cravings for salty food are caused by scattered energy and scattered thoughts. Salt grounds the mind in the body, rooting it in the present. I believe the ocean's salty air knitted me back together after months of defying death's grip.

Herbs with a salty flavour are used to soften and bring moisture to tissues. Just as salty tears wash away the hardness of grief and soften the lump of unspoken words in our throats, and just as they release fear's iron grip on our heart, salty herbs are offered when the body has become brittle and dry, and help to keep the body subtle and flexible.

Our bodies are made up of 78% water. A poetic anatomist might describe the body as an ocean wrapped in skin. Plasma, the clear liquid that red and white blood cells float in, is identical in mineral composition to the ocean. When herbalists speak of a salty taste they are referring to the taste minerals bestow on plants. These minerals are called electrolytes in the body. Electrolytes (or minerals that make the earth solid and able to contain water) control the movement of water in the body. They pull water from the plasma into the interstitial fluid and control the flow of water into the cells. Then electrolytes move the water from the cells to the interstitial fluid and back to the plasma, in a rhythm that is as ancient as ocean tides.

Living on the prairie I have come to have a deep respect for rivers. I have spent many afternoons sitting on a windswept hilltop, watching a river wind through the landscape. A master carver, the river shapes its path deeper and deeper into the landscape with each passing day, year, decade, century-- since time had no meaning. In spring, rivers overflow their banks which is not so good for family photographs stored in basements! Silty waters wash the photographed memories away. But the land is deeply nourished by the water and the minerals it carries. Plants flourish in flood plains, and our bodies thrive on these mineral rich plants.

When the snowstorms do not blow through the winter and the spring rains do not come, rivers do not flood, and the land dries up and cracks; crops are poor and if the rain never arrives, animals are slaughtered. They become too costly to feed. Life is sparse without the movement of water and the minerals its carries.

The eclectics, herbalists who practiced in North America during the 18th century, called drought conditions within the human body atrophy. Matthew Wood writes in The Practice of Traditional Western Herbalism:

It applies to an underfed, withered, weak condition....since undernourished tissues have less energy to function. Atrophy should also be associated with dryness because fluids carry food. Without them, there is no nutrition. This includes both water and oil, both of which move foodstuffs to the cells and waste products out of them. Well-nourished tissue holds more water and oil.

When contemplating offering salty herbs, consider whether the "landscape" of your client resembles hard, cracked soil. If this is the case, offer the salty taste to soften and bring moisture to the soil of the body.

In Traditional Chinese Medicine salt is added to kidney/adrenal tonics in order to draw the medicine to the kidneys. Salt is also used to stimulate detoxification, relieve dryness and cool the blood.

Sour Taste

Those who suffer with heartburn often describe a sour taste in their mouth. Sour is the taste of regurgitated food. There are different reasons for food to be regurgitated, such as low stomach acids, or a weakness in the pyloric sphincter that closes the stomach off from the esophagus. The result is the same: a sour taste in the mouth.

Understanding the sour taste when approached from different herbal traditions can be confusing. Those who practice Ayurvedic medicine consider the sour taste hot and dry. Traditional western herbalists consider it dry and cooling and refer to the sour taste as astringent. TCM practitioners attribute the sour taste to the wood element. Wood is the element that generates growth. They are all right. To understand the sour taste, let's begin by looking at sour foods.

Sauerkraut, miso, vinegar and yogurt are considered sour foods. All these foods support digestion. Sauerkraut and miso are high in digestive enzymes while vinegar mimics the chemistry of the stomach. The abundant bacteria in yogurt are necessary for digestive processes to take place in the gut.

In Ayurvedic medicine digestion is the activity of fire. It is the stomach's fire that transforms food into nutrients the body can use. In Ayurvedic thought, because sour foods support digestion, sour herbs are classed as warm.

In Western Herbalism an efficient digestive system does not store heat. The stomach heats up, purifies and breaks down the food, releases it into the small intestine, and cools down. The western herbalist concerns himself about not letting the fire get out of control. From this point of view, sour foods support an efficient fire in the digestive system and are therefore essentially cooling.

Traditional Chinese Herbalists understand the activity of the sour taste as essentially helping the body break down the earth element (food) to use it for growth of the body. Growth is the activity of wood.

All traditions consider a sour taste drying. If the digestive tract is too wet the fire does not burn hot enough and creates stagnancy in the gut and poor absorption of nutrients. TCM refers to this condition as "damp". The sour taste dries up a wet digestive tract.

It is important to note that western herbalists include the action of astringency under the sour taste, whereas Ayurvedic practitioners consider astringency as a separate flavour. For our purposes, we will consider astringent herbs as having a sour taste that makes the mouth pucker. These herbs, many being from the rose family, contain a class of chemicals called tannins.

Raspberry Leaf (Rubus spp) is an astringent famous for supporting the uterus' expansion during pregnancy and contraction following labour. In TCM raspberry leaf is offered in prostatic hypertrophy. Herbalists at one time referred to prostatic hypertrophy as a boggy prostate. In other words, the prostate is leaky. Raspberry leaf, being an astringent with an affinity for organs in the pelvis, dries up the capsule the prostate lives within, resolving its bogginess.

Boggy could also be used to describe critical situations associated with pregnancy. In the early stages of pregnancy, a leaky uterus is the sign of an imminent miscarriage.

Post labour, a uterus that does not contract is at very high risk of hemorrhaging. Raspberry leaf's astringency, or sour taste, reduces bleeding and supports the uterus in returning to its post pregnancy size.

One of the ways I like to think of the actions of astringent, sour tasting herbs like raspberry is that they maintain the integrity of the containers within our body such as the uterus, bowel, bladder, and blood vessels.

The plant chemicals responsible for tightening up and maintaining a container's membrane are called tannins. Plant tannins were at one time used to tan the hides of animals. Strong teas of tannins were painted over the hide to make tough leather impervious to water. The tannins bound the loose proteins that previously bound the animal's skin to its flesh.

Too Many Tannins

I recall British herbalist, Kerry Bones, lamenting the state of British guts. He was sure the poor digestion suffered by many of his British clients was due to drinking large amounts of strong black tea. Black tea (Camellia spp) is very high in tannins. He felt that the tannins in the tea have over time de-sensitized the gut lining, turning it to leather. A leathery gut lacks the fluid movement of peristalsis and is too tough to absorb many nutrients.

On the other hand, the sour taste of astringent herbs is extremely useful in drying up leaks of any kind within the body: hemorrhage, diarrhea or a runny nose. The astringent or sour taste binds that which is loose.

Umami Taste

The word umami comes from the Japanese language and is used to describe a meaty or savoury taste. A Japanese professor named Kikunae Ikeda in 1906 initially proposed an official classification of this particular taste, similar to the underlying flavours of tamari. In 1985 the scientific community acknowledged umami as the imprint glutamates and nucleotides leave on the tongue.

Glutamate is an amino acid commonly present in proteins. Within the body glutamate performs many tasks including protein synthesis, ammonia detoxification and guiding learning processes in the brain.

Nucleotides make up DNA. and are present in every cell of every living thing on this planet. It is in the DNA where the history of life on this planet is recorded. Our DNA is the imprint of our ancestors. When the tongue tastes nucleotides, it is sampling the DNA present in the food. Perhaps as the tongue become familiar with the nucleotides contained in the umami taste, it gains knowledge about the genetic history of the food it is absorbing.

Although the human body, makes its own nucleotides, it also uses food sources of nucleotides to build and repair cells that are used up quickly. These include cells that make up the gut wall and the immune system.

I remember the year I graduated from herb school I had the opportunity to give a talk about the benefits of using herbal medicine in long term care facilities. It was a brave and bold idea at the time. Planning the talk I was excited to enlighten the room full of doctors and nurses on why herbs needed to be introduced to our seniors.

The day before the talk, at the same conference, the keynote speaker who wasa medical doctor of some type, delivered a talk titled "Facts, Fiction, and Myths about Herbal Medicine". When he projected an image of a cartoon witch with green skin, a black pointy hat and warts, onto the oversized screen at the front of the packed room, I knew I was in trouble. He then went on to ridicule and denounce herbal medicine and herbalists as nothing but quackery. Through his two-hour presentation he listed the numerous effects of several herbs and threw up his hands, eyes towards heaven, asking, "How can a single plant do all that?" He obviously did not know anything about herbal medicine.

Nettle (Urticaria diaocia) is one of the plants he cited as offending his sensibilities.

Here are just a few ways herbalist use nettle's in the apothecary to relieve pain and stiffness in joints, quiet down allergic reactions, reduce childhood eczema, rebuild of atrophied muscles, moderate blood sugars and build blood, relieve anemia, heal the gut wall, slow the bleeding from fibroids and control postpartum hemorrhage. These actions do not include nettle's invaluable nutritive support in pregnancy or in recovery from chronic disease.

Nettle can do all this because it provides the body with essential minerals and proteins needed to strengthen the its resistance to disease, rebuild tissue, and improve the elimination of waste. Although frequently used in cleansing formulas, Nettle is essentially a herb that rebuilds and restores the body's natural vitality. Being that up to 40% of its dry weight is protein, nettle has an umami taste.

Considering the fact that DNA is active in

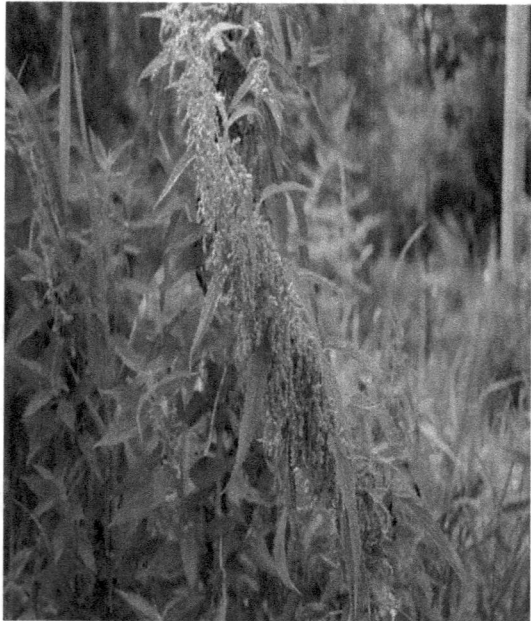

Nettles   Mark Arneson

every cell of the body and nettle is a rich source of nucleotides, it does not take a doctorate to understand how nettle can relieve the stress of illness on the body and free up the body's resources to speed the healing process along.

Adequate protein is essential for vigorous health. Many estimates suggest that the diet of a healthy person should be approximately 30% protein. Protein has an important role in building the messengers your immune system uses to direct its fights against infection and other illness. Antibodies are made from protein. Hormones are made from protein and essential fatty acids. It is well known that when a woman is severely malnourished her moon cycle fades. Digestive enzymes are made with protein, and blood and muscles are built from protein.

Simply put, nettle's high protein content supports the body in its return to health. That is not even mentioning the chlorophyll or flavonoids this healing plant offers, nor its profound effect on quieting down the histamine response when chronic inflammation causes debilitating pain in the body.

A little secret about nettles - if there is a lack of protein in the diet there are frequently cravings for simple carbohydrates. Have your client drink nettle tea throughout the day and her cravings will vanish.

If I had attended the good doctor's seminar at this point in my career as an herbalist, I would have stood up and said just that.

Review
Earth

Taste: Sweet or Umani
Creates a moist, cool climate and grounded mind
In excess leads to heaviness and sluggishness.
Physiological effect: rebuilds the body after prolonged stress, illness or malnutrition.

Psychological effect in balance: generous and comfortable in life.

Psychological effect imbalance: stingy, lack of confidence in support and stubborn.

Herb with a sweet taste: oats, licorice, slippery elm

Herbs with an umami taste: nettles, mushrooms

Water

Taste: Salty

Creates a moist environment, cohesion is an activity of water. In   excess: cold and boggy.

Physiological effect: carries away wastes, increases nutrition, soothes and softens hard lumps

Psychological effect in balance: reflective, able to see others clearly, go with the flow.

Psychological effect imbalance: brittle, rigid and angry.

Herbs: kelp, celery seed, red clover (some herbalists place nettles in this category.)

Fire

Taste: Pungent or sour (astringent)

Creates a warm, dry environment, in excess dries out tissues.

Physiological effect: stimulates digestion, circulation, the mind   and immune   system, dries up excess moisture, enhances sexual energy, can relieve pain caused by stagnancy, warms cold hands   and feet..

Psychological effect in balance: Brings passion and confidence to   life.

Psychological effect imbalance: Hot headed or frigid.

Herbs: Ginger, peppermint, rosemary. Sour: rosehips or hawthorn leaf and flower

Air

Tastes: Bitter or Sour

Creates a lightness of being, enhances movement, cools and
carries actions of other elements. In excess: flighty or over
thinking, flitting pain throughout the body.

Physiological effect in balance: Bitter wakes up digestion,
cools,   stimulates the parasympathetic system, cleanses the
liver. Sour   dries up excess dampness, often high in minerals
and wakes up   the mind and cleanse canker, resolves loose
stools

Psychological effect in balance: Able to touch life with a sense
of   equanimity, creative and active

Psychological effect imbalance: unfocused and overwhelmed.

Herbs: Bitter: Dandelion leaf and root, Mugwort, Burdock.
Sour: raspberry leaf, blackberry leaf.

The Physiology of Assimilation

"If more of us valued food and cheer and song above hoarded gold, it would be a merrier world." — J.R.R. Tolkien

Relying on the natural life force to do the healing, therefore healing is the input to that life. Life acts on well-digested nutrients to produce the health of the body, and create higher creative expression of life. - Treatise on Vitalism

The Oxford dictionary defines the word assimilation as: *to take in and understand fully.*

It is rooted in the Latin word assimilare, meaning to make similar or to make alike. When assimilation is referred specifically to physiology it means: *to absorb and digest.* Assimilation implies that we become the food we eat and the food we eat becomes us.

The physiology of assimilation is one of the primary considerations for the herbalist. She not only assesses the client's diet, but also how well the client's body is able to absorb food. If the food is not being absorbed in the small intestine, then the medicine she offers will also have a difficult time being absorbed. Therefore, a herbalist needs to turn her mind to the question of absorption for every client she sees.

In this chapter we will consider the following ways to improve the body/mind's ability to absorb of nutrients.

- Love. It is all about receiving the goodness of life.
- The elemental nature of the alimentary tract: fire, water, air and earth.
- The form of the alimentary tract equals its function.
- The alimentary tract is a composite of physiological systems.

Receiving the Goodness of Life

Ponder the Sufi story

There was once a man who was a little bit good and a little bit bad. He died. At the gates of heaven, St. Peter, reviewing the man's life, mused "This man is neither good, nor bad, he could go to either heaven or hell." So he offered the man a choice: heaven or hell.

Like the man did throughout his life, he hummed and hawed, weighing his options, "Harps are not my style but nor are eternal flames." So he asked St Peter, "Can I sample each and then choose?"

St Peter, in an agreeable mood, asked, "Which would you like to visit first?" The man opted for hell.

In hell, everyone was gathered at a bountiful banquet of the most delectable, scrumptious, tasty food imaginable. There were tender carrots fresh from the garden, sweet peas cuddling in their pods sprinkled with fresh mint, subtly seasoned meats, and wine that tantalized the tongue with the taste of black cherry. There were slivers of pungent

Four Ways to Improve Absorption of Medicine

•Take on an empty stomach
•Include circulatory stimulants in the formula: lobelia, cayenne, rosemary
•Add a herb high in flavonoids to the formula: rose hips, hawthorn berries, chamomile
•Add a dab of honey

ginger dipped in dark Belgian chocolate, violet petal syrup drizzled on sweet velvety ice cream, and more and more and more. There was not only food. Jasmine flowers were strewn across the table, roses burst from vases, and divine music filled the air.

The people at this vast feast were not happy. They wore gloomy frowns their skin was grey and their eyes lacked radiance. They sat with hunched shoulders, surveying the feast thinking, "I never get what I want", or "Everyone else has what I want", or "If only I could get my hands on this feast it would be all mine". Thoughts like this ran endlessly through their heads. They could not stop plotting and planning while their tummies rumbled with hunger and their hearts ached with desire. In short, the people of hell were miserable.

Why were the people at this wonderful feast so discontented?

Lying alongside each plate were chopsticks, very long chopsticks; they were to be used to enjoy the feast. Unfortunately their length did not allow one to pick up a bite of food and pop it in one's own mouth. Spending eternity staring at the banquet made the people of hell very unhappy.

The dead man turned to St Peter and shuddered, "An eternity of unfulfilled desire-- I don't think hell is for me." So off they went to visit heaven.

In heaven there was also a feast being celebrated. It was indistinguishable from the feast the man found in hell. Everything was identical, from the peas in their pods to the jasmine flowers. Yet at heaven's banquet the people laughed and sang, their cheeks glowed with healthy radiance, their eyes sparkled with joy and their hearts burst with happiness.

The jubilant celebrants also had very long chopsticks but they did not lie like twigs on frozen snow on the feast table as they did in hell. The chopsticks flew through the air with the deft handling of the euphoric crowd who with care placed the tastiest, most delicate morsels of food in the mouths of those who sat on the other side of the table. In heaven, the chopsticks were used to feed each other. Heaven was an eruption of joy.

More on the Goodness of Life

It was January first. The forest was silent under deep snow. It was a cold morning, the sky a bright winter blue. I was sitting in a cosy wooden cabin meditating with a group of friends. Later we planned to have a New Year's feast. There is something beautiful about meditating in a forest on a crisp winter's day; perhaps it is the stillness that winter brings, slower routines and snow sparkling like thousands of diamonds. It is probably all of these splendors of nature and more. This particular day I remember with great clarity. In the stillness of the moment angels appeared to me. They hovered with smiling eyes watching my friends and I. Then one spoke:

"Every bite of food comes to you with love." Then they were gone.

There is a saying amongst alternative health practitioners: you are not what you eat but what you assimilate. Perhaps this expression could be reworked: you are what you love.

Let's leave behind the mystical side of life and see how a reductionist comes to the same conclusions.

A Happy Gut is A Happy Brain

The gut has its own nervous system called the enteric nervous system (ENS). Enterologists, people who study the ENS, refer to the ENS as the second brain. The first brain is the fatty mass in your head!

The ENS is composed of approximately 100 million neurons. Some of these neurons talk to the central nervous system (CNS): the first brain in the head and in its tail-- the spinal cord. Some confer with branches of the anatomic nervous system (ANS) called the parasympathetic nervous system. (Recall the relationship between the bitter taste and the vagus nerve of the parasympathetic system.) Mostly, the ENS is not interested in networking outside of its personal domain. It prefers to work within in its own territory which is the alimentary tract. The ENS prefers to think for itself without much input from the "head brain". Most of the nerves in the ENS only chat with other nerves within the ENS.

To talk to each other the nerves of the ENS use neurotransmitters. Every neurotransmitter found in the brain is found in the guts. One of the favoured neurotransmitters the ENS uses is serotonin.

The alimentary tract makes 90% of the serotonin in the body because it needs this feel good neurotransmitter to function.

In the brain serotonin helps regulate mood, appetite and sleep. It is also active while we are learning and retrieving memories. (This is an important point to remember.)

Drugs called serotonin re-uptake inhibitors (SSRIs) are frequently prescribed by doctors who hope to ease mild to moderate depression suffered by their patients. SSRIs keep serotonin active in the brain. A sense of hopelessness is depression's predominant mood. Those I have spoken to who have had success taking SSRIs tell me that suddenly they can see possibilities in life where before the drug they saw none.

Depression often presents with a lack of appetite, poor memory and sleep, constipation or irregular bowels. Most of our serotonin is made in the gut. Here it coordinates the ripples, contractions and relaxation of the muscles lining the digestive tract as food and waste products move through the core of our body in a process called peristalsis.

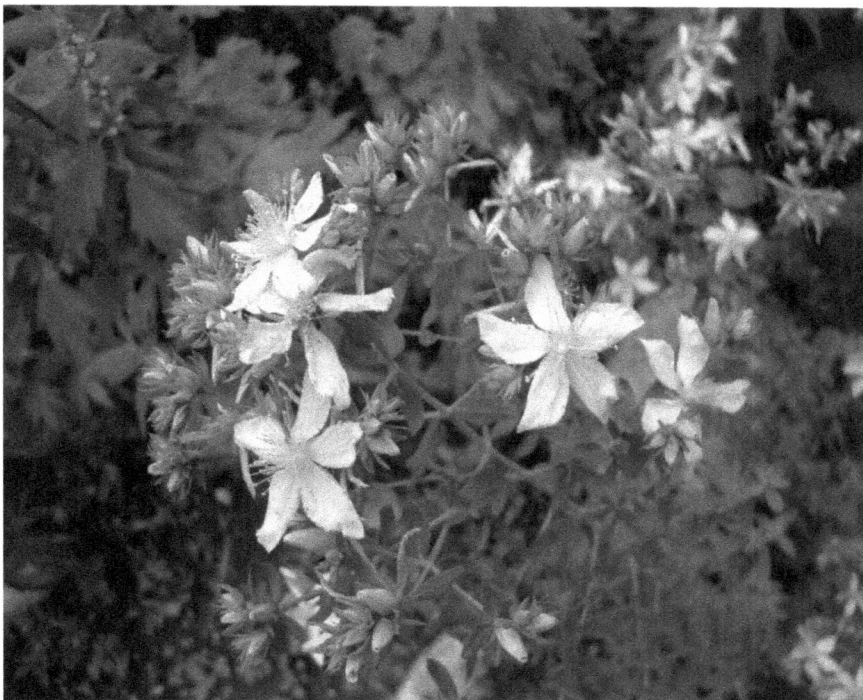

St. John's Wort   Abrah Arneson

St John's Wort *Hypericum perfolatum*

St. John's is well known for its effects on serotonin levels in body. It has a similar effect to the class of pharmaceutical drugs called SSRI which include: Zoloft, Celexa and Prozac. The over the counter supplement 5-HTP also acts like St John's in the body. If a client tells you they have had unpleasant reactions to an SSRI, be careful with St John's. Begin with a low dose and watch the client carefully. Although St John's has an effect similar to SSRI drugs, it is fundamentally different. St John's is plant medicine. Plant medicine is much more complex than a pharmaceutical medicine. For example, besides having an antidepressant effect, St John's Wort is a hepatic and also has anti-viral action. St John's can be used to treat viral hepatitis. Traditionally depression was treated with bitters and hepatics. In my practice I have successfully relieved depression with St John's Wort after SSRIs have been tried and failed to bring the desired result.

Let's return to the angels and their wise words, "All we eat comes from love." What makes human beings happiest? Is it being loved, having someone to love? Perhaps a child, lover, friend, dog or cat? Love opens our minds to possibilities like having children, making a career change, returning to school, and learning something new. All these endeavors require hope. New beginnings are the antithesis to depression.

Love allows us to open ourselves up to others and allows us to receive others deeply into our lives. Love makes it possible to mingle one life with another until it is no longer possible to separate the two individual lives. Is this not like the act of eating? Once enjoyed, the strawberry is no different from our body. Eating is the act of weaving different life forms to create one.

Eating is an act of love. The beginning of a meal is a moment rich with possibility. The expectant pause before biting into a plump red cherry is a promise of juicy sweetness. Munching on a handful of potato chips satiates the craving for salty crunchiness. A cool glass of water quenches our thirst. Food offers fulfillment, much the same way as love does.

Watch a one year old eat a freshly picked strawberry warmed by the sun. Her eyes are wide with awe and wonder. Her fingers reach with tentative anticipation. When the berry's sweetness bursts in her mouth, she smiles. As the strawberry travels down her gullet, serotonin is released from the ENS, helping its passage through the body. It is not surprising that a warm and full belly offers up sighs of satisfaction.

That is not all. Researchers suspect serotonin is a growth hormone in the gut for the very young. In his book *The Second Brain*, Dr. Michael Gershon suggests that serotonin is intimately involved in the formation of the ENS during gestation and quite possibly continues on into the third year of life. Serotonin gives the gut brains.

Let's consider the infant's and toddler's digestion. He begins life only being able to take in one type of food - mother's milk. Sometime around six months of age his mother senses he needs more than her breast milk. One day she offers him mashed sweet potato. He explores the potato's taste, caressing it with his tongue. Afterwards his mom watches him for signs of disturbance in his guts. She waits about 4 days before introducing the next food. Then she gives him a teaspoon of avocado. Between the introductions of each food, the brain in his gut grows.

If it is true that serotonin grows the brain in the gut, one could hypothesize that just as in the first brain, serotonin helps the gut learn each food, or more accurately, the chemistry of each food. This is why it takes times to introduce food to a child and requires patience. It is a learning process for the gut.

Enterologists (scientists who study the gut and its brain) hypothesize that this critical period of developing intestinal intelligence influences the bowel later in life. They suggest serotonin establishes the personality of the bowel. If the flow of serotonin in the gut is impeded during early life, the ENS develops glitches in its communication system resulting in irregular bowel movements and weak digestion.

In her clinic the herbalist meets many volatile gut personalities: Irritable Bowel Syndrome, Constipation, Crohn's and Ulcerative Colitis. Each of these

Herbs Traditionally Used to Influence Both Digestion and Mood

There are a number of herbs that have a long history of being used to create a sense of well being in both the brain and the gut.

Lemon balm *Melissa officinalis*
Mugwort *Artemisia vulagaris*
Damiana *Turnera diffusa*
Peppermint *Piperita menthe*
Chamomile *Matricaria recutita*

conditions profoundly affects the bowel's motility that serotonin is responsible for regulating.

Because of serotonin's role in the early development of the ENS, enterologist Dr. Gershon recommends that the infant's digestive tract be treated well. He amused me though when he wrote, "Unfortunately, no one knows what the immature enteric nervous system considers to be good treatment."

Any mother knows the love offered during breast-feeding is the greatest pleasure the infant knows. The question to ask may be: what came first: the loving embrace and warm sweet milk or serotonin? I suspect it is the loving embrace that aids in the making of serotonin in the infant's gut and the subsequent development of the ENS. It is the love given while breast-feeding that enables the child to receive and assimilate nourishment throughout his life. At least this is what the angels teach!

The Elemental Nature of the Alimentary Tract: Fire, Water, Wind and Earth

- It's Like Being a Good Cook

When the body is in good health..... the function of digestive warmth is to nourish the body, to prevent disease, and act as a support for exerting effort. It is the digestive warmth that enhances one's vitality, produces the splendor of the body and strengthens the bodily constituents. - Dr Yeshi Donden, His Holiness The Dalai Lama's personal physician for over 50 years.

As a child I remember going to my grandmother's apartment for dinner. She was a generous cook. The tables overflowed with food, homemade and delicious. Everything was perfect but for the vegetables. My grandmother boiled vegetables for a very long time. Soggy broccoli fell apart when stabbed with a fork, green beans limped their way to my mouth and mushy carrots reminded me of my brother's baby food. My grandmother cooked the vegetables until all the windows in her apartment steamed up. None of the goodness in the vegetables ever made it to the dinner table. It all remained in the water in the pot.

When cooking, if the elements water, fire, earth and air are in correct proportions the food's nutrition will be preserved and easily assimulated by the body.

Fire warms the food, exciting it to release its nourishment. Water softens the food and acts as a solvent drawing out nutrients, carrying them into the body.

The air element controls the movement of food through the alimentary canal.

The earth element is represented by the food we eat. If the food is of poor quality or insufficient, the earth element is out of balance. If the food is too rich or there is an overabundance of it, the earth element remains out of balance.

A Cold, Wet Gut

While living in Asia, I became accustomed to drinking warm teas sweetened with cardamom to cool off on steamy, hot days. Then while in hospital, the nurses encouraged me to drink warm water. "It is

Flatulence

When a client complains of flatulence, the air element is out of balance in the gut. Flatulence can be resolved by using herbs that have both a bitter and carminative action. Peppermint is a good choice.

Peppermint *Mentha piperita* is warming and soothing to the digestive tract. It calms nausea and eases bloating and gas. Peppermint is particularly helpful in treating irritable bowel syndrome (IBS). A cup of peppermint tea wakes up the senses after a meal has left you feeling sluggish and dull. Sluggish digestion can interrupt sleep. Peppermint tea before bed will ease tension held in the digestive tract, release the sense of heaviness and promote a good night's sleep.

good for your digestion," they said. I was having severe stomach pain after being fed through a tube threaded through my nose and down into my gut for over a month. The tube lacked the warmth of a meal shared with others.

My Chinese nurses knew drinking iced water and sodas puts the fire out in the gut. It dampens down the digestive process. I have not met one individual who drinks several cold drinks a day and does not have a challenge with cramping, painful guts and poor absorption of nutrients. Cold liquid creates a cold, wet gut.

A cold, wet gut brings to mind images of leftover oatmeal: gelled, unappetizing sludge. When the digestive system is too wet, the fire element is weak. Water extinguishes fire. Too much water weighs down the digestive process. Mucous membranes become a swamp-like environment where stinky flora and fauna live. The fine, delicate villi lining the small intestine become boggy. The enterocytes, the cells making up the villi and responsible for absorbing nutrients, swell and lose their ability to discriminate between what is to stay in the guts and what is absorbed into the blood stream. Traditional Chinese Medicine refers to a soggy gut as damp spleen.

Damp Spleen

When an organ is referred to in Traditional Chinese Medicine, it is not the specific organ that is being named. It is activity of the organ that is being referred to.

For example, when speaking of the spleen, a TCM practitioner is naming all processes within the body, whether within the small intestine, a blood vessel, or a cell, engaged in the activities of transformation and transportation. Processes are closely associated with absorption and metabolism.

In TCM spleen activity is responsible for making blood. The small intestine plays a vital role in making blood, selecting nutrients and moving them through the gut wall and into the blood stream. It is the nutrients absorbed by the small intestine that give blood its life.

When the stomach fire is burning low and the small intestine is slough-like, nutrients become bogged down in soggy membranes. Just as the broccoli's goodness was left behind in my grandmother's pot after sitting in water all afternoon, few nutrients pass into the blood when the gut is cold and wet.

A Western Point of View: A Phlegmatic Gut

Nicholas Culpepper, the 16th Century British herbalist, referred to a wet digestive tract as an imbalance in the phlegmatic humour. He described a phlegmatic gut as wet, cold and sticky. Think of mud.

The digestive system under the influence of the phlegmatic humour resembles a mind caught in depression. Depression is heavy with water, cold to life and stuck in repetitive unhappy thoughts. The phlegmatic gut feels full with very little food. Not having the fire to transform food into nutrients, the food sits in the guts, undigested and fermenting. Fermentation draws the water out of the food. The water settles in the gut and in humoural language, a phlegmatic imbalance arises. Just as the depressed mind has no ability to absorb life, the phlegmatic gut has no ability to absorb nutrients. People with wet guts experience fullness in the belly, bloating, perhaps nausea and diarrhea.

Besides being associated with pouring icy drinks down the gullet, dampness in the gut is often caused by excessive sugar in the diet.

A perfect example of what sugar does in the gut occurs when we make medicinal syrups.

To make a medicinal syrup, you begin with a watery decoction to which sugar and heat is added. On a quiet simmer, some water evaporates while the rest is absorbed into the sugar. The decoction becomes thicker and thicker, until it oozes from the spoon. The herbalist then offers the thick, sweet syrup to sooth a dry, hot sore throat, not to increase the dampness in a cold gut.

One of the most useful pieces of advice to offer to people with phlegmatic guts is to cut back on sugary foods including fruit juices, pop, sugared yogurts, candy, ice cream, etc.

To treat a wet, cold gut, two types of herbal actions are employed: carminatives and astringents.

Carminative Herbs (Also called Aromatics)

Aromatic plants open and relax us. - The Wild Medicine Solution, Guido Masé

When the kitchen in a home is warm and fragrant with the scent of wholesome foods cooking, those who live in that house are content and happy. Carminative herbs, fragrant and warm, comfort the body's kitchen and the digestive tract. As the digestive tract warms up, the excess water dissipates just as the sun dries rain soaked gardens.

Ginger (*Zingiber officinale*) is a hot carminative. Ginger's pungent volatile oils excite depressed wet tissue and normalize digestive processes.

People with damp, wet guts tell their herbalists that they feel full all the time, suffer with painful bloating and gas, and often have nausea in the morning. Looking at the client's tongue the herbalist sees a lavender to purplish colour and thinks immediately of ginger.

There are many ways to take ginger. My favourite and easiest is to add a couple slices of fresh root to a cup of green tea. I recommend clients enjoy a cup of this twice a day, particularly in the morning if they have nausea.

Fresh ginger is not as pungent as dried ginger. The water in fresh ginger dilutes the hot volatile oils and I find clients tolerate fresh ginger root better than dried. This is my personal preference. I suggest you try both fresh and dried and experience for yourself the difference.

Ginger is also useful for calming cramping below the navel, whether the cramps are coming from reproductive organs or the digestive tract. To quiet cramps, try a poultice over the area to relieve the pain.

Poultice Using Ginger

To a 1/4 cup of castor oil (You can find it in any drug store, along with witch   hazel,   castor oil is one of the last remnants of the apothecary in modern   pharmacies)

Add 5 drops (ggt) of ginger essential oil

Pour over a piece of flannel. I use a clean dishcloth.

Place over abdomen.

Over the cloth, place a warm hot water bottle.

Leave on 20 minutes.

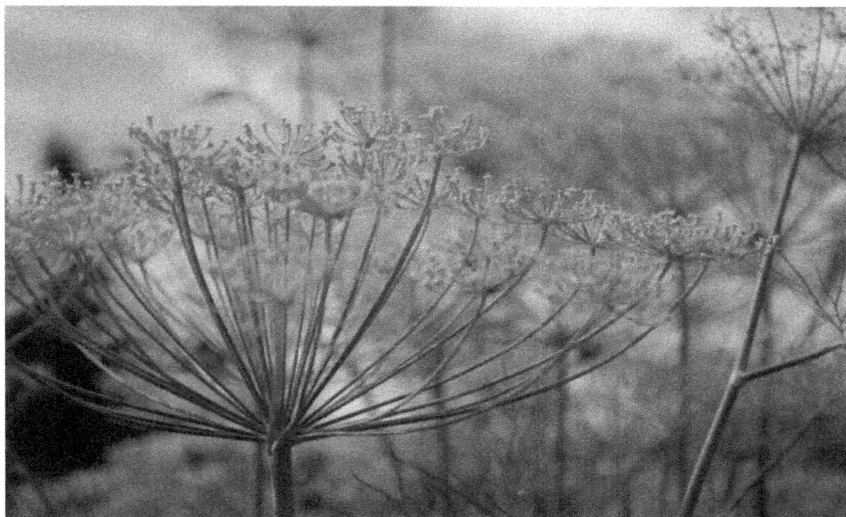

Dill   Mark Arneson

Dill (*Anethum graveolens*) seed is a gentler carminative than ginger. It is not as warming but still effective. Culpepper recommends dill seed to digest "raw and vicious humours". In other words, dill seed dries up a phlegmatic gut. Remember stronger medicine is not always the most effective. This is particularly true when offering herbal medicine to children. Dill seeds are commonly used to make gripe water, a traditional remedy used to ease colic in infants.

Dill is an over-looked remedy in the modern herbal apothecary, perhaps because it is so common. It can be found in any prairie garden with its feathery leaves swaying in the breeze.

I always prefer a herb I can grow, harvest and make medicine with to herbs that I need to bring in from far away. Dill is not as tasty as other carminatives such as cinnamon, cardamom or anise, but it is just as effective in getting a stalled digestive tract moving.

To catch the dill seed from plants in your garden, wait until the plant begins to die back and the seeds are starting to dry. Each morning taste the seeds. When the sweet pungency of the seed fills your mouth, place a paper bag over the seeds and their umbrella-like spokes. Fasten the bag to the stem with a paper clip or twist tie. Cut the stem leaving enough room to hang it from a string. Take the dill plant with the bag over its seeds into the house, and hang it from your drying string. As the seeds ripen they will fall into the bag.

Gripe Water

To one tablespoon of dill seeds add one cup of boiled water. Cover. (You do not want the volatile oils to evaporate into the air. You want them to stay in the pot. They are the medicine.) After 10 minutes, strain and let cool to room temperature. Give baby a teaspoon of the tea and mom can drink the rest of the cup.

You can make more than one cup at a time, but it can only be stored in the fridge for 24 hours. Then you need to make a fresh infusion.

If you leave a couple of plants in the garden, they will self-seed and in the following spring you will have several dill plants happily gracing your garden.

Astringent Herbs

To understand astringent herbs you need to taste them. Go into the garden and introduce yourself to a raspberry plant and ask permission to pick a leaf. Chew on it for a while. Let its greenness mix with your saliva. Notice its taste, but pay particular attention to what the leaf does in your mouth. Astringency is not so much a taste as an experience.

As you chew the raspberry leaf the moist surfaces of your mouth will dry under the influence of the astringent plant's tannins. Then in response to the tannin's dryness, the body will produce saliva. After a moment or two of chewing the leaf, your mouth will feel fresh and clean, as the old saliva has been replaced with new saliva. This is a good example of the body seeking balance. As the raspberry leaf dries, so the body moistens.

Astringency dries up excess moisture in the body. In response the body will release fresh secretions, diluting the thick mucus lining a cold, wet gut. This process encourages the sticky fluids to flow.

There are many, many astringent herbs. The prolific rose family offers medicinal plants with astringent properties. This includes two of the most commonly used astringent herbs in the apothecary: raspberry leaf (*Rubus idaeus*), and blackberry leaf (*Rubus villosa*). A prairie herbalist may want to add the wild rose to this list (*Rosa acicularis*).

The tannins found in the raspberry and blackberry leaf are water-soluble. Therefore the easiest form of medicine to offer them in is a tea. Medicinal teas made with these plants will dry up a wet digestive tract. If a stronger astringent is required, decoct a root from either plant.

Lynwood Tall Bull, a Cheyenne herbalist, tells a story of his mother carrying a root from the wild rose plant in her purse. When the family went camping, she would take the root from her purse, unwrap it and make a tea with it. The rose root was a gift from her mother. For many years the same root was used to make tea.

Traditionally, blackberry is the herb of choice to dry a wet digestive tract. Raspberry is considered not as efficient and more specific to supporting the uterus from becoming boggy. In a pinch, raspberry leaf will help a phlegmatic gut.

One more useful astringent....

Meadowsweet (*Filipendulum ulmaria*) leaf is an astringent. Generally because astringents are drying, they are contraindicated when the digestive tract is hot and dry. Recall

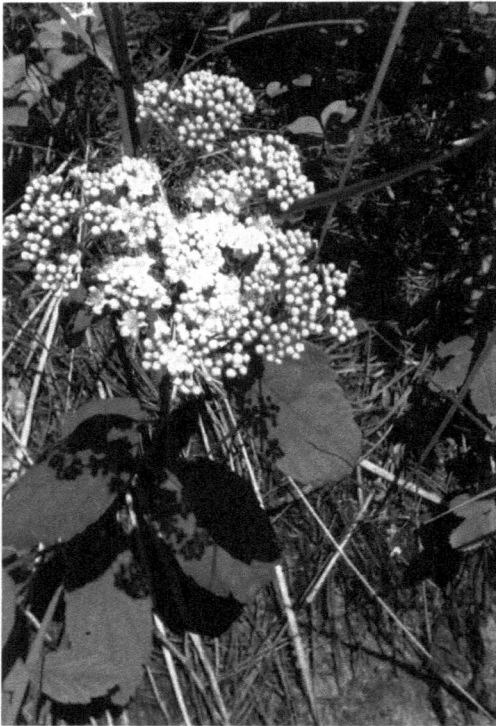

tasting the raspberry leaf. First it dried up the surface of your mouth and in response saliva was produced to counter the dryness. Meadowsweet is a mild astringent compared to other members of the rose family. Meadowsweet's astringency can be used to encourage the stomach and small intestine to release their own moisture. This not the primary medicine

Meadowsweet   Rosalee de la Forêt

meadowsweet offers an overheated gut.

Meadowsweet balances stomach acids. If the stomach acids are too low, which is frequently the case when a mushy, carb rich diet is preferred, meadowsweet leaf increases the stomach acids. When stomach acids are too high, as frequently seen in a diet high in animal protein, meadowsweet brings them down.

A tea made with 2 parts marshmallow root, 1 part meadowsweet leaf and 1 part melissa will sooth a hot, dry stomach and improve absorption of nutrients in the small intestine.

One more herb worth mentioning....

Horseradish (*Armoracia rusticana*) is another garden herb useful in relieving a cold, wet digestive tract. A small bowl of horseradish was always found on my grandmother's table when she served roast beef. The heat contained in the plant's root warms the stomach and supports digestion of protein rich food.

The extreme pungency of Horseradish stimulates peristalsis by encouraging the secretion of bile. Western physiologists consider bile essential in the digestion of fats. Eastern physiologists consider the bile to be the source of the fire element in the body. In either case, the horseradish's ability to encourage the flow of bile and warm up the stomach and small intestine improves absorption of nutrients.

Be careful offering it in tincture form as it can be very irritating. It is best to encourage a client with a sluggish digestive tract to use horseradish as a condiment with their supper.

A Hot, Dry Gut

A good cook pays attention to the stove. She does not get on the phone to her Mom and forget about the rice simmering on the stove. Nor does she try to cook the food too fast, turning up the temperature on the stove. In both cases the result is too much fire. The delicious food becomes burnt, unappealing, and impossible to digest. The pot, crusted with the charred food, requires soaking in water and baking soda followed by a vigorous scrubbing.

Just as the sun dries up the land on a hot summer's day, excess fire in the gut dries up mucous membranes and the moist, warm gut becomes a scorched environment. Without the water element to soften food, draw out its nutrients and carry them into the enterocytes lining the villi, everything eaten becomes a burning pain in the belly. The wind element (responsible for the flow of nutrients through the alimentary tract) becomes unpredictable and the bowels swing from constipation to diarrhea.

When the digestive tract suffers with heat the tongue will be red. In extreme heat the tongue takes on a flame shape and is pointed. Often I find those who have used pharmaceutical drugs that manipulate serotonin over a number of years show this shape of tongue.

The primary task the herbalist faces with a hot, dry gut is to cool the heat down. I often find cooling down the gut also means cooling down the head. A hot gut often accompanies anxiety and flares of anger. My favourite herb in this situation is lemon balm (*Melissa officinalis*).

Melissa, as I fondly refer to this lovely, gentle plant, is a cooling carminative. While most carminatives are warming herbs, melissa cools. She will cool down a hot belly, a hot head and hot blood.

Let's pretend that a man, age 45, comes into your office. At first you think his rosy cheeks are a picture of health, and then he begins to tell you about his many health challenges. His guts burn relentlessly, so much so that he cannot eat. He flies off the handle at the slightest provocation. He is worried about having a heart attack as his father died of one at his age. You feel his pulse and it is hot, thick and tight. When you palpate his abdomen it is hard to the touch. He has sudden unexpected tears when you express your concern. This is a case for melissa.

Melissa calms the heart, relaxes the mind and eases heat from the digestive tract. Melissa is a traditional antidepressant and it is my favourite plant when anxiety walks hand in hand with depression and an overheated digestive tract.

In laboratory studies, melissa inhibits the uptake of thyroid stimulating hormone (TSH) by the thyroid gland. Therefore melissa is contraindicated for those struggling with a hypothyroid.

If the herbalist understands melissa's cooling and calming medicine, they know that the herb is a poor choice for those struggling with a low thyroid. A low-functioning thyroid is a cold condition. Nothing moves: bowels, digestion, mind, and emotions because the metabolism that is controlled by the thyroid is sluggish. A low thyroid is like a fire that is buried in ashes. Cooling herbs like melissa are not offered to a client struggling with a cold condition. This is a classic example of how understanding a herb's energetics (temperature) will protect you from making a client's condition worse instead of better.

There are three more things I love about melissa.

1. I grow it my garden. The fresh herb makes a beautifully calming tincture.

2. It has both immediate and long-term effects on the body. It is immediately cooling while over time it restores the nervous system (an action called *trophorestorative*).

3. It is pleasing to the tongue.

Demulcents Herbs

The stomach hates being hot and dry. It depends on the moisture of its mucous membrane for its health and support in absorption of nutrients. Water contained in the membrane softens food, facilitating its absorption. The mucous membrane protects the stomach from the burn of stomach acids.

A hot, dry gut feels hard when palpated and can be painful for the client. Food sits in it like a lump and can cause heartburn that keeps one awake at night. The belching is embarrassing and the bloating accompanying the heat is uncomfortable. As time passes ulcers develop in the stomach, esophagus and duodenum. An over-heated gut can develop into cancer.

Demulcent herbs soothe hot, dry stomachs.

Plantain *(Plantago spp.)* Again, wander into the back yard and find yourself the common weed named plantain. It will be growing on a path used to cross your garden. Introduce yourself. It is a friendly plant and probably will not mind you picking one of its leaves.

Squish the leaves in your hand. Notice the moisture contained within plantain's leathery outer surface. This moisture is called mucilage and is common to all plants with demulcent actions.

Plant mucilage is composed of heteropolysaccarides, or in other words various forms of sugar. This sugary, water loving plant constituent is commonly called

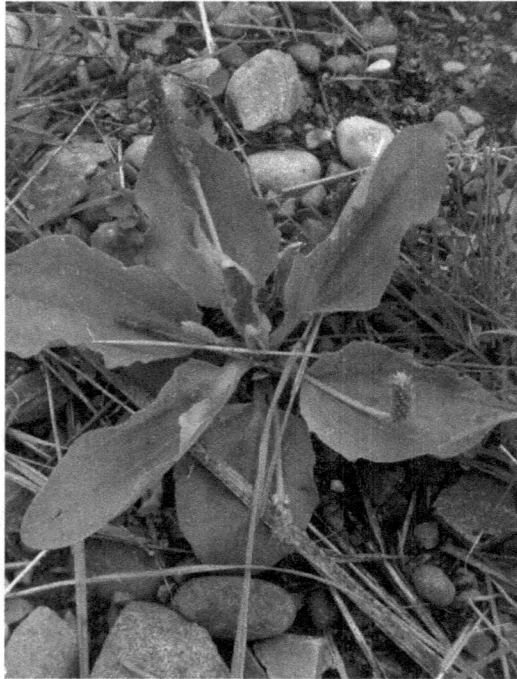

Plantain   Rosalee de la Forêt

pectin or gum. For simplicity herbalists lumped these complex sugars together under the term mucilage.

How do you know a plant has mucilage? Chew on it. As the plant mixes with your saliva a slimy gel forms in your mouth. This gel is called mucilage and carries demulcent properties that sooth, moisten and soften hard, dry surfaces in the body. (Demulcents, when used on the hot, dry eczema, are called emollients.)

Plantain is an excellent demulcent for a hot, dry digestive tract. Mexican herbalist, Jaime Barre, taught me to offer it as a tea to those with stomach cancer. Cancer has a furious appetite and it demands food continuously. To keep its hunger appeased, cancer grows many, many blood vessels in a process known as angiogenesis. The web of blood vessels serves the cancer with an endless supply of nutrients. Because blood carries heat, the excessive blood flowing to the cancer creates a hot tumour. Plantain's demulcent action cools down the burn of cancer.

Marshmallow (*Althea officinalis*) is an easy plant to grow in moist areas of your garden. All parts of the marshmallow plant make copious amounts of mucilage - flower, leaf, and root. This is why the plant enjoys

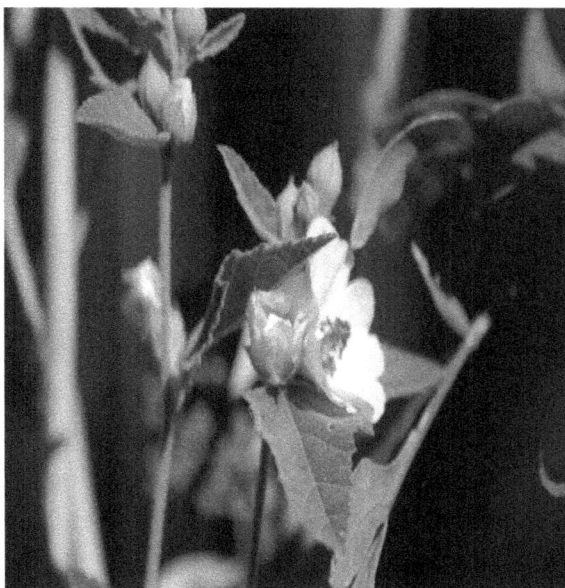

Marshmallow   Mark Arneson

moist earth; it needs water to make its healing mucilage.

I use marshmallow whenever a client tells me of burning in the body. This could be a burning in the guts, bladder, or throat. Marshmallow, both the root and leaf, soothes any irritated mucous membrane in the body.

Traditionally, marshmallow is prepared as a cold infusion to ease the fire element in the body. Add a teaspoon of marshmallow root or a tablespoon of the plant's leaf to a cup of cold water. Cover the cup and put it in the fridge overnight. In the morning, the polysaccharides in the mucilage will have been drawn from the plant into the water, forming a viscous medicinal cold tea that will soften and soothe hot, dry surfaces in the body.

Slippery elm (*Ulmus rubra*) bark is a nutritive demulcent. Historically slippery elm was offered as gruel during convalescence. It was given to those recovering from an illness that wasted their body, mind and spirit. It nourishes the body, soothing irritation within the alimentary tract and calms a fraught nervous system.

Although where I live elm trees self-seed, in the eastern half of the North American continent the graceful elm is endangered. Thousands of trees died with the spread of Dutch elm disease during the last century. For this reason, it is important to offer this medicine only when no other demulcent will do.

A couple of summers ago a 56-year-old man came to me. He had been stricken with an E.coli infection, and within two weeks he lost 35 pounds. His body was weak and his spirit disheartened. Even though he was free of the bacteria when he came to see me, he continued to have loose stools with blood. Three times a day I had him take two tablespoons of slippery elm in a smoothie with plain yogurt and a banana. He also freely drank a bone broth that included nettle leaf. Within a week, his bowel movements normalized. Beginning with rice, slowly whole foods were introduced. Today, he has completely recovered and has gained back the weight he lost including 5 more pounds.

I have also seen slippery elm regulate bowels suffering with inflammatory bowel diseases such as crohn's disease and ulcerative colitis. When there is a chronic history of loose stools mixed with fresh blood, I find slippery elm an essential element in the treatment.

In some herbals you will find that slippery elm is contraindicated in pregnancy. This is not because of the plant's healing properties. First Nations People at one time used twigs from the elm tree to induce abortions. An elm twig was inserted into the vagina up to the cervix and attempts to break the amniotic membranes were made. Missionaries considered the abortions immoral and the elm tree became associated with abortion. For this reason, slippery elm use continues to be discouraged during pregnancy.

Form Equals Function

The bowel just is not the kind of organ that makes the pulse race. No poet would ever write an ode to the intestine. To be frank, the popular consensus is that the colon is a repulsive piece of anatomy. Its shape is nauseating, its content disgusting, and its smell bad. The bowel is a primitive, slimy, snakelike thing. Its body lies coiled within the belly, and it slithers when it moves. In brief, the gut is despicable and reptilian, not at all like the brain, from which wise thoughts emerge. Clearly, the gut is an organ only a scientist would love. - The Gut has a Mind of Its Own: The Second Brain - Michael D. Gershon, MD

When assessing the health and disease of a client, the herbalist needs to ask herself if the health challenges relate to the form of the body or its function or both.

The herbs we have just explored can be classed as either acting on the form or the function. Astringents and demulcents affect the tissues that make up the digestive tract. Astringents tone tissues while demulcents soften them. Carminatives and bitters have a more pronounced effect on the function of the gut. Carminatives calm and regulate the movement of smooth muscle tissue in the gut, while bitters encourage peristalsis and the secretion of digestive juices from the stomach, liver and pancreas.

A herbalist's practice of plant medicine is greatly enhanced by a thorough and on going study of the alchemical processes in the gut. It is important to understand the role each digestive organ and tissue plays in these fundamental processes of life.

The following is a brief introduction to the form and function of the human gut.

Sometimes I compare the human body to a donut - a fleshy ring with a hole in the middle. The long hollow tube that runs the length of the human torso is called the alimentary or digestive tract. It is a living landscape of flora and fauna. It is as multicultural as Toronto or Vancouver. It is an alchemical vessel where the most refined processes of purification and chemical transformation take place.

The alimentary tract is referred to as a lumen. Lumens are stacked layers of cells surrounding a hollow tube and are one of nature's repeating structures. Besides being the form the alimentary tract takes, lumens are found in leaves, stems, trunks, and roots such as the dandelion's hollow stem or the channels that run the length of the mighty oak's trunk. Through plant lumens, nutrients and water flow from roots to leaves and from the leaves to the roots.

The red worms my husband feeds vegetable peelings to in a box in the basement are wiggling lumens. In goes vegetables and out comes compost.

The human's lumen, or alimentary tract, performs the same function as the red worms and plants do. It transports the raw materials of life from outside of the body to the inside. Once inside a lumen, the raw materials of food and water transform in ways we barely understand. And after the transformation has taken place, lumens discard the left over wastes. (It is not really wastes, just another kind of food humans do not find particularly palatable.)

In some ways one can define life as being able to transform one life form into another. In health, when something enters a lumen, it leaves in a completely different form. This is the purpose of the lumen in nature.

The Journey Through the Lumen

The mouth represents one end of the human lumen. In the mouth the transformation of food begins. While teeth macerate the food, the tongue assesses its chemical make-up while mixing it with digestive enzymes provided by saliva. The enzymes begin the work of breaking down cell walls and releasing nutrients. The tongue, as skilful as a baker making dinner rolls, kneads the food into a swallowable bolus.

When the bolus reaches the back of the tongue, the body's hunger takes over from the conscious mind and the bolus is gulped down. A mild contraction by the pharynx propels the bolus onto the second leg of its journey.

The pharynx's contraction begins a wave that ripples through the entire digestive tract. Slipping down the slimy oesophagus, the bolus arrives in the stomach.

In the stomach the tasty food that was divided into vegetables, chicken and rice on your plate meets the formidable pepsin: a combination of hydrochloric acids and a hormone called pepsinogen. Pepsin burns protein's tough cell membranes, releasing inner nutrients liquefying the bolus in the process. The bolus leaves the stomach in a new form called chyme.

The pyloric sphincter, a tight band of muscles at the lower end of the stomach, squirts chyme into the small intestine. Inside the small intestine your dinner mingles with an unusual crowd that welcomes its arrival.

Herbal Probiotics
Herbs that contain complex sugars act as food for the indigenous micro flora. These herbs are marshmallow, chickweed and calendula, just to name a few. Feeding micro flora is another activity of demulcent herbs.

The small intestine houses 100,000,000,000,000 bacteria. There are more bacteria making their home in your gut then there are people living on this beautiful planet.

Like big cities, your gut is a multicultural environment driven by commerce and the exchange. You, the one who walks around thinking you are not bacteria, are part of the equation. The indigenous micro flora (the scientific name for the bacteria in

Notes on a Multicultural Environment
Multicultural environments are about ideas, sharing knowledge and different ways of living. At their best they are dynamic, creative environments where commonalities and differences bring about an inspired life.

A multicultural gut is adaptable. Capable of receiving a wide variety of information, its able to discriminate between that which is useful and that which needs to be abandoned. A multicultural gut transforms itself according to food eaten. To achieve balance in life, a diverse diet is needed. A bland, repetitive diet dampens the environment and slows down the exchange of nutrients between the gut wall and your insides.

The ability to experience and digest new foods and ideas could be a metaphor for health, both physical and mental.

your guts) needs you to provide adequate housing, the correct pH balance, sufficient O2 levels, food and a transit pass. You on the other hand, the landlord, require the bacteria to break down the chyme and prepare the food you bought, cooked and ate for assimilation. This is called a mutualistic relationship.

Other organs come into play with the chyme's arrival in the small intestine. Bile from the liver traveling by way of the gallbladder spurts into the small intestine through the bile duct. Bile is essential for the absorption of fats (including fat-soluble vitamins) and encourages peristalsis. Because bitter herbs like dandelion root (*Taraxacum radix*) and vervain (*Verbena officinalis*) encourage the secretion of bile and stimulate peristalsis, they can have a laxative-like effect on a sluggish alimentary tract.

The pancreas delivers two substances into the small intestine. One is alkalizing bicarbonate to neutralize the acids that accompany the chyme into the small intestine. Bicarbonate saves the small intestine's tender villi from being seared by stomach's acids. (The indigenous micro flora prefers the alkaline environment created by the bicarbonate.)

The other pancreatic secretion is a medley of digestive enzymes: amylase (which break down carbohydrates), lipase (fats) and protease (proteins).

As the chyme becomes intimate with the indigenous micro flora, it passes over the villi. The villi, another type of lumen made by stacks of enterocytes, absorb nutrients from the processed chyme. Within the villi, the water-soluble nutrients are passed into veins where they are shipped to the liver for processing. The fat-soluble nutrients are ushered into lymphatic vessels contained within the villi called lacteals. The fatty nutrients pass into the lymphatic system becoming a substance called chyle. The chyle eventually passes into the blood stream and travels to the liver for processing.

What is not absorbed by the small intestine(mostly fibre, water and minerals) passes through the ileosecal valve and into the colon. In the colon, water is reabsorbed by following salt through the wall of the colon in a process called osmosis. As the chyme becomes denser, stool is formed and eventually the waste products of digestion are excreted at the lower end of the lumen, known as the anus.

The Alimentary Tract is a Composite

The wise herbalist studying physiology keeps focused on the interplay between various systems. Perhaps it is helpful to think of the study of the body from the point of view of Jung's four functions (recall chapter one).

- The study of anatomy involves knowing the form of the body and is related to the sensing function. What you see is what you know.
- The study of physiology involves understanding how the form functions and requires the use of the thinking function. What you know is what you think.
- The feeling function understands the relationship between the form and function.
- When all the bits and pieces of anatomy and physiology are put together, the "whole-ness" of the body, the miracle that it is, is understood by the intuitive function at play.

The alimentary tract is a perfect example of different systems working together to process and assimilate food for the body. Although considered a significant member of the gastrointestinal system of the body, the alimentary tract is a composite of several physiological systems. It is composed of skin and muscles and is self-regulated by an intelligent nervous system. The circulatory system and lymphatic system are essential for both the health of the alimentary tract and the delivery of the nutrients it assimilates to the rest of the body.

The endocrine system which manages the body's fight and flight mechanisms controls the on and off switch for many of the alimentary tract functions. Even bones, shaped like teeth, participate in the assimilation of food within the alimentary tract.

When our digestion is efficient and the systems of the body function harmoniously we feel enlivened by the food we eat. One could say that good digestion is good health. However when the systems become imbalanced, digestion is troubled and we slowly (or quickly) become malnourished. Malnourishment due to poor digestion is the root of many diseases, both acute and chronic, transient and lethal.

Herbal medicine shines when the herbalist understands the alimentary tract is a composite of systems. Let's explore the digestive system's composite nature by looking at a few plants that help bring it back into balance.

Bayberry (*Myrica cerifera*) is a pungent herb with astringent actions specific to the lower digestive tract (the small and large intestines). Bayberry's pungency stimulates circulation within the abdomen, increasing the supply of fresh oxygen and nutrients to the digestive tract and aiding in the removal of metabolic waste. These processes are critical for the health of any organ in the body.

Bayberry bark's astringent effect brings tension to relaxed bowels. When the muscles of the bowel lose tone, peristalsis becomes sluggish. Herbalists call this condition a relaxed condition or a sluggish bowel. A relaxed bowel tends towards constipation with poorly formed stools.

A relaxed bowel causes stagnancy of the bowel's contents. In traditional North American herbalism the stagnant material is referred to as canker. Left for an extended period of time, canker results in "canker sores". Bayberry increases circulation and promotes the dilution of the canker. This supports the body eliminate the offending canker and creates a healthy bowel environment.

Bayberry is medicine for the bowel's mucous membrane, musculature and circulatory system.

Oregon grape root (*Mahonia aquifolium*) is a moist, bitter, cooling herb that has effects on the bowel, liver and lymphatic system. It is also an antibacterial herb. It is favoured for treating eczema that is caused by a hot and dry leaky gut.

The alimentary tract, although contained within the flesh of the body, is considered to be the outer surface of the body. It is open to the outside world at both ends of its tube. The lining of the alimentary tract is made with the same tissue as the skin. Both are composed of epithelial tissue. Designed for covering outer surfaces, epithelial tissue is made of tightly packed cells that do not have their own blood vessels. Epithelial tissue is designed to keep stuff out of the interior of the body.

Epithelial cells (both skin and the alimentary tract lining) are fed from within the body. Nutrients diffuse into epithelial cells through the connective tissue that binds them to muscles. In holistic herbal medicine, skin conditions are generally associated with leaky bowels. The leaks begin in weak epithelial tissue lining the bowel. Many of the herbs used to treat skin diseases like eczema also improve the integrity of the epithelial tissue in the gut.

Oregon grape is one of them. It moistens and soothes irritated epithelial tissue in the gut.

Oregon grape's bitter taste encourages secretion of bile from the liver. This improves absorption of fats in the villi's lacteals. Recall

Herbs Containing Anthroquinones
Turkey Rhubarb *Rhuem palmata*
Senna *Senna alexandrina*
Cascara *Rhamnus purshiana*
Buckthorn *Rhamnus catharticus,*
Yellow dock *Rumex crispus*
Aloes   *Aloe spp.*

the lacteals are part of the lymphatic system. The improved absorption of fats encourages movement within the lymph system.

Historically oregon grape was considered a blood maker. Recall the relationship between the activity of the spleen and the small intestine in TCM. Oregon grape improves the movement of chyme through the small intestine, enhances the absorption of fats, and encourages the elimination of wastes in the large intestine. Each of these activities enriches the blood.

Finally, oregon grape root contains a strongly antibacterial alkaloid called berberine. Berberine is effective against *Staphylococcus aureus, Candida albicans, Escherichia coli, Klebsiella pneumonia*, and many others.

Bugleweed (*Lycopus virginicus*) is a nervine with a dramatic effect on the thyroid. Bugleweed reduces the pituitary's production of thyroid stimulating hormone TSH that, in turn, calms an overactive thyroid.

One of the symptoms of a hyperthyroid gland is frequently loose stools. In extreme cases diarrhea can cause dehydration and malnutrition. Bugleweed's ability to quiet down the thyroid almost instantly results in regular bowel movements.

Please note that bugleweed's effect is symptomatic. It does not heal hyperthyroidism.

Liquorice (*Glycyrrhiza glabra*) is a plant I continually get to know. It is complex and rich in activity. The classic herbal *Bartram's Encyclopaedia of Herbal* Medicine lists the following actions for this sweet, juicy root: *expectorant, demulcent, anti-inflammatory, glycogen conserver, mild laxative, adrenal restorative, regulates salt and water metabolism, anti-stress, anti-ulcer, hepatoprotective, anti-depressive and modulates gastric juices.* Bartram refers to liquorice as the "Universal Herb" while TCM calls it "Grandfather".

Liquorice's demulcent actions sooth irritated membranes throughout the body, including the alimentary tract. Its ability to support the liver improves both peristalsis and absorption of nutrients. Through acting on the adrenal glands, liquorice quiets downs the stress response, allowing the alimentary tract to relax and prepare for food. Its laxative effect aids in the bowels in the removal of toxins. It heals ulcers in the lining of the alimentary tract. I strongly recommend spending a significant amount of time with this plant to gain a deep appreciation and understanding of its medicine.

Valerian (*Valariana officinalis*) is a bitter, pungent nervine and is best known as a sleep aid. I however find it most effect for tense, sensitive and cramping bowels. For those who eat their emotions (they bite their lip to contain their feelings as opposed to talking them out) valerian root is a comforting herb. It relaxes tension in the gut better than any other herb I have tried.

What I really like about valerian (other than the fact that it loves to grow in my garden) is one only needs a small dose to release abdominal tension. This in turn improves absorption of nutrients and elimination of wastes while providing emotional space to take care of difficult feelings.

A Quick Word About Diet

Although this is not a book about nutrition, a herbalist who does not understand the fundamentals of nutrition is like a silk flower. She may look good but she has no substance. There are thousands of books on nutrition. I advise you to get a few and read them. For our purpose though, I would like to just outline a few simple ways anyone can improve their nutrition.

1. Enjoy your food. Have gratitude and respect for where it comes from.

2. Eat breakfast sitting down. Think outside of the cereal box.

3. Have some protein at every meal.

4. Enjoy a wide range of foods. Give up a monotonous diet.

5. Eat according to the season: cooling foods like salads during the summer and warming foods like soups in the winter.

6. Choose organic foods. Plants sprayed with herbicides do not have the same opportunity to develop the life sustaining chemistry humans translate into medicine and food.

7. Choose carefully raised and compassionately butchered animals.

8. Avoid fad diets.

9. Listen to your body's nutritional needs and trust what it tells you.

Final Notes on Assimilation: Deficiency and Excess

To add to what is already full or to decrease what is already deficient, to penetrate further into what is already flowing

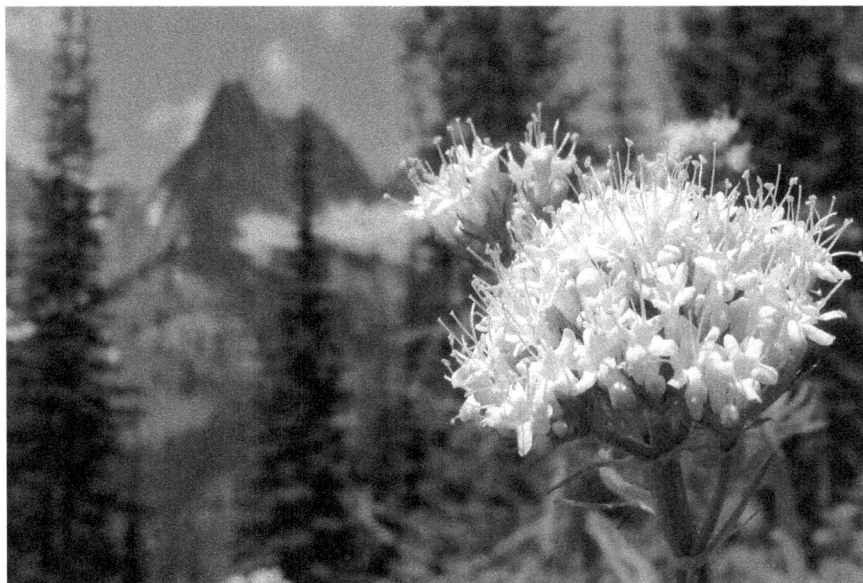

Valerian   Rosalee de la Forêt

freely or to congest what is already blocked, to cool what is already cold or to warm what is already hot, this is only doubling the disorder – Sun Si-mialo paraphrased in Western Herbs in Chinese Medicine by Thomas Avery Garran

Deficiency and excess manifest at many levels in life. Every health challenge is built on deficiencies and excesses. One never appears without the other. If health is defined as balance, a continually moving moment in life, observing the relationship between deficiency and excess can help us learn to walk in balance, harmony and health.

Assimilation is not just about food - it's about ideas, emotions, play, goals, spiritual beliefs, etc. When pondering the activity of assimilation in life, one is also studying the effect of deficiencies and excesses on all levels of being. The question to ask when looking at the assimilation process is: what is being absorbed and what is not being absorbed?

States of deficiencies can also be called stagnation. Pain - physical, emotional and mental - is caused by stagnation. Let's consider a few states of stagnation.

Physical: Pain causing stones in the gallbladder when there is stagnant or deficient secretion of bile from the liver. Drinking dandelion leaf and root tea improves the release of bile into the gallbladder and into the bowel, resolving chronic stagnant liver conditions.

Emotional: Constant sadness dampens life-creating stagnation. Rosemary is a pungent herb that lifts the weight of sadness and enlivens the mind and digestion.

Mental: Repetitive thoughts that circle round and round are mental stagnation. Often these are thoughts that attack self-esteem. Bitter herbs like skullcap ease anxious thoughts while improving the action of the liver and releasing the muscular tension, a result of punishing thoughts.

Examples of Deficiencies and Excesses through a study of the elements:

Element	Deficiency	Excess
Earth	Crumbling bones, unable to take a stand, sense of lack, a poverty of being	Hard, immovable masses, miserly, entitlement
Water	Hard, dry, hot, a lack of compassionate feelings, punishing attitudes	Wet, heavy, lacking tone, overly emotional, gushing, suffocating
Fire	Cold, lack of passion, excitement, drive	Hot, overly passionate, emotionally explosive
Air	Wet, stagnant, dull mind	Dry, excitable, flitting pain, fingers in too many pies

The Physiology of Circulation: An Ocean Wrapped in Skin

After assessing the client's ability to take in nutrients, herbalists move on to evaluate their circulation. Circulation is concerned with the delivery of absorbed nutrients (including oxygen) to the body's cells and the removal of metabolic waste from the body's tissues. Traditional herbalists believe circulation is the key to good health. When circulation is stagnant the supply of oxygen and nutrients to the body (or certain areas of the body) is interrupted and metabolic wastes build up. Starved and oxygen deprived organs and tissues open a portal for disease to enter the body.

The human body is 85% water. Water, the most malleable element, takes many forms in the body: blood, lymph, intracellular and extracellular fluids, inter-cranial and spinal fluid, tears, sweat, mucous, saliva and synovial fluid, and bile. Sometimes I think of the body as an ocean wrapped in skin.

In health, water flows. Springs gurgle, creeks tumble and rivers wander. The ocean's tides ebb and flow with the moon while the wind rides ocean currents, spinning saline waters from north to south and back again. In the body, rhythmic pulsations, fluctuations between warmth and cold, physical movement, and the pull of oxygen and nutrients across cell membranes keep water in healthy flow. Our minds also play a role in circulation. Stormy thoughts send hearts racing while blood boils. A peaceful mind quiets the heartbeat and the body is infused with the gentle warmth of bliss. The body's water, managed by finely tuned kidneys pumped by a tireless heart, courses through networks of blood and lymph vessels, mazes of extracellular matrix, and weaves in and out of cells carrying nourishment and waste.

Let's consider the body's circulation of fluid from a holistic point of view.

- The elements of circulation: fire, water, air, earth
- A Traditional View of Treating Illness: Samuel Thomson and Circulation
- Getting to the Heart of the Matter: Cardioneurology
- Understanding Circulation Through the Study of Trees: branching vessels
- The Liver: Cleaning and Nourishing the Blood
- The Kidney: Blood Pressure and Hydration

The elements of circulation:
Fire, Water and Air

Circulation of nutrients through the body involves the interaction between water, fire, air and earth. The fluid nature of blood represents the water element. The continuous movement of blood which is controlled by the body's nervous system represents the air element. The warmth blood carries symbolizes the fire element, and the earth element is embodied by the nutrients found in the blood.

Water Controls Fire

The water element controls, contains, and circulates the fire element in the body.

To understand the relationship between fire and water in health, we must first define two basic principles of water and fire.

Fire

Heat seeks cool. When a fire burns too hot, it devours oxygen circulating in the air, eventually burning itself out. In fire's thirst for oxygen rich air, the heat of fire always flows to cool areas.

Pine trees know this. They use this principal to protect themselves from fire. Pine needles are highly flammable. Pine resin, the scabs a pine tree forms when there is an injury to its bark, is also highly flammable. Forest fires raging through pine forests burn very hot. The hotter the fire the more oxygen it needs. When the wind is still, fire's ravenous desire exhausts itself in a pine forest. Unable to breath, the fire loses its virility and dies. The pine forest will sacrifice some trees to feed the fire's intensity and save the forest.

Think of it this way. On a hot summer's afternoon, parks are filled with people lying on blankets spread out under shade trees. People naturally do this to cool down. Dreaming under a big, leafy tree, the heat of the day flows from your body into the cool ground beneath the tree. Heat spreads to cool.

Water

Takes the path of least resistance. Water always flows into open spaces.

Fire, Water and Air During Stress

During the fight or flight stress response triggered by the adrenaline surges from the adrenal medulla (the inner portion of the endocrine organs capping the kidneys), blood rushes from the digestive organs to the heart, lungs and skeletal muscles. Carrying the fire of action, the blood provides the essential force these organs need to run or fight for life. After a stressful event flowing tears release adrenaline's fire and all its fury from the body/mind.

The body keeps a tight control on the fire element. In health the surface body temperature is 36.8 degrees Celsius while the core temperature of the body is 37 degrees.

When the fire element flares up too high in the body, whether spiking a fever, during vigorous exercise, or in a steam bath, the arterial vessels close to the surface of your skin dilate. Water, in the form of blood, seeks the path of least resistance and flows into the open, relaxed blood vessels towards the surface of the body. Because the surface of your body is naturally cooler than the interior, the heat contained in the blood flows out of the body into the cooler air surrounding it. To enhance this effect, the sweat glands of the skin open and the water element in the form of sweat releases more heat. As the sweat trickles over you, the temperature of the skin becomes even cooler, encouraging more heat to flow from the blood. The cooler blood circulating near the surface of the body eventually flows towards the core of the body relieving the excess interior heat.

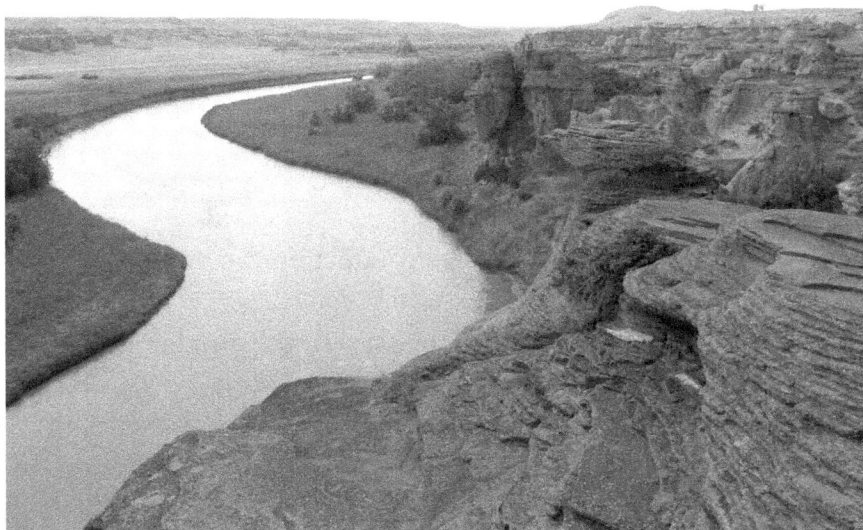

Milk River, Alberta   Mark Arneson

When the fire element in the body is weak, blood moves deeper into the body to guard the body's heat for survival. The fire element is essential for the health of inner vital organs, lungs, heart, liver, etc. An individual can survive the loss of fingers due to frostbite, but a cold heart is life threatening.

Air Controls Water

The air element controls the movement of the water element. Wind profoundly influences the ocean's circulation. Gentle ripples appear on the ocean surface under the wind's caress while a hurricane can whip up turbulence to 200 meters deep. The air element has a similar effect on the body's circulation.

The Branches of the Circulatory System

Interstitial fluid: The fluid the cells float in. It is like a gel and similar in chemistry to seawater. Some compare its movement through the body to tides in the ocean.

Arteries: Deliver oxygen and nutrients to the cells. Muscles within the walls of the arteries pulse in sync with the opening and closing chambers of the heart.

Veins: Removes CO_2 and wastes from interstitial fluid. The movement of fluid is controlled by a series of valves within veins and skeletal muscles surrounding veins. Movement of the body stimulates the flow of blood through the veins. Veins do not have their own muscles.

Lymphatic Vessels: Run alongside of veins and arteries. Lymphatics mop up what the veins have left behind. The skeletal muscles' movement controls the movement of lymph.

Physical exercise encourages the flow of the air element in the body. It is common knowledge that movement has a significant role in the circulation of body fluids and the overall health of the body. Running quickens the heart, strengthening its muscle while toning muscles that support venous return. Walking moistens stiff joints by increasing the secretion and flow of synovial fluid. Blinking moistens eyes. Hot yoga drenches skin. Sex stimulates a cascade of pleasure fluids. Powerful emotional surges release tears.

The air element is also represented by the heart's rhythm and the subsequent pulsation of arteries. Let's consider the pulse.

Imagine dropping a stone into a clear pool of water. Watch the water ripple in concentric circles. Within the body a similar phenomenon occurs with each rhythmic arterial pulse. Each pulsation causes ripples in the interstitial fluid (the saline fluid that suspends cells). The cells floating in the interstitial fluid bob like buoys on the ocean as the ripples come and go. The interstitial ripples are called pressure waves.

Structures within the body have different densities. For example, the liver, a lattice of tubes and canals, is thicker than the thin elasticity of the lungs and thinner than the powerful heart muscle. The density of each organ and the pressure waves stirred up by arterial pulsations create a microcirculation within the geography of each organ. Dense organs have a slow, shallow pressure wave. Organs with less cellular compaction have faster pressure waves with higher peaks and lower valleys.

Blood Pressure

Although the kidneys play a significant role in monitoring the pressure blood exerts on the walls of arteries as it flows, the nervous system is intrinsically involved as well.

For example, valerian, a commonly recommended sedative, may be the only plant a client needs to lower their blood pressure. Valerian blocks the re-uptake of GABA, a neurotransmitter that encourages relaxation of neurons. A deficiency of GABA is associated with anxious states of mind that lead to high blood pressure. For many, a low daily dose of valerian relieves anxiety and the high blood pressure that accompanies it.

The pressure waves offer a warm fluid massage to the body's cells. This movement is important for the overall health of the body. Think of it this way: stagnant water is murky, thick, smelly, and unpleasant. Flowing water is clear, clean, sings and is refreshing. Without the pulse humming throughout the body creating ripples in our ocean wrapped in skin, the water element becomes a swamp.

The Elements and the Pulse

Gently place the pads of your fingers tips over the radial pulse. To find the radial pulse, trace your finger from the joint where your thumb meets your hand to your wrist. On the small bump on the side of your wrist bone you will find a pulse. Then follow the radial pulse down the bump (epicondyle bone) to the small hollow. Find that pulse. Next continue to follow the pulse a little further up the arm. Find that pulse. On both the right and left arm these three pulses are used in most traditional forms of herbal medicine to assess the relationship between the fire in the body and the air element.

Pulse diagnosis is an art form that takes many years of patient observation to learn. Yet even a beginning herbalist can glean essential information about the state of the client's health by carefully listening to a client's pulse using her fingertips.

The following chart defines basic pulse characteristics frequently seen in a herbalist's clinic. To become familiar with this elegant and insightful form of diagnosis, I suggest you become familiar with the following pulses.

Pulse	Description
Vata (Air & Fire) constitution	Like a snake
Pitta (Fire) constitution	Like a frog

Pulse	Description
Kapha (Earth & Water) constitution	Like a swan
Cold condition	Slow and deep
Heat condition	Rapid and flooding (full)
Cold damp condition	Slow, slippery, frail and languid
Damp heat condition	Rapid and slippery
Wind condition	Taut and wiry

A Traditional View of Treating Illness Through Enhanced Circulation

Samuel Thomson was an American herbalist who practiced in the late 1700s and early 1800s. Thomson's methods of practice, called Thomsonian medicine, continue to have a significant impact on European and North American herbalists today.

Samuel Thomson's parents were homesteaders in New Hampshire. He was one of six children and whenever one of them became ill, the Widow Benton, the local herbalist, was called to doctor the family. Although Samuel Thomson claimed to be a self-taught herbalist, the basic knowledge and confidence in herbal medicine he gathered as a child influenced his entire career.

Some suspect Samuel Thomson's healing methods were also influenced by First Nation practices (particularly the practice of sweating out an illness) from those who lived near his home.

While treating life threatening infectious disease, Thomson observed the life-giving powers of fever. When Thomson witnessed death from infectious disease, he saw coldness settle into the body. The life giving heat of fever and death's coldness inspired his methods. Thomson based his practice of herbal medicine on the distribution of heat in the body via the circulation of fluids.

Thomson divided the body's circulation into four phases:

- Phase one: the interstitial fluid and local vaso motor control (pressure waves).
- Phase two: the heart, arteries, veins and systemic vasomotor control.
- Phase three: the lymphatic system (mops up whatever does not make it into the veins).
- Phase four: temperature regulation (hot or cold), peripheral blood flow (delivery of oxygen and nutrients to cells and removal of CO_2 and wastes), and sweating (removal of toxins through skin as well as temperature regulation).

Thomson assessed his patient's circulation through each of these phases and then prescribed plant medicine to enhance the delivery of nutrients and the removal of waste.

The Medicine of Diffusive Herbs

Thomson's two favourite herbs were cayenne *(Capsicum minimum)* and lobelia *(Lobelia inflata)*.

These two herbs are referred to as diffusives. Diffusives are used in herbal formulas to increase the absorption and distribution of other herbs in the protocol. Cayenne serves this function through its rapid and intense effect on circulation. (Think of biting into a cayenne pepper and the instantaneous runny nose and tearing eyes.) Thomson used cayenne when his patient's fire was burning low. When the fire burns low the pulse is weak, maybe difficult to locate, and the skin is pale, cool and dry to touch. In severe cases such as just before death, the skin can take on a waxy texture.

Lobelia achieves a diffusive effect by relaxing the muscles lining the artery walls. By relaxing the arteries a hard pulsation softens. A relaxed artery allows more blood flow than a tense, rigid artery. Thomson chose lobelia when fire burned too hot in a patient. This pulse is full, tense and hot. It is close to the surface of the skin and the skin may be flushed and moist.

Samuel Thomson on Diet

During the digestive process, blood flows to the digestive organs. Thomson saw this action as drawing on the resources his patients needed for battling illness. Thomson's advice during acute illness and convalescence was to simplify diets with

Circulatory stimulants are a class of herbs used to increase the movement of both the macro and micro-currents in the body. Each circulatory stimulant has an affinity with specific parts of the body, or densities.

Ginger (*Zingiber officinale*): Specific to the organs of the pelvis although useful for enhancing movement within the colon and small intestine. Ginger is also useful to warm the chest, in particular the lungs.

American prickly ash (*Xanthoxylum americanum*): Useful for enhancing circulation throughout the legs and arms, particularly when weak circulation is causing pain.

Cayenne (*Capsicum minimum*): Increases circulation within the heart muscle

Angelica (*Angelica archangelica*): Specific to improving circulation within the lungs but also very useful for increasing circulation within the liver and lower digestive tract.

Rosemary (*Rosmarinus officinalis*) Improves cerebral circulation. There is an old herbal expression attributed to Shakespeare (who I suspect had an interest in herbal medicine). Hamlet recommended "Rosemary for memory" for oall those suffering from denial in his life!

warming broths and watery porridge. He believed a bland diet allowed the body to easily receive absorbed nutrients while allowing the body's limited resources to fight off the attacking pathogen. Once the body had destroyed the pathogen and the patient's strength began to return, foods requiring greater digestive powers were reintroduced.

I find this useful advice for many conditions I see in clinic, including chronic disease. It is important to encourage the client to reintroduce a variety of food as their health returns.

Thomson Provoked Sweating to Remove Toxins from the Body

Doctors in the early 1800s overwhelmed by infectious disease, offered treatments to suppress the body's response to acute illness, and to fever in particular. Thomson was a great believer in encouraging and managing fever and was fiercely at odds with the orthodox medical doctors. Disliked by the medical elite, Thomson was a hero among many simple folk who were unable to afford the high costs of clinical doctors and used his treatments for their families and neighbors. Thomson's treatments were effective and not as violent and forceful as the use of mercury and other poisons frequently prescribed by the medical authorities of the day.

Thomson's methods of healing were simple. Provoke fever, using sweat lodge like practices, steam inhalations and wrapping the patient in many blankets to encourage sweating. Thomson believed toxins, called canker in his day, were released from the body with sweat.

Diaphoretic: Herbs used to manage fever

Thomson had a great respect and appreciation for the fire of fever. Knowing fever was a weapon the body used to kill pathogens, and understanding that raging temperatures could cause fire in the brain leading to mental debility or death,

Thomson carefully managed rising body temperatures with a class of herbs called diaphoretics.

Diaphoretics, acting through a variety of mechanisms, relax blood vessels near the surface of the body. When offered in large frequent doses these herbs raise the body temperature and help the body sweat. During fever, sweating signals the break in a fever and the death of the pathogen. A skilled herbalist like Thomson used diaphoretic herbs both to raise body temperature and to lower it. Favoured diaphoretics were boneset (*Eupatorium perfolatum*) and yarrow (*Achillia millefolium*).

Modern herbalists rarely manage fever. A body suffering with chronic disease has difficulty gathering the resources required to spike a fever. Some herbalists theorize that when a body can summon up a fever it is a sign of its overall health and fortitude. Yet when

Clinical Notes: It is important to note that Thomson was primarily concerned with treating infectious disease such as malaria and measles. These are acute illnesses. Today's herbalist mostly sees chronic disease in clinic.

Many herbalists believe that the journey to chronic disease begins with an acute illness. Because the modern model for treatment of acute illnesses caused by bacteria and viruses is based on suppression of symptoms (such as shutting down a fever with aspirin) herbalists believe that the body never truly recovers or overcomes the infecting pathogen. The acute illness is driven deeper into the body only to surface later as a chronic condition. Chronic illness generally manifests with inflammation, fatigue and depression (all the symptoms of acute illness).

For today's herbalist, reviewing protocols for traditional treatment of acute illness offers clues in relieving chronic illness. In many cases the treatment is similar except that lower doses of medicine are offered over an extended time.

the body cannot rise to the challenge of infection with a fever, it is an indication that vital resources are low and more than likely the time to recover from the acute illness will be lengthy. If the infecting pathogen is not overcome by the body's immune response (such as fever) it is possible a chronic illness will develop. Rheumatoid arthritis (RA) is an example of a chronic condition that frequently begins with an infection. Frequently RA follows a lung infection.

Although not battling acute illness daily, modern herbalists do continue to use diaphoretics. I find diaphoretics particularly useful when the blood has become stagnant and pools deep inside the body as in the case of uterine fibroids, liver heat (the liver is congested with stagnant hot blood) causing migraine headaches, frequent urinary tract infections or hot, dry bowels. When blood pools in the pelvis you will find red bumps on the back of the tongue. If the blood is congested in the central area of the torso, such as the liver, the middle area of the tongue will be red.

Yarrow (*Achillia millefolium*) is my favourite diaphoretic for clearing stagnant blood and enhancing circulation throughout the body. Yarrow moves stagnant heat from the interior of the body to the surface, thinning out thick congested blood and returning a healthy flow of the body's water and fire elements. I offer a tea or a tincture of yarrow flowers, my preferred plant part, for this purpose. Unlike when treating acute illness to encourage and then break fever when frequently high doses of hot, hot yarrow tea are offered, I use low doses given twice a day to clear the congested blood. In most cases, yarrow will begin to show results by the end of a week of treatment.

Yarrow is also useful for superficial areas of congested blood. I offered yarrow to a woman who had a 25-year-old bruise on her hip. It was a dark patch of skin left behind by a horse's sharp kick. She was 75 when I saw her. "It has never healed," she said, mumbling about the damn horse. A tincture of yarrow three times a day cleared up the bruise over a period of two months. I have seen yarrow do this many times. Remember yarrow for conditions with stagnant blood and when healing is stalled.

Linden Flower also called Lime Blossom (*Tilia europa*) is another diaphoretic used in the modern apothecary. Linden is a peaceful plant. It is calming to the mind and soothing to the digestion. Linden eases excess fire from blood. I think of linden as sheltering the body/mind from surging storms caused by stress and its effects on the mind, digestion and blood vessels.

Linden flower is a pleasant tea that relaxes the heart and the muscles lining the walls of the arteries. Linden flower is unique in its ability to heal damaged blood vessels. Blood raging through tense arteries is not mindful of its effect on blood vessels and can cause collateral damage to the more delicate blood vessel. Linden heals both the rage in the mind and the damage in the blood vessels. Some herbalists believe it removes the plaque from arterial walls. David Hoffman suggests linden flowers are the "only demulcent" for the circulatory system.

Getting to the Heart of the Matter

The French have a beautiful expression, "*Bon courage*", which translates to "Go with good heart". The origin of the word *courage* comes from the French word for heart, *coeur*. As the French say "bon courage", English speakers say, "Follow your heart." I do not think there is any better advice for living life well lived.

Borage (*Borago officinalis*) There is a very old saying amongst herbalists, "borage for courage." Originally from the Middle East, Borage has been very effective at traveling the world and finding a home in many gardens. An unkempt looking plant with big floppy, fuzzy leaves beloved by spiders, it thrives in North American gardens. Borage's saving grace is its lovely star-shaped sky blue flowers. Extremely adept at self-seeding, perhaps borage grows where there is a need for courage.

Will Worthington; writer of "The Druid Plant Oracle" has this to say about borage's ability to in still courage: "True courage requires a strong and generous heart, and it involves looking beyond your own needs to perceive the greater good of those around you."

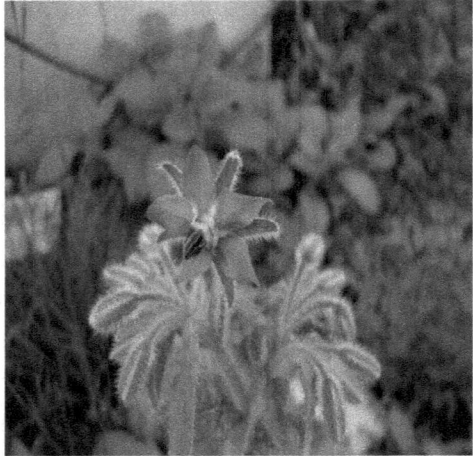

Borage   Mark Arneson

In today's apothecary Borage is classed as an adaptogen.

Adaptogens help the body/mind adapt to long-term chronic stress. Stress creates friction in the body/mind. In the body stress manifests as excess heat while in the mind it creates anxious heated thoughts. Borage's cooling nature calms the heat of chronic stress and soothes the mind.

Stress builds up in the body/mind when we lose our sense of connection to the people around us and the daily tasks we perform. Stress devours the pauses in every day that offer moments for connection and reflection. Under stress life loses its subtle meaning. Without purpose and meaning we lose courage and anxiety takes over.

In Europe wine steeped with borage flowers and young leaves is given to those who are so deeply exhausted they can no longer rest. When restless and unable to find meaning, borage offers the courage to stop, rest, and reconnect with our heart's desire.

Enjoying a good heart is a key to finding balance within one's emotional, spiritual, mental and physical life. A good heart is the essential ingredient for a happy and healthy life.

The Heart and Mental Health

Let's begin with looking at how the heart creates mental health with a story from Jack Cornfield's book *The Wise Heart*. It goes like this:

At a small psychiatric hospital in the States, there was a parking lot designated for physicians. In the parking lot, the physicians were asked to use an honorary payment system and put a dollar in a box each time they used the lot. Grad students studying at a nearby college set up an experiment in the physician's parking lot. Without notifying the physicians, a camera was set up on the box to monitor who paid and who did not. After a period of six months, the students looked at who had paid and who had not paid and their rate of success in treating their patients. It was found that the patients whose physicians regularly paid the parking fee recovered from their illnesses quicker and had fewer relapses.

When a heart is generous it automatically creates activity that supports life. It does not matter if the actions involve helping those who suffer with debilitating depression or paying a volunteer parking fee. Every act is done with the same intention: harmony within one's self, family, workplace, and community.

As a healer, it is essential to return continuously to the generosity of the heart and develop faith in the wisdom of courage.

Spiritual Health

My Celtic ancestors believed that life contained within us wasn't limited to our human experience but extended to the experiences we had when we were other life-forms: animals, birds, fish, stones, or plants. These were all considered living beings capable of independent action and thought. The wise people were expected to be able to reach back not only into the memories of their current life, but also into their memories of all their other lives. Colonization changed all that: I was cut off from my roots. I lived a childhood being told that creatures and plants were alive but only humans had real souls. It was when I came to the West Coast and met people of the Coast Salish tribe that I heard stories of metamorphosis that were like the stories my people shared centuries ago, stories that indicated that humans are not the peak of evolution but part of a shifting interchangeable web of life. - The Lost Language of Plants, Stephen Harrod Buhner pg 254

The greatest medicine plants have given me is the unshakeable knowledge of life's interdependence and boundless generosity. This understanding is the foundation of my spiritual life.

There is a sadness in my heart some days. Before my life became rooted in plant medicine, the sadness in my heart lingered for days, months, and years.

It is the sadness I feel when I see an empty package of potato chips carelessly tossed into the small forest where my dog and I walk every morning.

It is the sadness I felt standing on a hillside surrounded by stumps of ancient fir trees, crushed shrubs and smaller plants squished into the ruts left behind by heavy machinery.

It the sadness I felt when I watched a teenage girl change from her sneakers to stilettos to walk the streets. Her body, her commerce.

The same sadness filled my heart when my neighbour told me he drowned the kittens born three days earlier in his tool shed. The sadness in my heart swells when I see disrespect for life whether it be plant, animal or human. This sadness is like an old grey blanket. Wrapped in it, I feel alone, disconnected and frightened. The grey blanket of sadness is woven with threads of disconnection and spun by the disassociated techno age we live in. When the sadness threatens to smother me I walk in a forest.

Dappled green light, the ruffle of leaves, red berries gleaming like jewels, and chickadees darting in and out of sight with their joyful call, all nourish my spirit in ways the most elaborate spiritual ceremonies fail to do.

Some people consider plant medicine primitive and not up to our technological age. Roots nourished by soil, worms and bacteria, dug by hands with dirt under fingernails and washed in the cool water of a nearby stream is too primitive for our time. Plant medicine is too messy and unpredictable. Nothing in wild plants is stable. Like life, plant medicine is too full of surprises.

Our techno age does not really enjoy surprises. Medicine needs to be made in controlled settings, sterile, and isolated from the messiness of life. Medicine, like life in our techno age, needs to be predictable and controlled.

I have noticed that the emotions plant medicines from the forest or the garden evoke are very different from the medicine made in sterile settings.

Many people take the medicine dissociated from life's fertile soil and isolated in sterile environments with fear. It may be fear of death, authority, disease, loss or even fear of the medicine. Plant medicine rarely evokes the same fear. Often people take plant medicine with a sense of enthusiastic optimism. It is almost like humans have an intuitive knowing that life nourishes life. Deep inside the human spirit it is known that plants care for us. It is impossible to separate human life from plant life. Human life is completely dependent on plant life for food, housing, clothing, air and medicine. Plants are boundlessly generous and willing to help humans. Even after being trampled on.

For this reason, plant medicine restores my faith in life again and again. faces. Living touching the earth and dreaming on the stars brought a certainty to life, even when it was full of surprises. Knowing nature assures the human's anxious spirit of life's goodness. Living with the knowledge of the planet's boundless generosity assures our isolated self that we all have a place in the web of interdependence.

Primitive people understand their connection to planets and the natural world. Their nights were not lit with computer screens. Their days were not spent hurling through space at 100 km an hour, their feet off the ground. They walked the earth. Their day's activities were determined by changing seasons, warmth and sun and rain and snow. They slept under the stars. At one time, humans knew the scent of medicinal roots, the taste of spring water and the names of the moon's many

Consider this incantation sung by Gabon Pygmy of Africa.

All Lives, All Dances, & All is Loud

The fish does....HIP
The bird does...VISS
The marmot does...GNAN
I throw myself to the left,
I throw myself to the right,
I act the fish,
Which darts in the water, which darts
Which twists about, which leaps-
All lives, all dances, and all is loud.
The fish does....HIP

The bird does...VISS
The marmot does...GNAN
The bird flies away,
It flies, flies, flies,
Goes, returns, passes,
Climbs, soars and drops,
I act the bird-
All lives, all dances, and all is loud.
The fish does....HIP
The bird does...VISS
The marmot does...GNAN
The monkey from branch to branch,
Runs, bounds and leaps,
With his wife, with his brat,
his mouth full, his tail in the air,
There goes the monkey! There goes the monkey!
All lives, all dances, and all is loud.

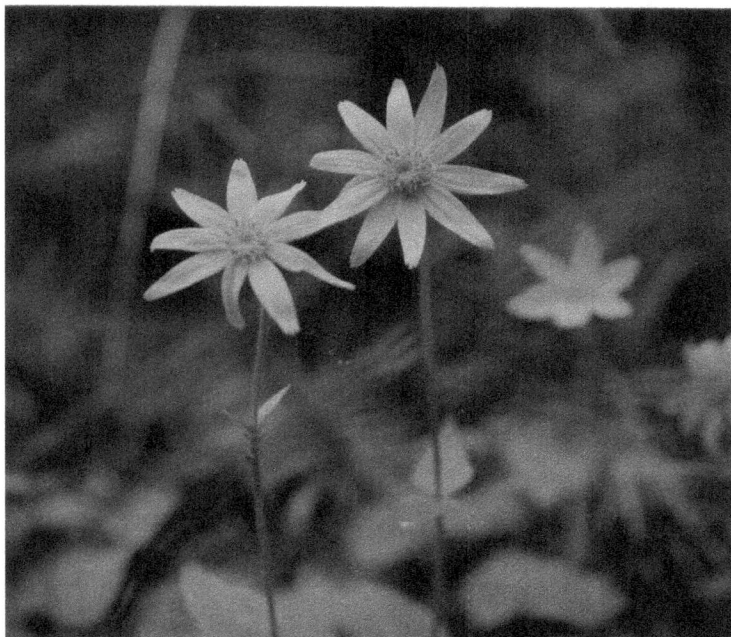

Arnica   Mark Arenson

Spiritual Health

When assessing the spiritual health of the heart, consider the client's ability to take emotional risks, be vulnerable, and not know the answer and remain in the unknown.

Years ago, in a fit of altruism, I took a vow to help those who I believe I cannot help. Since then, every so often someone comes along who completely overwhelms me. I perceive their needs as daunting. Generally they are physically ill, angry, poor, and have no boundaries. When they show up at my door and begin to rant and fume, I think to myself, "this is too hard," and become impatient. Impatience does not have a generous heart. Then a little voice in my heart says, "Remember your vow." So I try to help them (which is really helping myself).

The challenge I have with these folks is not just their unpleasant nature, but also the fact that I do not know what to do for them. I have found the key to helping people I find challenging is to ask the question, "How can she help me?" Perhaps she will teach me to establish better boundaries, or to return to my heart to listen deeper. I have found difficult people are my greatest teachers. It is easy to love those who agree with you, share the same values, speak your language, or look like you. Loving those who challenge your views and ideas, or who threaten you with their foreign appearances, customs or smells challenges us spiritually.

Physical Health

For centuries those who studied the human body believed the heart was simply a muscle of the circulatory system. Over the last fifty years, physiologists have learned that matters of the heart are much more complex. The study of cardioneurology, the interaction between the heart and the nervous system, has revealed that the heart often determines how the brain functions. Endocrinologists have classed the heart as an endocrine organ and consider it as important in the regulation of stress hormones as the adrenal glands. To support the complex inner workings of the heart, herbal medicine is more than suitable. Let's begin with studying the heart and its many mysteries.

Cardioneurology

The facts: The heart has its own intrinsic nervous system made up of approximately 40,000 neurons that communicate with the brain and the automatic nervous system.

The Vagus Nerve

The parasympathetic nervous system is responsible for calm feelings, good digestion and a smooth heartbeat. The mnemonic for the parasympathetic system is "rest and digestion." The sovereign of the parasympathetic nervous system is the vagus nerve or the "wandering" nerve. This nerve journeys from the brain, makes a stop at the heart, and then moves on to the digestive organs. The relationship between an open, relaxed heart and good digestion is easy to understand when considering the thread that binds them: the vagus nerve. Recall the relationship between the vagus nerve and the taste of bitter herbs: the bitter taste stimulates the parasympathetic nervous system via the vagus nerve. The heart and brain's primary pathway of communication is the vagus nerve. An open heart is essential to be able to absorb and digest meaning in life. Motherwort (*Leonurus cardiaca),* a bitter herb, supports the absorption of nutrients and calms heart palpations.

Dopamine: The heart makes and transmits dopamine. Dopamine is the harmonious neurotransmitter. When the heart releases dopamine the brain secretes endorphins.

Low levels of dopamine in the brain cause hand tremors and lack of coordinated movement. The muscles just do not do what the brain tells them to do.

Herbs influencing dopamine levels in the body:
Kava kava *Piper mysticum*
Chaste berry *Vitex agnus castus*
Marijuana *Cannabis sativa*
St John's Wort *Hypericum perforatum*
Rhodiola *Rhodiola rosea*

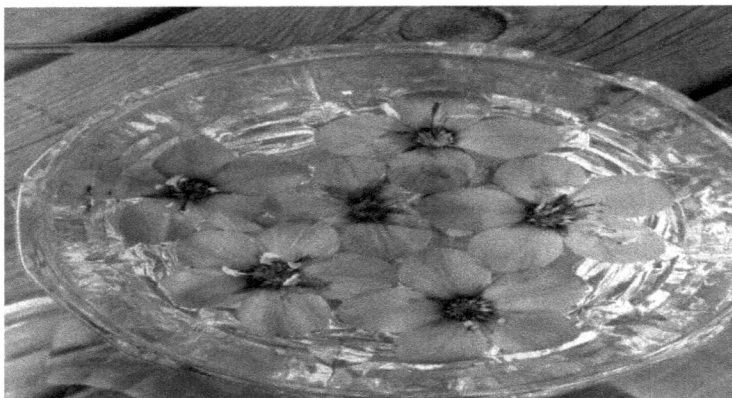

Flower Essences

Flower essences are used to shift entrenched attitudes and release the emotion underlying physical disease. Flower essences contain the vibration of the plant. Some call this vibration the spirit or the energy of the plant. They are in some ways closer to homeopathic remedies than tinctures and teas.

Borage flower essence instills courage.

To make an essence:

Collect your supplies; I like to do this the night before making the medicine. You will need: a crystal bowl, spring water, brandy, a clean bottle and label.

In the early morning, just as the dew is about to dry, gently approach the plant you wish to make an essence with. Ask permission of the plant to make medicine with its flowers. Fill the crystal bowl with spring water and using a leaf or chop sticks (you do not want to touch the flowers with your fingers) delicately pick enough flowers to cover the water in the bowl. Place the bowl in direct sunlight and let sunlight; flowers, water and crystal mingle for 3 hours. I strongly suggest you sit with bowl while the medicine mingles, offering your good heart energy into the mix. Carefully remove the flowers. Fill the jar half way with the water, top it off with brandy. Label. Take 4 drops 4xs a day when you require courage.

Parkinson's is a disease associated with low dopamine levels. One of the primary symptoms of Parkinson's is a mask-like facial expression. They cannot show the heart's emotions on their faces. Dopamine creates harmony between the heart, facial expressions and the ability to move towards your heart's desires. A lack of dopamine creates a hesitancy in movement.

Dopamine also encourages a robust libido. One could say that dopamine supports the affairs of the heart.

Noradrenalin: Noradrenalin is both a neurotransmitter and a hormone. When released from the adrenal glands it is called a hormone and is responsible for the fight or flight stress response. The heart, like the adrenal glands, produces and releases noradrenalin, but when the heart releases noradrenalin it is called a neurotransmitter and acts on the sympathetic nervous system (SNS). The SNS responds to the adrenal gland's fight or flight call to action. Whether noradrenalin is coursing through the blood stream as a hormone or leaping across synapses as a neurotransmitter, it increases blood flow to the heart, lungs, and skeletal muscles and speeds up the heart rate. Noradrenalin triggers the secretion of cortisol from the adrenal gland's cortex. Cortisol is the ageing hormone. Cortisol pushes the body to work harder. The harder the body/mind works, the more stress is experienced. Stress pushes the heart and the adrenal glands to release more noradrenaline. As physical and mental stress increase, metabolism speeds up causing the production of free radicals or loose oxygen molecules. I think of free radicals as sparks circulating through the body, causing minute burns in the tissue. Free radicals are part of the ageing process and are particularly damaging to blood. Noradrenalin and cortisol are released during feelings of anger, anxiety & competition.

When the parasympathetic nervous system turns on and the heart releases dopamine, the mind and body relax and the anti-ageing hormone DHEA (dehyrdoepiandrosterone), is released. The body begins to heal any damage caused by the free radicals.

Noradrenalin preserves life in the most desperate situations. It is not however, a long-term solution to life's many challenges.

The Heart as an Organ of The Endocrine System

In 1981, the heart graduated from simply being the muscle behind circulation to a complex endocrine gland when it was discovered it secreted hormones. The endocrine system includes the thyroid the hypothalamus and pituitary in the brain, the adrenals, ovaries and testes, and pancreas.

Atrial Natriuretic Factor (ANF) was the first heart hormone discovered. At first it was believed that the right atrium (the chamber that pumps deoxygenated blood into the lungs) released ANF when there was an increase in blood pressure. It was found that ANF eased the pressure on the walls of the heart's chambers by increase the release of sodium from the kidneys and dilating blood vessels throughout the body. Shortly after the discovery of ANF, its name was changed to Atrial Natriuretic Peptide, and three other similar acting hormones were discovered, all made and release by the heart.

Current research suggests ANP has a detrimental effect on cancer cells, particularly pancreatic cancer cells. It is also suspected as having a role in regulating the thyroid and adrenal glands hormones.

Oxytocin: Oxytocin, the love hormone, is made and released into circulation by the heart. Oxytocin is a bonding hormone; it makes us feel connected and generous. Oxytocin is the pleasure hormone that triggers the euphoria of orgasm. (It is interesting that a man's heart only releases oxytocin during sex when he is in love.) Compassionate actions stimulate the flow of oxytocin from the heart. I have a friend who claims healers are oxytocin junkies!

Deep breathing causes the diaphragm to massage the vagus nerve. A happy, massaged vagus nerve stimulates the heart to release oxytocin.

Other ways to stimulate the release of oxytocin are being trustworthy, knowing you can be counted on, hugging, a good belly laugh, walking in nature, reaching out, calling a friend, or even liking someone's picture on Facebook.

Entrainment: The Heart Seeks to Harmonized

If there are several grandfather clocks in a room and they have all been set with a different rhythm, over time they will synchronize with the clock that has the loudest "tick tock". This phenomenon is called entrainment.

The heart is the dominant rhythm in the body. It not only controls the rhythm of the pulse and pressure waves in the organs but it also sets the rhythm of brain waves. When the heart is pounding, brain waves speed up. Speedy brain waves are called beta waves. Under the influence of beta waves, thinking becomes scattered and in the worst-case scenario, thoughts are tense and frightened. A steady, serene heartbeat encourages the flow of alpha waves in the brain and produces calm thoughts and a clear mind.

Oxytocin and Labour

Oxytocin plays a significant role in labour and the bonding between mom and baby immediately following childbirth. During labour oxytocin eases the pain. When combined with the surge of endorphins (opiate-like neurotransmitters) that are released with each contraction, mom survives the pain of labour. With the birth of her child, the sudden relief from pain and the infusion of a cocktail of feel good hormones (oxytocin and endorphins) Mom falls into the bliss of unconditional love. She snuggles and coos with her newborn when seconds earlier she was pleading, "Get this thing out of me!"

Spiritual rituals around the world take advantage of entrainment. The heart will entrain powerful rhythms in its environment such as rhythmic chanting and drumming. A steady drum beat or recitation of mantras slows the heart and as alpha waves begin to flow peaceful states of mind arise. With peaceful thoughts, the body experiences bliss. Alpha waves create a safe internal psychic environment where new understandings, ways of being, and perhaps mystical experiences can arise.

On a more practical note, studies have shown that gently beating the heart's rhythm on a drum helps an anxious child sleep.

The Pump

Just as the relationship between the heart and the endocrine system was not understood until recently, it was not until the 1600's that Europeans understood the heart as a pump. For much of human history, the heart's four chambers and their relationship was a mystery.

The heart receives non-oxygenated blood into its right chambers from the venous system. It pumps this "blue" blood into the lungs where the iron molecules in the blood pick up oxygen. From the lungs, the "red" blood flows back into the heart to be pumped out of the left chambers into the aorta from where it flows through the arterial circulation to the rest of the body, delivering oxygen and gathering up carbon dioxide.

It is important to note that the first arteries branching off the rich freshly oxygenated blood to the heart. The heart feeds itself first. When the heart stops beating, death is imminent. This is a tidy metaphor for taking care of one's self first so one can move through life with "bon courage".

Hawthorn: The Great Heart Tonic

In Celtic traditions, the Hawthorn (Crataegus oxycantha) *was the tree that grew atop the hollow hills that were the entrance to the realm of Faery -- their thorns protecting against those who would come blundering through, but their flowers and leaves and berries feeding and nourishing the heart to allow it to open to another way of being, a way described in some lines of the Feri tradition of witchcraft as "kinder but less civilized."* - Sean Donahue

The hawthorn tree is the medicine for the heart.

Throughout the lands of the Celts, the hawthorn is referred to as "gentle bushes". "Gentle"is a reference to the faeries who one avoids naming directly. The ancient Celts cautioned against disturbing a hawthorn tree. Willful destruction of the hawthorns brought grave misfortune. This belief is still alive and well among the Celts.

Earlier in this century, a construction firm ordered the felling of a faery thorn on a building site in Downpatrick, Ulster. The foreman had to do the deed himself, as all of his workers refused. When he dug up the root, hundreds of white mice - supposed to be the faeries themselves - ran out, and while the foreman was carting away the soil in a barrow, a nearby horse shied, crushing him against a wall and resulting in the loss of one of his legs.

Even as recently as 1982, workers in the De Lorean car plant in Northern Ireland claimed that one of the reasons the business had so many problems was because a faery thorn bush had been disturbed during the construction of the plant. The management took this so seriously that they actually had a similar bush brought in and planted with all due ceremony! http://www.druidry.org/library/trees/tree-lore-hawthorn

It is not surprising that causing harm to the great plant tonic of the heart causes ruin. Ignoring yearnings and songs of the heart brings similar misery.

The Druids taught that caring for a hawthorn tree allowed one to speak with the faeries. The faeries only speak the truth. Within the realm of the faeries it is not possible to speak an untruth. To lie is to be expelled from the faeries land.

There is a saying: the heart never lies. To lie is stressful. An article from Psychology Today reported a study involving liars and non-liars. The participants in the study were divided into two groups, one group given permission to lie, and the other group

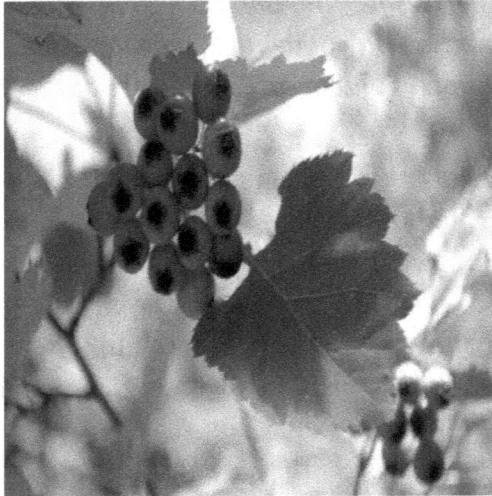

Hawthorn   Mark Arneson

offered strategies that help to avoid lying. The group that did not lie found their relationships improved, they slept better, had less mental and physical tension, fewer headaches and sore throats. Other studies have shown lying increases blood pressure and heart rate. In short, the faeries seem to be onto something: lies stress the heart.

TCM practitioners favor the hawthorn flower for an anxious heart. In France, a tea of hawthorn flowers is offered to treat insomnia. French herbalist Maurice Messegue writes, "I myself make use of the hawthorn for nervous spasms, arteriosclerosis, angina and obesity and it is one of my favourite tranquilizer herbs." Hawthorn flowers stimulate the parasympathetic nervous system, allowing the heart to rest. A quiet heart creates a quiet mind. A quiet mind leads to thoughtful speech.

The hawthorn's berries, leaves and flowers are a gift to a tired heart. A tired heart, whether from a long life or too much stress, struggles to push blood out of the left arterial chamber and into the aorta. A tired heart cannot fulfill its duty to the rest of the body so it tries to work harder. Like all muscles in the body, when a tired heart works harder it becomes bigger. Unlike the spiritual heart of the Grinch Who Stole Christmas, when the heart muscle grows, it loses its efficiency. The extra muscle mass fills the chambers of the heart and leaves less room for blood to flow. Less blood passing through the heart means less blood is pulsating through the body. In turn, the body asks for more blood, and the heart tries harder. It continues to grow bigger and more inefficient. A vicious cycle develops that leads to all sorts of health problems including congestive heart failure.

Hawthorn is the remedy for this tired heart. It increases the force of the heart's pumping action without causing the heart to enlarge. It also enhances the heart's ability to relax. When the heart relaxes during the pause between heartbeats, it fills with blood. A relaxed heart has more blood to offer to the body.

When hawthorn is added to a high blood pressure formula, do not expect immediate results from it alone. Hawthorn is a long-term herb with long-term gentle effects. Mistletoe (*Viscum album*) is a much more efficient herb for lowering blood pressure. The addition of a small amount of mistletoe tincture to the formula is usually enough to bring most cases of high blood pressure down. (If mistletoe does not work, try valerian). But do not under-estimate the long-term effects of hawthorn.

I think of the story of the rabbit and the tortoise when I compare the two herbs. Mistletoe is the rabbit. It brings instantaneous results. Hawthorn is the tortoise. The tortoise did not "wow" audiences with his speed, but he not only won the race, he also lived for another 225 years.

Lastly, hawthorn berries are high in flavonoids and offer up a sour taste. Recall that the sour taste is cooling in nature. Hawthorn berries are very specific when there is heat around the heart or congestion of blood in the heart. You can know this by looking at the tongue. The very tip of the tongue represents the heart. If the tip is bright red, try adding hawthorn to the client's formula.

Understanding circulation through the study of trees

Branching vessels

My cherished friend Corky Larson, a Cree Elder, says "If you want to know what to do, look at the trees." She says in the fall when the trees let go of their leaves and

Mistletoe and the Druids

Mistletoe is part of the winter solstice ceremony which welcomes the return of the light. Mistletoe symbolizes the end of a difficult time and of creative new beginnings. To the druids, mistletoe represents fertility, guidance and inspiration.

send the sap (a tree's blood) deep into the earth, it is time to let go of the summer's exuberance, harvest root vegetables, fill the freezer with winter soups and stews, and turn inward for winter's long dream. In the spring when trees dress themselves in fresh green lleaves, it is time to leave behind the dreamtime, shed winter's protective clothing, seek fresh greens to cleanse our blood of winter's cold and begin an outward adventure.

In *The Earthwise Herbal: A Complete Guide to New World Medicinal Plants,* Matthew Wood takes an in-depth look at the practice of southern American folk herbalists and their methods of assessing blood. In this succinct form of medicine blood is likened to the sap of trees. The question the southern folk herbalists asked was, "Is the blood too thick or too thin, too

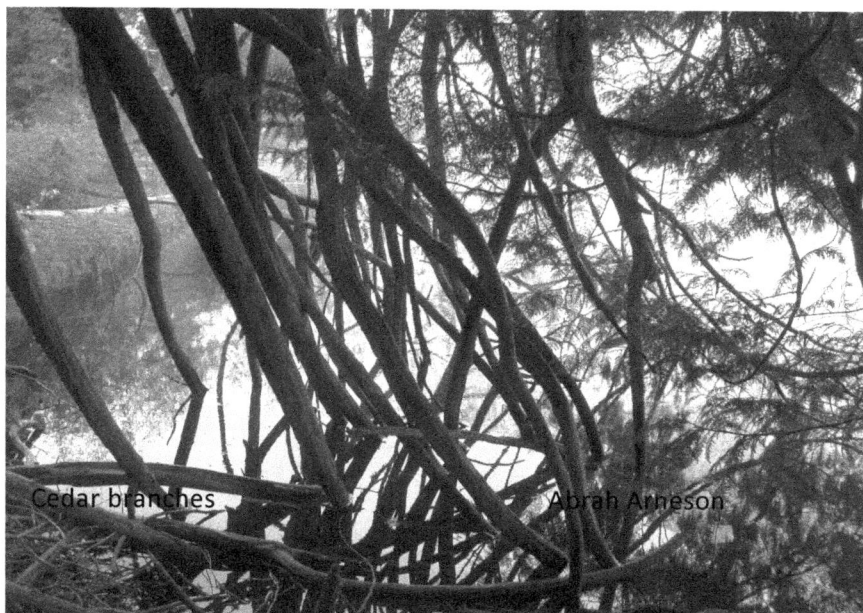

Cedar branches   Abrah Arneson

hot or too cold?" Once the herbalist understood the quality of the patient's blood, she offered the appropriate herbs.

Thin Blood

Thin blood is generally cold. It's too thin to carry heat any distance. Remember that water conserves the fire element. If the blood is too watery, it cannot contain the fire element.

Thin blood lacks nutrients (earth element) and tends to leak from blood vessels. The patient's energy is low, their muscles lack strength, and their skin is pale. Thin-blooded people often suffer with low blood pressure and dizziness. It is my experience that thin-blooded people tend towards anxiety with depression. This is in part due to the poor nutrition their blood provides to the brain and the rest of their body. These individuals frequently suffer with hypoglycemia.

Nettle (*Urticaria dioica*) is a perfect herb for thin-blooded people. Nettle is not only rich in minerals, but it high is in protein that will help resolve the hypoglycemia, anxiety and depression. Nettle is a traditional herb used for increasing blood pressure.

Raspberry leaf (*Rubus idaeus*) is another useful herb to nourish the blood. It is high in minerals, particularly calcium. Raspberry leaf also has an astringent action. The leaf's tannins improve blood vessel integrity for thin-blooded people. Often when I listen to a client who has thin blood, I have the impression that their life force is leaking out of them. The folk herbalists say that blood vessels have a hard time containing thin blood. Their vessels are leaky. The astringent action tightens leaky blood vessels. Raspberry leaf is also known for improving blood vessel integrity in the uterus and helping the uterus contain life.

Thick blood

Thick blood is heavy and has a challenge rising. This results in poor circulation in the brain. The mind becomes sluggish, the memory poor and creativity dull. Thick blood pools in the pelvis causing hemorrhoids and varicose veins. Women with thick blood suffer with heavy periods. Thick blood pushes on blood vessels. The excess tension thick blood exerts on blood vessels causes high blood pressure.

Thick blood is sluggish and has difficulty flowing through the capillary's narrow pores. This leads to poorly nourished and dry tissues. Although thick blood contains heat, it is slowly dispersed into the surrounding tissues. The body is cold. Toxins build up in thick blood.

Herbalists use alteratives to clean up and thin out thick blood. Alteratives are a class of herbs once referred to as blood cleansers, blood purifiers or blood sweeteners. These "unscientific" names were dropped in the 19th century when it became clear that if the blood is poisoned the body dies. Blood purifiers were reclassed as alteratives. Some herbalists believe this strange word "alterative" reflects the fact that these herbs alter the blood.

Despite the references to blood, alteratives have more of an effect on the interstitial fluid. Think of the blood stream and the interstitial fluid like this:

The blood is the river of life. The interstitial fluid is the ground water. The river's water seeps into the ground water, dispersing nutrients into the earth. At the same time, ground water flows back into the river, dispersing minerals. There is a dynamic exchange between the two.

I once lived in a place where someone had long ago buried a tractor. The well water tested for lead and other heavy metals. We could not figure out the source of the heavy metals until we learned of the buried tractor. The tractor's metals were slowly seeping into the ground water and into the well. The heavy metals also flowed into the nearby creek. The creek eventually flowed into the Trent canal system after merging with several lakes. All these bodies of water received some of the heavy metal leaching from the tractor. The dispersal of the metals over a large area weakened their toxic effect. However, because of the proximity of the tractor to the well, the well water was not fit to drink.

In many ways there is a similar dynamic in the body, between the blood and the interstitial fluid. The alteratives do not so much clean up the blood, but disperse and help off load the toxic buildup in the interstitial fluid. They do this by interacting with the lymphatic system, kidneys, and liver. Alteratives clean up stagnant water.

Most alteratives have a warming quality or a sweet flavour. Few are drying and many are moistening. Some are bitter. Alteratives are a diverse group of herbs with wide ranging effects on the body.

Three of my favourite alteratives demonstrate this clearly:

Oregon Grape Root

(*Mahonia aquifolium*) is a bitter, moistening root that supports secretion of bile from the liver and efficient bowel movements. It is an important remedy for dry, itchy, inflamed skin.

Red Clover (*Trifolium pratense*) has a sweet taste and a cooling, moist quality. A tea or tincture (particularly of fresh flowers) is a dynamic lymphatic cleanser, softening stubborn hard, swollen lymph nodes. It is an important remedy for many childhood ailments and clearing up cysts in the body.

Burdock (*Arctium lappa*) is a bitter sweet herb, with a milky appearance when tinctured. Deeply nourishing (reflected in its milky appearance) burdock root is an excellent choice for any formula to help the kidney release its toxic load. Chronically dry skin indicates the need for burdock root.

Essiac Formula

6 ½ cups of burdock root (cut)*
1 pound of sheep sorrel herb powdered
1/4 pound of slippery elm bark powdered
1 ounce of turkey rhubarb root powdered

Mix these ingredients thoroughly and store in glass jar in dark dry cupboard.

Taking a measuring cup, use 1 ounce of herb mixture to 32 ounces of water depending on the amount you want to make.

I use 1 cup of mixture to 8 x 32 = 256 ounces of water. Boil hard for 10 minutes (covered) then turn off heat but leave sitting on warm plate overnight (covered).

In the morning reheat to steaming hot and let settle a few minutes, then strain through a fine strainer into hot sterilized bottles and sit to cool. Store in a cool dark cupboard. Must be refrigerated when opened.

This recipe <u>must</u> be followed <u>exactly</u> as written.

Alteratives are traditional herbs chosen to help the body overcome cancer. At one time, it was thought cancer was caused by a toxic buildup of interstitial fluid. It was believed that eventually the stagnant toxins seep into the cells, disrupting DNA processes and firing up a cancerous growth. Think of tumors as hot, hard, and solid. Softening, soothing, and cooling alteratives were and still are considered by many herbalists the best herbs for treating cancer. The famous Essiac cancer formula is made with alterative herbs.

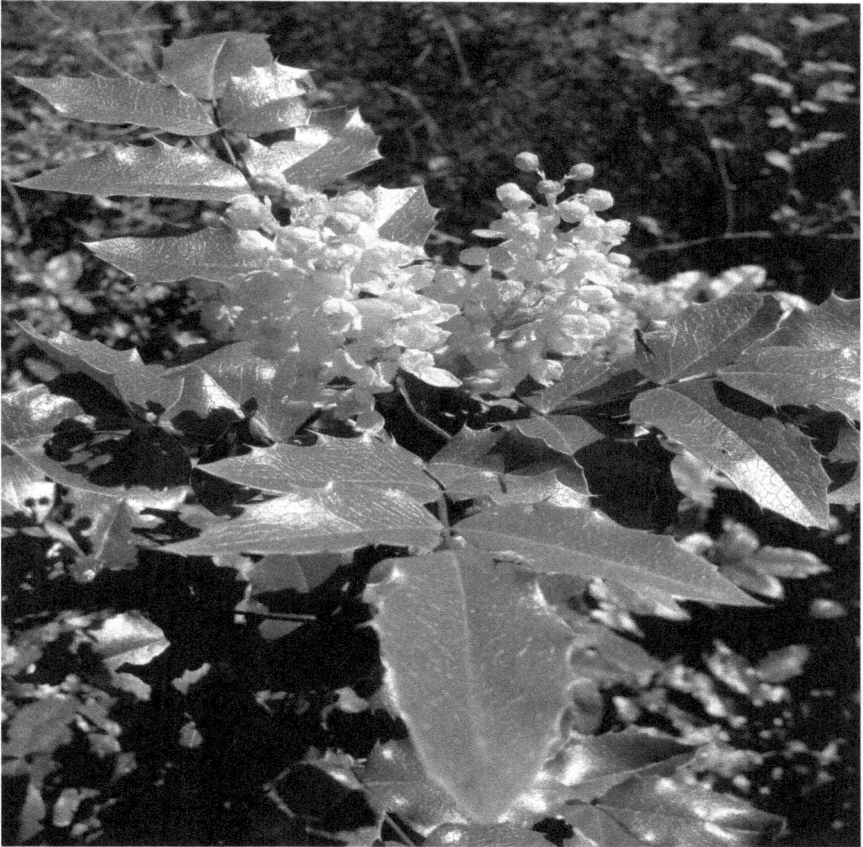

Oregon Grape   Rosalee de la Forêt

Herbalists offer alteratives to ease cysts, chronic infection, eczema, arthritis, and autoimmune conditions. All these conditions require that the herbalist aid the body in eliminating heat and moistening dry tissues. Remember alteratives are used for thick blood that contains heat and allows little nourishment to flow into tissues.

Thyroid disease

One the most common health challenge herbalists see is thyroid disease. Traditionally, a sluggish thyroid was treated as bad blood. A very effective alterative used to reset a low functioning thyroid is black walnut husk (*Juglans nigra*). It nourishes the thyroid with iodine while gently cleansing the body.

Echinacea - A Superb Alterative

Ask anyone when to take Echinacea and they will say, "When you have a cold; it stimulates the immune system." Looking closely at herbal medicine, one finds many plants that stimulate the immune system: astragulus (*Astragulus membranaceus*), boneset (*Eupatorium perfoliatum*), poke root *(Phytolacca decandra)*, old man's beard (*Usnea spp*) and garlic (*Allium sativa*), just to name a few. There is nothing special about immune stimulation in the world of plant medicine. To understand echinacea's unique actions within the body one must go back to its original use.

First Nations applied a spit poultice made with echinacea's root over rattlesnake bites. It stopped the spread of snake poison to other tissues. Interestingly, snake poison, bacteria, viruses and cancer all spread through the body in a similar manner, by secreting an enzyme called hyaluronidase that breaks down hyaluronic acid.

Hyaluronic acid is a fine web of sugar molecules that give structure to the extracellular matrix. The extracellular matrix is the scaffold that defines the space between cells. It provides both structural support for tissues and a canal-like system for interstitial fluid to flow through.

Echinacea angustifolia dismantles one of the primary methods a pathogen uses to travel through the body: hyaluronidase. Neutralizing hyaluronidase isolates the pathogen to a specific area and allows the immune systems weaponry to focus in a very concentrated manner on the germ. Echinacea stops infection, poison or cancer from eating its way into the circulatory system and spreading to other tissues.

The Liver: Cleaning and Nourishing the Blood

In the practice of over-the-counter herbal medicine, the liver is viewed as an organ of detoxification. This is true. But this large blood-rich organ is so much more.

The Liver and Circulation

Circulation is all about delivering nutrients and oxygen to the cells of the body and the removal of metabolic waste. This life giving activity occurs when the water and earth element are in harmony. The liver processes all nutrients (earth element) to be dispersed by circulation. The liver also sorts through the metabolic waste delivered to it by circulation and prepares it for either recycling or disposal.

How the liver keeps busy:

- Carbohydrate metabolism: turns carbs into sugars and stores them
- Fat metabolism: turns fat into sugars for energy, prepares fat to transport hormones, converts fat into bile that carries toxins out of the body through the bowel
- Protein metabolism: breaks protein down into amino acids that are used for making blood (both red and white blood cells), hormones, muscles,

neurotransmitters, almost every part of the body.
Note: The kidneys remove the toxins produced in
this process.

- Processes toxins: this includes endogenous
  (metabolic) toxins, environmental and food toxins,
  drugs and alcohol
- Breaks down hormones: sex, thyroid and adrenal
  hormones.
- Makes bile salts: these help us digest fatty foods
- Storage: Vitamins A, D, E, K & B12, and sugar as
  glycogen and fat
- Eats up and spits out worn out red and white blood
  cells and dead bacteria

The Liver and Traditional Chinese Medicine

Many contemporary healers believe that each organ has an
affinity with a particular emotion. This insight into the body
and emotions comes to the West by way of Traditional Chinese
Medicine or TCM, although there is a long history of this belief
in the West as well. The liver in TCM is the home of anger.

TCM practitioners are trained to see flow. Western healing
traditions prefer to work with fixed states of being (or one
could say diagnosis). In TCM, the elements flow one into
another, just as seasons do. Each season has a different balance
of the elements. For example: fire manifests very differently in
summer than in winter. For this reason TCM practitioners
check to be sure the flow of the elements within are in harmony
with the flow without. For example wearing inappropriate
clothing for the day's weather will create an imbalance in the
fire element in the body.

Each element is assigned a specific organ that in turn has a
dominant emotion. One of the easiest ways to assess the flow
(or non-flow) of a client's elements is to discover her preferred
emotion. When the element within an organ is imbalanced, the

emotion becomes the dominant form of expression. For example, when the water element is imbalanced, the kidneys express fear. When the lungs are suffering, metal is imbalanced and the overriding emotion is sorrow. When the liver manifests an imbalanced wood element, the liver barks angry demands.

I am never satisfied with this seemingly simple formula: liver imbalance equals anger. So let's take a closer look. The element associated with the liver is wood (similar to the earth element's governance of growth and storage but also recall the metaphor of trees and healthy circulation). Wood is the element of spring. New life unfolds during the spring. The spring is a time of creative freedom. It is a time to make one's desires known and put forward an effort towards fulfilment. It is time to plant seeds.

When a person's creative freedom is stifled, the result is frustration. If the frustration ensues, anger will arise. Underneath anger, jealousy festers. "After all, why should anyone have what they want, if I can't," goes the inner dialogue. In short, anger is frustrated desire. Blood is strongly linked with desire, often desire tainted with anger. Commonly used idioms demonstrate this: in cold blood, blood on your hands, boiling blood, etc.

Now let's think about what the liver does. It sorts out that which is useful to the body and that which is not useful. It does this by filtering the blood. When the liver's filtering system is congested, blood stagnates. The nutrients blood carries to the body are bogged down in the liver's filtration system while the toxins the body needs to eliminate linger like unwelcome, irritating guests.

Because the blood carries the fire element in the body, when it becomes stagnant in any area of the body that area becomes hot. This is true of blood congestion in the liver. Anger is closely associated with the fire element. It either rages like a forest fire or is frozen like ice. When the liver is thick with stagnant blood, it is a hot, bloody organ. Creativity in life is destroyed by too much passion, just as fire destroys wood. TCM practitioners refer to this condition as "liver heat".

So how does this influence circulation? Heat rises. The blood, being the carrier of heat, rises as well. Think of the warmth of spring drawing the tree's sap from the earth. Being overheated from too long a stay in the liver, heat rises quickly and goes straight to the head. There are several signs of this type of angry heat: reddening of the face, cheeks with webs of broken blood vessels and migraine headaches.

Prolonged liver congestion is detrimental to the heart. Liver congestion creates thick, hot blood. From the liver blood travels through a large vein called the vena cava to the heart to become oxygenated. When blood is thick and hot, many healers believe it damages the delicate heart valves. The thick hot blood also pushes against the chambers of the heart increasing blood pressure. As the oxygenated blood is pumped from the heart and into coronary arteries, thick blood is slow to diffuse into the already overworked muscle, creating further stress on the heart.

Anger, as liver heat, strangles the heart, both metaphorically and physically. Besides the following plants, a holistic protocol for liver heat should include watching comedies and hanging out with fun people. TCM teaches that joy is the emotion of the heart.

Peace on Earth

When the liver is healthy it promotes a sensitive happy state of being that is able to dialogue with easy to resolve conflict. A friend of mine believes that if every human on the planet did a liver cleanse, we might become closer to world peace.

Thistles: Herbs for liver heat

There are many thistles that grow on disturbed soil. Many

of them offer soothing medicine for liver heat.

Blessed Thistle (*Cnicus benedictus*) is named after St. Benedict, the patron saint of poison antidotes. Blessed thistle grows in the dry, arid soil surrounding the Mediterranean Sea. (Remember excess fire dries up the life force contained in the earth element.) Traditionally used as a diaphoretic, Blessed Thistle was used to remove virulent infection from the body such as malaria, small pox and influenza-- all conditions that accompany raging fevers.

It is blessed thistle's action on the liver that differentiates it from other diaphoretics and makes it so useful for infection.

Blessed thistle stimulates the secretion of bile in the liver. Bile carries heat and toxins from the liver, relieving congestion. The increased flow of bile improves the liver's efficiency and enhances circulation through the body. Blessed thistle is the herb to turn to when treating hepatitis or a stubborn infection clinging to the body.

Low doses are preferred for this healing, cleansing herb. Blessed thistle becomes an emetic when higher doses are offered.

Milk thistle (*Silybum marianum*) is another European thistle. It does however enjoy the milder climates of coastal BC. It is easily identified by the large milk-like splash on its leaves. Milk thistle's seeds have a sweet, oily coat containing a plant constituent called silymarin. This chemical protects liver cell membranes from oxidation by free radicals. Free radicals are loose oxygen molecules that burn tissues. In hot conditions of the body, such as liver heat, free radicals are furious and burn through the body starting fires and destroying healthy cell membranes. Milk thistle is specific to protecting the liver from free radical damage. It soothes and heals a hot liver. Traditionally milk thistle was used for chronic liver congestion involving the spleen and cirrhosis of the liver. It is an excellent remedy to relieve gallstones and the spasmodic pain associated with them.

In the practice of iridology, brown spots on the iris of the eye indicate liver weakness. If a client has used pharmaceutical or recreational drugs over an extended time, these patches of brown are known as drug spots. I see plenty of brown spots in clients' eyes even when there has not been drug use. I always include milk thistle in a formula when there are liver spots on the iris.

Canada thistle's (*Cirsium arvense*) medicine lives in the plant's roots. Although it does not have the lengthy recorded history of its use in medicine as its European cousins, Canada thistle's chemistry suggests liver protectant properties as well. Its root is high in rutin, an alcohol soluble flavonoid. Rutin is well known for its ability to scavenge free radicles and is favoured for a stressed out liver.

Studies have shown Canada thistle lowers blood pressure, and has antispasmodic and anti-inflammatory activity. Its high levels of rutin suggest these actions.

Canada thistle stalk and root are emergency wilderness food. Peel the outer skin of the stalk and you have a moist, crunchy veggie. The root, dug up in autumn or just as the snow flies, can be eaten raw or cooked.

The **Sow thistle** (*Sonchus arvensis*) has a yellow flower head and grows vigorously in disturbed soil. The flowers are a sweet treat when hiking on a hot day. They are chewy like bubble gum. The sow thistle is also very high in flavonoids and is an effective scavenger of free radicles. Throughout South East Asia, the sow thistle is called *Tempuyung* and is offered as a tea to break up both kidney and gall stones.

Kidney and Circulation

While in herb school I had the opportunity to take cadaver anatomy. The memory of holding a kidney remains vivid. It was like squeezing a sponge, but not quite. The kidney retained a fleshy feel while fluid seeped to its surface. The kidney is essential in coordinating the circulation of the water element in the body.

The kidney is a multitalented organ that performs many life-giving activities for the body:

- Manages water in the body
- Eliminates urea and other metabolic and exogenous wastes
- Manages and maintains the pH balance of the body
- Manages and maintains the electrolyte balance of the body

The kidney's role in elimination of metabolic wastes and maintaining the body's pH balance is explored in the chapter on elimination. In this chapter we are primarily interested in the kidney's role in circulation.

The kidney is in charge of maintaining the fluid balance in the body. This is a huge job as the body is approximately 85% fluid. Like all those who carry heavy responsibilities, the kidney does not act alone.

Most people notice the more water they drink the more they pee. On the days I get my recommended eight glasses of water, it is almost like all the water I drink goes straight from my mouth into my bladder. This is not the case.

Under the command of the endocrine system, the kidney controls the flow of fluids through and out of the body in three ways.

The Kidney and Low Blood Pressure

There a some very busy days when I am lucky if I get to supplement my morning coffee with two glasses of water. How is it I do not become dehydrated on these days? How does the body conserve fluid?

Method #1

It all begins in the brain with a small endocrine gland called the hypothalamus. The hypothalamus monitors the blood pressure exerted on the inner surface of blood vessels. When fluid intake drops, so does the blood pressure.

If the hypothalamus senses the pressure on the walls of the blood vessels is low, as when there is very little fluid intake, it signals the pituitary gland (another small endocrine gland in the centre of the brain) to release antidiuretic hormone (ADH).

ADH flows through the blood stream to the kidney. Upon reaching its destination ADH lets the kidney know the pressure on the inner surface of the blood vessel is low. The message ADH carries to the kidney is: store water. The kidney then makes less urine.

Method #2

The kidney is able to limit the loss of fluids

Kidney Anatomy Facts
- Two kidneys, right and left
- 11 cm long, 3 cm thick and weighs 150 grams
- Embedded in fat and held in place by fat
- Delicate system of capillaries called glomerulus
- Fragile nephrons
- Capped with adrenal glands

Kidney Physiology Facts
- Blood in glomerulus move in and out of nephrons
- Nephrons filter the blood
- Drain into ureters which fills bladder and empties through the urethra

from the body by conserving salt. Water loves salt. Think of the ocean, most of the world's water is bound with salt. Water follows salt. When less salt is expelled from the body via the kidneys, the body retains water.

The signal to slow down the absorption of sodium (salt) into the nephrons (tiny tubes that carry urine to ureters and onto the bladder) comes from the adrenal glands. Each kidney has one adrenal gland sitting on top of it like a toque. The medulla, the interior of the adrenal gland, releases a hormone called aldosterone that insists the kidney stop expelling salt from the body and store water.

Liquorice (*Glyzzhiriza spp*) can be used to increase blood pressure. It can act on the kidney like the hormone aldosterone.

There is a condition called aldosteronism in which the adrenal glands secrete excessive amounts of aldosterone leading to excess absorption of sodium. This raises low blood pressure to high blood pressure and carries significant risks of heart disease and stroke.

In some people long term use of liquorice causes pseudoaldosteronism. This condition is exactly like aldosteronism, only the cause is liquorice. Once liquorice is no longer taken, the condition resolves. No one is sure why liquorice affects some people this way. A study in Japan suggests it is the interaction between specific gut flora and liquorice that determines the development of pseudoaldosteronism.

The upside of liquorice's unusual action on blood pressure is that it can be used to increase low blood pressure.

Method #3

The third method is an interaction between the enzyme renin which is made in the kidneys and a hormone called angiotensinogen made in the liver. When angiotensinogen meets renin it is broken down and becomes angiotensin 1. As angiotensin 1 circulates in the blood it interacts with an enzyme found both in the lungs and kidney and becomes angiotensin 2. Angiotensin 2 is made to conserve fluid in crisis situations such as severe bleeding and hemorrhaging. Angiotensin 2 constricts blood vessels and creates a sense of thirst and cravings for salt. It also stimulates the secretion of aldosterone from the adrenal glands.

Drugs called ACE inhibitors that mimic the effects of angiotensin 2 are commonly used to lower high blood pressure.

Hydration, Dehydration and Diuretics

In Holistic Anatomy, Pip Waller explains how chronic dehydration can be misdiagnosed as high blood pressure and using ACE inhibitors with diuretics only makes matters worse. *When the body is dehydrated, it may do all kinds of things to try and set things straight. Sometimes it panics and tries to hold onto water, leading to symptoms such as edema (excess water in the tissue spaces) and high blood pressure. The orthodox treatment for these conditions will be diuretics-drugs that take water from the cells and force the kidneys to excrete it. Of course, if the problem is actually caused by dehydration this treatment will make the situation worse. Actually, a better treatment could be to start drinking more water. Two side effects of diuretics are dizziness and drowsiness. These are actually caused by the brain*

Electrolytes

- Electrolytes are trace minerals that conduct electricity within the body. The primary electrolytes are sodium, potassium, chloride, bicarbonate, calcium, magnesium and phosphate
- The interaction between these electrolytes drives nerve impulses (sodium and potassium) and muscle contractions (calcium/magnesium)
- These substances interact with each other as magnets attract polar opposites or repel the similar
- Loss of electrolyte balance results in the symptoms of dehydration and possible seizures in children and the elderly

being dehydrated, causing cells to shrink. This can cause confusion that makes a person forget to drink or eat, exacerbating the problem...especially among older people.

There are many causes of dehydration: extreme vomiting or diarrhea, lack of fluids, fever, and crying for a long time. Many serious illnesses cause dehydration: diabetes insipidus and mellitus, and kidney disease. Then there is what is called endogenous causes of dehydration. Endogenous means causes from outside of the body. This includes diuretics traditionally prescribed by allopathic doctors. Pharmaceutical diuretics are offered for one single purpose: to forcefully remove fluid from the body to lower blood pressure. (Remember dehydration increases blood pressure.)

It is important that an herbalist does not confuse the actions of pharmaceutical diuretics with plants that are called diuretics. Although the word diuretic is derived from the Greek word to urinate, its modern usage in herbal medicine is much more complex. Essentially when an herbalist says a plant has a diuretic action, she means the plant affects the kidneys.

Many, many medicinal plants increase urination but are rarely offered by the herbalist to initiate this activity. For example nutritive herbs such as nettles, alfalfa, dandelion leaf, parsley, kelp and chickweed are diuretics. These herbs are used to rebuild depleted resources after a long illness, poor lifestyle choices or simply as part of healthful daily living. Each of these herbs has a high mineral content.

Symptoms of dehydration:
Dry, sticky mouth, thirst
Decrease urine output
Dry skin with no elasticity
Headache
Constipation
Dizziness or lightheadedness
Sunken eyes (infants fontanels)
Low or high blood pressure
Lack of sweat
Rapid heart rate and breathing

Minerals, including sodium and potassium, are part of the body's electrolyte system. Electrolytes play a role in nerve impulse transmission and blood pressure regulation. The kidney maintains the balance of electrolyte levels in the body. Introducing herbs that are high in minerals increase electrolyte levels in the body. This in turn increases urination as the kidneys maintain a steady electrolyte balance for the body.

Dandelion Leaf (*Taraxacum officinalis folia*) is often viewed as a first class diuretic that rivals Lasix, a commonly prescribed pharmaceutical diuretic used in heart disease. The use of Lasix can lead to depletion of potassium. The heart needs potassium and low levels can cause heart failure. Along with Lasix, people are prescribed a potassium supplement to counter the negative effects of the drug. Herbalists suggest dandelion leaf as an alternative to Lasix because the plant is high in potassium. Many suggest that taking dandelion has a diuretic effect while increasing potassium levels.

In clinic, I have found dandelion leaf to be an unreliable diuretic. Some people find they "pee like a horse" (I live in horse country), while others report little change in their urination. I suspect dandelion's diuretic properties depend on the mineral, and in particular the potassium levels, of the body at the time when treatment with dandelion leaf is begun. I have noted when people who have a diet high in green vegetables (a source of potassium) take dandelion leaf tea, they experience a diuretic effect. Those who eat fewer veggies do not experience an increase in urination. The dandelion's diuretic action occurs in relation to the electrolyte levels in the body. In this way dandelion leaf is a paradoxical herb. Its medicinal action reflects the body's need. Sometimes dandelion leaf increases urination for some while for others, there is little change.

Because nutritive herbs change the body's circulation of fluids through balancing and increasing electrolytes in the body, I often use them to increase low blood pressure.

Low Blood Pressure

In clinic, I see many clients with low blood pressure. Most of them say, "I have always had low blood pressure." Frequently, besides the extreme athletes, these clients lack passion and drive. Most are thin, cold and have an air of fragility about them. Sometimes they suffer with anemia. Remember in TCM the sound for a kidney imbalance is the sigh. Clients with low blood pressure sigh. It is like they have no energy for life. One of the keys to improving their overall wellbeing is increasing their blood pressure.

Offering mineral rich herbs, particularly nettles along with circulatory stimulants will increase blood pressure and bring warmth to life that previously was lacking. An example of a tea formulated to increase blood pressure is:

Nettles   2 parts
Rosemary   1/2 part
Licorice   1 part
Yarrow   1 part
Peppermint to taste.

The diuretic action is explored further when we take a look at elimination.

Physiology of Defense:
It's All About Healthy Boundaries

It is common wisdom in our society that we 'catch' colds. In other societies and other times infection and fever were considered to be possession by evil spirits. Our science tells us one truth, their beliefs told them something different. Who is to say what is truly so? To a medical herbalist and most practitioners of holistic medicine, we do not catch infections; rather we let them in. - David Hoffman The Herbal Handbook: A User's Guide to Medical Herbalism. page 182

During the study of circulation we explored the traditional herbalist's focus on the delivery of nutrients and oxygen to the cells of the body and the removal of metabolic wastes as one of the keys to good health. We played with the premise that if circulation is deficient then the body/mind is weakened and disease finds a ways in. When circulation is hampered and disease enters the body, the immune system comes to the rescue.

The immune system is all about boundaries. It protects our bodies from foreign invaders. The health of the immune system is closely linked to circulation, the nervous and endocrine systems and the quality of your food. The immune system is more complex and aggressive than any military arsenal on the planet.

The first time I studied the immune system I was shocked to learn that with each breath, bite of food, and every time I enjoy sex, my body furiously attacks foreign invaders. Stomach acids fry bugs hitching a ride on the back of food. Mucous membranes lining respiratory passages act like quick sand trapping germs that swirl in on the air currents of my breath. My skin is crawling with hungry bacteria that vigorously defend their territory within the nooks and crannies

Nonspecific and Specific Immune Activities

The immune system actions are classed as specific and nonspecific. Nonspecific actions are either boundary related, such as the skin and mucous membranes, white blood cells called killer cells or macrophages that destroy anything not known as self, or physical responses that remove bugs from the body such as snot, diarrhea and emesis.

Specific immunity involves specialized B-Cells that target specific pathogens. When the body battles a pathogen-- in particular a virus-- it stores information on the virus' weaknesses in memory cells that live in lymph glands. When a virus enters the body, information on its makeup is presented to the memory cells by the messengers. Upon recognizing the virus, the memory cells begin the production of B-cells designed to destroy the infecting virus.

of my voluptuous body. Skin bacteria ruthlessly evict squatters or unwelcome neighbors. My vagina spews acid on germs my partner carries. My body knows who I am, whom it likes and whom it does not.

When my body's initial boundaries of skin, stomach acids and mucous membrane are crossed, then weaponry of the immune system takes charge and things get really nasty. In Paul Bergner's summary of the immune system weaponry, he imagines a science fiction battle in which the planet (the body) defends itself against invaders (antigens or more commonly referred to as germs):

The alarm is raised (phagocytes, white blood cells that eat germs) and the planet is put on war footing (fever and inflammation). The army, (T-helper cells) declares martial law and orders are then sent throughout the planet to set up weapon factories (plasma cells) that will manufacture weapons deadly to this particular invader. Within a few hours, billions of genetically engineered invader-specific weapons (antibodies) are being produced. These are rapidly circulated to every corner of the planet. The army institutes the draft (proliferation of more T-helper cells) and mobilizes local attack by foot soldiers (attracts and activates phagocytes). It sends out special-forces troops (T-killer cells) to destroy any cities or towns of the planet in which the invader has established a foothold.

Afterwards, mop-up operations (more phagocytes) remove the debris of battle and clean-up crews (the last stages of inflammation and fever) rebuild and fortify any cities or towns that have been damaged. - The Healing Power of Echinacea and Goldenseal pg. 66.

To encapsulate Bergner's not so fictional story, the body knows how to defend itself.

When disease penetrates the body, herbalists offer the immune system support to aid its cause. Herbalists do not become commandeering generals who take over the battle. Herbalists are more like strategists; they support the body in its battle. The number one principal in aiding a fight against a pathogen is to go in the same direction as the body is taking. How do herbalists do this?

During the initial phase of infection herbalists offer medicine to:

- Support fever with diaphoretic herbs
- Encourage inflammatory processes responsible for the delivery of the immune system armory and support staff with circulatory stimulants and lymphatic herbs
- Offer herbs that help the body build white blood cells
- Use anti-microbial herbs that assist the immune system in killing off the offending pathogen
- Provide demulcent herbs to line mucous membranes
- Make calming nervine teas to calm and cool the mind
- During the final phase of infection herbalists offer medicine to:
- Support the cleanup of debris left over from the battle between the immune system and the pathogen with lymphatic and circulation stimulatants
- Perhaps offer a stimulating expectorant to clear out any lingering mucous from the respiration tract
- Provide a gentle liver cleanse and mild laxative to remove debris from the battle through the bowel
- Continue to encourage sipping of calming tea so daily life does not take over before the final stages of healing are done

That is a quick summary of the immune system and how herbal medicine can help get you back on your feet quickly.

Now let's peer more deeply into the complex workings of the immune system and the plants that nourish and support it.

In this chapter we will explore:

- The Elements and the Immune System
- Boundaries: The Lover and the Warrior
- A battle with many fronts: The common cold.
- Cold vs. Hot or Acute vs. Chronic
- Friend or Foe: Our relationship with bacteria

The Elements and the Immune System

Defining health as balance does not work well when we explore health and the immune system. When working hard, the immune system throws the elements out of balance. Fire burns hot. Water overflows as pus, snot, diarrhea, emesis or urine. The air element is either dampened down by the water element or becomes stirred up by fire. Traveling on the air element, pain flits through the body or penetrates deep into muscles and bone. The earth element weakens as the immune system suppresses the appetite to conserve the body's energy.

The immune systems excesses are uncomfortable, painful and are far from convenient. However, as illness passes and the immune system quiets down, the elements return to balance and life becomes "comfortable" again.

When considering the actions of the immune system, health needs to be defined as the ability of the body to respond and adapt to changing inner and outer environments. A healthy immune system heats up and flows when the wellness of the body is threatened. As the threat passes the fire element cools down and the water element is contained.

When the immune system cannot respond to the changing environment within the body either by igniting an immune response or by putting out the immune system's fire, chronic disease develops.

Boundaries: The Lover vs The Warrior

Your body sparkles with more cells than stars in the Milky Way. Every day 60 billion of your cells die, while 60 billion are born. For every cell in your body there are ten bacteria. Every 90 seconds your immune system creates millions of antibodies, each one woven together with 12 hundred amino acids. Every hour 200 million red blood cells are regenerated. Your immune system can recognize every cell and every bacterium that belongs in your body! Those that do not belong, it destroys. The complexity of the immune system's knowing blows my mind!

So what does being a lover have to do with complex knowing?

Always working in the background while you tie your shoes, sip your coffee while discussing daily events with a friend, walk the dog or make dinner, your immune system is monitoring every cell twinkling under your skin while tracking everything entering your body. To do this the immune system requires the following from you:

- A relaxed attitude towards life
- A good night's sleep with sweet dreams
- Nutritious food, including adequate protein (those 12 hundred amino acids used to make antigens are made with protein)
- A good stretch several times a week (like the old saying: stretch like a cat and live for nine lives) and a walk in fresh air every day.

Succinctly put, for the immune system to remember every detail of its enormous task it needs you to take care of yourself. Self-love keeps yourself together. This is where the lover comes in. To love yourself is to love life. To love life lifts the burden of struggle from your shoulders, refreshes the senses with this remarkable planet's beauty, and creates an atmosphere of enjoyment all around you.

Loving yourself means that you decide what supports your well-being and what does not, just as your immune system does. Self-love sets up boundaries for your relationships, addictions, attitudes and time. Self-love is what the immune system requires. When we can rest in self-love, we become exceptional communicators.

The immune system is a system of communication. It is constantly relating with the environment you are living in. The immune system excels at the language of boundaries.

A good boundary is permeable. Boundaries are not impenetrable walls. Boundaries are mutable. Boundaries shift depending on the situation, the environment, and our personal needs. (Recall the immune system is what helps us adapt to changing environments.) Good boundaries are interested in what is on both sides of the line. This creates informed decisions. Communication is required to maintain good boundaries.

An example of the immune system's dialogue with its environment is breastfeeding mothers. Mom's body is in contact with all the germs in her environment, most of which her immune system handles without her even being aware she is "infected".

Baby's body is in contact with all the same germs, but he does not have a full-grown immune system. He has no boundaries. Baby relies on antibodies made in Mom's body to protect him. Mom's antibodies, responding to the changing environment, travel through her breast milk and into baby's body. Over a period of four months, the knowledge gathered by Mom's immune system is transferred to baby and builds his immune system. Mom's immune system provides baby with a protective boundary. One could say the immune system is an inheritance of your maternal ancestors.

Becoming a lover of life is the best preventive medicine you can take. When the heart is open to life, time loses its intensity and minor set backs are easily let go. A closed heart shrinks time and we become hypersensitive to the everyday irritants. Communication and listening becomes impossible. Being a lover eases stress from our lives and supports a smooth functioning immune system.

Let's take a look at what stress (or struggle) does to the immune system.

What is Stress?

Stress is the body's response to demands. The body does not differentiate between good stress and bad stress. Planning a wedding or negotiating a divorce triggers the same stress in the body.

The General Adaptive Syndrome (GAS) **GAS** —outlines physiological response to stress in three phases.

Alarm response (Fight, flight or freeze) This is the initial response to stress whether it is meeting a bear in the woods, a car accident or a loud unknown noise.

Dialogue between the brain and the adrenal glands durning the alarm response involves: nerve impulses from the hypothalamus trigger the release of noradrenaline from the adrenal glands, while the limbic system fires up provoking reactions (as opposed to a thoughtful response from the cerebral cortex)

Physiological responses to the alarm phase:
- Increased heart rate
- Increased blood pressure
- Constriction of superficial blood vessels to redirect blood to muscles, lungs, heart and brain.
- Constriction of spleen, decrease immune function
- Sweating

- Release of glucose from the liver.
- Dry mouth, decrease in peristalsis and gastric secretions

Resolution to the alarm phase involves:

- Fleeing the situation- flight
- Igniting -fight
- Taking a few deep breaths massages the vagus nerve with the diaphragm encouraging the PNS
- Drinking a glass of water moistens mouth signalling body everything is okay

Resistance reaction occurs when stress is prolonged and constant., for example: a week before exams, the period of a job search, the week or two before moving house.

Dialogue between the brain and the adrenal glands involves communication between the hypothalamus and the pituitary about the on going stress. The pituitary than releases stimulating hormones that ignite a response from the thyroid, adrenal cortex, the pancreas and the liver. Each stimulated organ releases hormones revving-up the metabolism in hopes of providing more energy to contain the stress-inducing event

The physiological response includes:

- Increased blood pressure
- Water retention
- Revved up glucose production by proteins breaking down
- Cells absorb more glucose while blood glucose remains the same
- Delayed healing of wounds and inflammation

Resolution to the resistance phase involves:

- Prolonged relaxation with a balanced diet, good sleep and fun.
- Herbs such as adaptogens and nervines to support relaxation. These plants counteract the effects of the

stress hormones such as immune suppression and interrupted sleep.

- Using adaptogens can prolong this stage of GAS.

The final stage is **Exhaustion Phase** when the resources of the body are depleted.

Due to the prolonged bath of stress hormones from the adrenal cortex the immune response is suppressed the insulin secreting cells of the pancreas burn out, muscle mass is lost

The Pericardium: The Heart's Protector

The heart is contained in a sack called the pericardium. A thin layer of fluid fills the space between heart and pericardium. This fluid ensures there is no friction with the heart's movement and the rest of the bits and piece of your body contained in the rib cage.

In TCM the pericardium is considered an organ or energy within the body that protects the heart. The heart is considered the King of the body/mind and there is no differentiation between the heart's pumping action and emotional intelligence.

The TCM practitioner says the heart houses Shen, the spirit of the mind/body complex. The best definition of shen I have seen is the light that twinkles from your eyes and the charisma of your personality.

The pericardium in TCM protects the house of shen, or the heart, from emotional attacks.

A revered historical doctor of TCM Liu Wan Su wrote, "Not only does the pericardium provide the heart with physical protection, its energy also protects the heart from damage and disruption by excessive emotional energies generated by the other organs, such as anger from the liver, fear from the kidneys, and grief from the lungs. A weakened pericardium is a powerful disruptor of internal energy balance and a major cause of disease."

In today's modern language, the pericardium supports self-esteem essential for a healthy immune system.

becoming difficult to regain, ulcers erupt in the chronically dry digestive tract, ongoing tension in blood vessels causes loss of elasticity, etc.

Several diseases are symptoms can accompany the exhaustion phase:

- Irritable bowel syndrome
- Ulcerative colitis
- High Blood Pressure
- Rheumatoid arthritis
- Migraines, increased asthma attacks, type two diabetes
- Anxiety and depression
- Autoimmune disease such as Lupus and interstitial cystitis

At this stage, chronic illness sets in. Herbs specific illness to the illness and to aid the body in recovering from exhaustion are used.

The Warrior: Stress as Part of Life

Love is essential medicine but there is no denying that there is stress in life. Some people believe it is the stress in life that makes us strong. There is a certain truth in this statement. First Nations say, "Strong medicine grows in harsh environments."

Yet I cringe every time someone says to me, "If it does not kill you, it makes you stronger." This expression brings to my mind images of people armored, pushing forward at all costs and never surrendering. Then finally exhausted and embittered, they collapse and seek a miracle herb that allows them to regain control.

We are now entering the arena of the warrior. Being able to call upon an inner warrior is an essential element of life. The warrior is able to speak her truth even when it may not be agreeable to others. The warrior stands up to injustice. Sometimes one needs to call on warrior fortitude to walk with integrity. (Integrity is another word to describe the immune system.)

Being a warrior is stressful. Confrontation is the arena of the warrior. Few people thrive on confrontation. Yet being a doormat or simply being blown about by the wind of other people's emotions is detrimental to your ability to love yourself. Engaging your inner

warrior can be an act of self-love. The immune system knows this. It routinely blows up harmful pathogens as an act of self-love.

The challenge with warrior energy is that once it is harnessed it becomes invigorating. Some people find a cause worth fighting for and make it their raison d'être. They thrive on the fight and forget to balance the rigid principled (or not so principled) attitudes with enjoyment of beauty, sensual delight and just hanging out. Life becomes a fight. Remember, confrontation is stressful. Constant confrontation demands enormous resources from the body. Prolonged confrontation leads to burn out and a door opens for chronic illness to enter the body/mind.

Some people believe that the immune system is a warrior. I do not think so. The immune system has a feel for every cell of the body. It intimately understands what the body needs and does not need. This sounds like love to me.

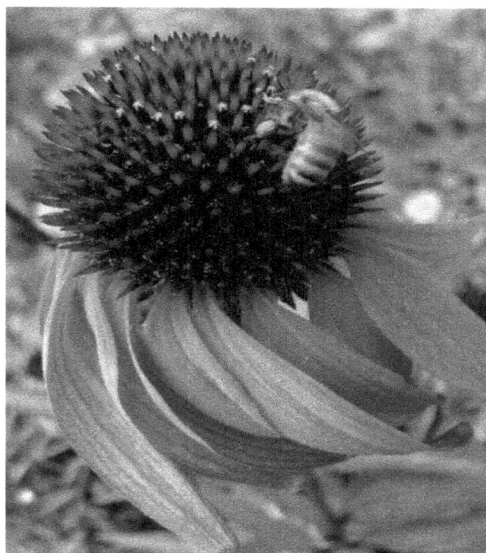

Echinacea   Rosalee de la Forêt

The immune system is able to become a warrior and take charge of the whole body, as we will soon learn. However, once the battle is done, it falls into the background and lets you get on with loving your life.

Echinacea and Autoimmune Disease

Autoimmune disease is caused when the immune system can no longer recognize the difference between proteins that are part of the body and proteins that belong to pathogens. This confusion between self and other causes the immune system to attack the body.

Some healers believe the underlying cause of autoimmune diseases is an inner war that cannot be resolved. They say, "The body is at war with itself." Perhaps this is true in some cases, but I do not think this belief reflects all autoimmune diseases.

Perhaps autoimmune diseases occur when the essential core of who we are becomes misplaced in the messiness of life and the underlying cause of autoimmune disease is not enough self-love. Caught up in life's struggles, one is no longer able to discriminate between the battles that need to be fought and the battles to let go of. During the exhaustion phase of stress one forgets boundaries and allows the discipline of self-care to fall away. This weakens a sense of self. Maybe the undercurrent of autoimmune disease is a weak sense of self that leads to an over-protective warrior energy. Echinacea is a remarkable plant that helps the immune system finds its footing again, or one could say its sense of self.

Often the pain associated with autoimmune diseases first asserts itself during the exhaustion phase of stress. Is the immune system fatigued during the exhaustion phase and no longer able to distinguish between self and pathogen? Think about times when you have been extremely tired: up for several nights with a sick child, during long distance travel or perhaps working night shifts. Consider how confused your thinking became with each sleepless night. Recall how emotionally raw you felt, reacting to every little irritant like the very core of your being was being attacked.

Many suspect that the seed of an autoimmune disease is a deeply penetrating infection the immune system has struggled with for years. The immune system, after battling constantly for an extended period of time, falls under the spell of fatigue. It loses the plot of self and becomes unable to choose it battles. The warrior takes over and the lover can no longer stop the fight.

A little echinacea tincture will help the immune system wake up to the reality of the unrelenting battle. Echinacea stimulates the immune system and helps it resolve its inner conflict: the deep infection. The resolution of the infection leads to remission of the disease.

The herbalist must be very careful using echinacea in cases of autoimmune disease. It is important not to over stimulate an already exhausted immune system. Very small doses over a short period of time are all that is need. It's sort of like taking a few sips of strong coffee after a night shift to wake up long enough to drive home safely. Too much coffee will keep one awake and further irritate the nervous system; just the right amount will keep one from falling asleep at the wheel.

A Battle on Many Fronts: A Study of the Common Cold

Let's look at how the immune system works by studying the common cold.

Symptom 1. Nasal Stuffiness or Runny Nose: The Immune Power of Mucous

The mucous membrane coats the inner surfaces of our body: mouth, nose, sinus, pharynx, trachea, bronchi, esophagus, stomach, small and large intestine, vagina, urethra, bladder and ureter. Its function is to protect our body from infection in a number of ways.

- The membrane oozes with gooey mucous that captures pathogens and escorts them from the body.

- Mucous' slimy texture limits the pathogens' ability to get a hold on the tissues that lie beneath, thus preventing secondary infections such as a bacterial infection in the nasal sinuses following a cold.

- Mucous is more than irritating slime; it is rich in IgA antibodies. IgA antibodies are found on all body surfaces. Their job is to cling to germs and call for back up. IgA antibodies are good friends with the white blood cells called Killer T-Cells. When the Killer T-Cells show up, they shoot missiles into the cold virus exploding it from within. At this point, the cold is on its way out.

- An herbalist encourages a runny nose. A stuffy nose is not a good sign for a quick return to health. When a virus sneaks into the respiratory passages mucous needs to flow.

Steam inhalations to Encourage a Runny Nose
Fill a kettle full of water, put it on the stove and bring it to a full boil.
While the water is warming, gather a large bowl, large towel and choose an essential oil (Tea Tree, Eucalyptus or Thyme). When the water boils, pour it into the bowl, add two drops of essential oil and put the towel over your head and the bowl. Breathe deeply.
 When you need to come up for air, pop your head out from the towel. When ready breathe in the steam again.
Try to do this 3 times a day until the cold resolves.

Symptom 2 - Body Aches and Fatigue

Have you seen the ads on TV for antidepressants that list the many symptoms of depression, including body aches? Low serotonin levels in the muscles, not just the brain, cause the body aches in depression.

When you have a cold, the immune system commandeers the body's serotonin. Specialized immune cells called dendritic cells use serotonin. These powerful immune cells hunt down invaders that have never before infected the body. Once the unknown invader is discovered, dendritic cells educate the rest of the immune system on how to destroy the invader. The Dendritic cells' messenger is the happy neurotransmitter serotonin. Dendritic cells send serotonin speeding to T-cells revving them up for battle.

During a cold, bodies ache because the immune system ushers serotonin out of the muscles to help with its fight. The body aches experienced with a cold have the same cause as body aches accompanying depression.

The immune system also recruits serotonin from of the brain during illness. Lower serotonin levels in the brain cause fatigue, lethargy and an "I don't care" attitude. During a cold, low serotonin levels leave the ego on the couch, dosing on and off between movies. While the ego moans on the couch, the body rests. A depressed, dull mind ensures the immune system

Easing Body Aches

Soaking in a warm bath with a 1/2 cup of epsom salts and 8 drops of sweet birch essential oil comforts the body during a cold. The warm water relaxes the body. Epsom salts are high in magnesium. The skin easily absorbs magnesium. Increased magnesium levels in the body enhance muscle relaxation and resolution of inflammation. Sweet birch essential oil furthers the action of magnesium.

receives all the necessary resources required for the quick destruction of the virus. Getting up, getting dressed and trying to carry on as if you do not have a cold only prolongs the depressed state and physical aches as the immune system fights the ego for resources.

Symptom 3 - Sore throat and hoarseness

The sore throat is caused by inflammation and suggests the virus is trying to roost more deeply in your respiratory tract.

Once the virus enters your body, the immune system employs inflammation to seal off the infected area, kill the bug and clean up the resulting mess (dead virus pieces, white blood cells and collateral damage) while rebuilding healthy tissue.

The signs of inflammation describe the process: redness, swelling, pain and heat.

This is a very short synopsis of inflammation.

- Cells damaged by the virus release histamines and serotonin to signal they need help. This is the beginning of body aches.
- This creates a rush of blood to the area carrying weapons and soldiers (white blood cells). An increase in blood supply where the pathogen is seeking lodging results in localized redness and heat.
- Blood vessels become porous to allow support staff, weapons and soldiers to infiltrate the damaged area and kill the invading pathogens. This is the cause of swelling.
- The soldiers, including natural killer cells, blow up any cells they do not recognize while macrophages (also called "big mouths") eat all foreign looking cells. Helper T-cells send messages to B-cells in lymph glands about who the pathogen is and what specialized poison (an antibody) will kill it.

- The support staff includes a variety of substances performing the role of messengers and herders. For example: corralling pathogens into a clump and serving them up to the macrophages for a snack.

Pain is the result of inflammatory substances such as prostaglandins and bradykinin that direct the traffic during the battle. The raw nerve endings caught in the middle of the battle also contribute to inflammation's pain.

Remember, the inflammation process has a beginning, middle and end. After the battle, inflammatory process assists with the clean up and promote healing.

Herbal Anti-Inflammatories

Many herbs are referred to as anti-inflammatory. Plant anti-inflammatories do not act like over-the-counter or prescribed anti-inflammatories drugs such as NSAID, antihistamines and steroids. Unlike these drugs, plant medicine does not shut down the inflammatory processes.

Nature's anti-inflammatories moderate the inflammatory process in many different ways. Saying a plant is an anti-inflammatory is practically meaningless. The word anti-inflammatory gives the student of herbalism little direction on how the plant heals. To understand a plant's anti-inflammatory action it is necessary to understand where and how the plant acts in the resolution of the inflammatory process.

Throat Spray for Sore Throats

25 mls Rose hip syrup (made with honey)
25 mls Elderberry syrup (made with honey)
15 mls Echinacea tincture
5 mls Thyme tincture
25 mls distilled water

Combine herbs and water in a spray bottle. Shake well. Spray onto back of throat frequently until inflammation resolves.

Calendula *(Calendula off.)*is one of the most useful anti-inflammatories in my apothecary. It has many anti-inflammatory activities.

Calendula is a demulcent. Demulcents bring moisture to dry, hot surfaces (a surface can be on the inside of the body). This cooling action is anti-inflammatory. Demulcents limit the damage to the area

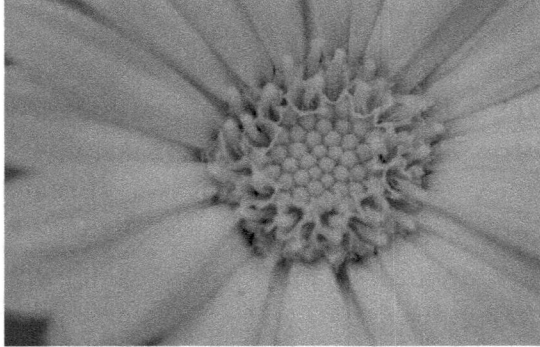

Calendula   Rosalee de la Forêt

surrounding the infection and help reseal the site of the battle with a mucous membrane. Marshmallow (Althea officinalis) and plantain (Plantago spp.) are two other demulcents.

Calendula's bright orange flowers are high in flavonoids. Flavonoids scavenge free radicals. Free radicals are a by-product of the immune system's war with a virus. Loose free radicals can cause collateral damage by irritating adjoining tissues and spreading inflammation. Calendula's flavonoids bind free radicles rendering them harmless.

Calendula flowers are sticky. They are covered in a resin. Like most plant resins, calendula's is anti-microbial. When encountering pathogens, the resin penetrates virus cell membranes and destroys them from the inside out. This results in fewer pathogens and less inflammation.

Calendula contains tannins. Tannins bind proteins. When there are small tears within the body or on the skin, loose proteins break free of damaged tissues. Tannins, whether in calendula or black berry leaf or plantain, bind these exposed proteins and close the tear with a scab. Scabs are a weaving of protein. Plantain is a demulcent herb with astringent actions as well.

When you read that a plant is anti-inflammatory, please explore the plant a little deeper and see if you can discover all the ways in which it supports the resolution of inflammation in the body.

Symptom Four - Fever

In the chapter on circulation we briefly explored fever. Let's take a deeper look at the immune response fever.

Fevers have always been one the most common causes of death, and some like plague, smallpox, typhoid and cholera, have been notoriously destructive. In the cramped unhygienic conditions of pre-twentieth century European cities and towns, epidemics of fever, or pestilence, have decimated populations and caused untold hardship....

Coincident with the rise of urban culture was the development of the use of mineral medicine as medicaments. Preparations of compounds of arsenic, mercury, sulphur and other toxic elements were increasingly used to suppress the febrile and other symptoms of severe infections.....A new tradition of allopathy, symptomatic prescribing, was born. The Essential Book of Herbal Medicine - Simon Mills

Many people still shudder at the thought of a fever. The fear that the fever will rage out of control has led to the practice of shutting it down with aspirin. Fevers demand respect. When helping someone through a fever, it is very important not to treat it casually, and to keep a finger on the fever's pulse.

Fevers are ignited when a metabolite, produced by a pathogen, is presented to the hypothalamus. The hypothalamus responds to the metabolite by turning up the body's temperature. When the hypothalamus initially turns up the temperature, the body feels cold and blood flows into the inner regions of the body. To preserve life the body will always choose to keep vital inner organs warm over the surface of the body. No one has ever died of frostbite on the tips of the fingers. When hypothermia penetrates deep into the body cooling the essential organs, life is threatened. Once the fever is initiated, the change in temperature and redirection of blood flow to the interior causes shivering, pallor and a feeling of coldness on the surface of the body.

When the body reaches the temperature set by the hypothalamus, there is no dominant feeling of being hot or cold. As the number of pathogens triggering a feverish response decline, the thermostat of the hypothalamus is turned down, causing peripheral circulation to open and blood to flow from

Herbal Teas for the Common Cold

There a number of very common herbal teas used to treat the common cold. These herbs support the efforts of the body. They do not stop the work of the immune system.

Tea #1

1 part Yarrow (*Achillia* millefolium)- diaphoretic, antibacterial, bitter

2 parts Peppermint (*Mentha piperita*) - calms the mind/body, anti-microbial

2 parts Elder flowers (*Sambucus nigra flora*) - diaphoretic, relaxes the body

Tea # 2: For a cold trying to settle in the chest

2 parts Sage (*Salvia off.*)- anti-microbial, diaphoretic, bitter, warming

1 part Boneset (*Eupatorium perfoliatum*) - diaphoretic, antibacterial, bitter, anti-viral

1 part Hyssop (*Hyssops off.*)- expectorant, anti-microbial, diaphoretic

the vital organs to the surface of the body. Skin becomes hot andflushed and sweat glands open releasing cooling perspiration.

Once there is balance between the temperature of the body and the hypothalamus, there is again no sense of being too hot or too cold.

Managing a Fever

The trick to managing a fever is maintaining the body temperature between 38 and 39 degrees C. At this temperature blood is pulsing quickly and delivering a frenzy of killer immune cells to the infected area. Many pathogens find it difficult to live at this temperature for any length of time; this also helps the body's cause.

To support the body in maintaining a safe temperature during fever, herbalists use diaphoretic herbs. Diaphoretics are heat producing and sweat inducing herbs. They both cool and heat the body at the same time.

Catnip (Nepeta cataria) is a diaphoretic that calms the nervous system. Irritability and restlessness accompany fever. Catnip tea quiets the mind and is likely to bring refreshing sleep while encouraging the fever and its resolution. Catnip has a strong scent and like any strongly scented herb, it is high in volatile oils. Volatile oils are nonspecific destroyers of germs. The only challenge with

A quick summary on how to follow a fever's progress:
- At between 38-39 degrees Celsius (101-102 F) the immune response is in the heat of battle. (Note: brain damage occurs when a fever reaches 41.6 degrees Celsius or 107 degrees F.)

Symptoms of a fever rising: feeling cold, shivering, pallor

Symptoms of a fever coming down: feeling hot, flushed skin, sweating

Symptoms of a fever resolved or peaking: there is no sense of feeling hot or cold catnip is its taste. It is a bitter. A little honey in catnip tea helps it go down.

Elderflower (Sambucus nigra) is a better tasting diaphoretic that is often preferred over catnip. It too has a diaphoretic effect and calms the nerves. Elderflowers are not as strong as catnip in bringing on sleep.

When using a diaphoretic tea to manage fever, offer frequent sips and be sure it is as hot as the patient can stand it. Continue to offer the tea throughout the course of the fever.

Fever and Chronic Disease

During a chronic disease, the body has difficulty generating a fever or seems to maintain a low-grade fever that never really peaks or resolves. In this case the herbalist offers a circulatory stimulant to give the body's febrile response a little motivation. Herbs like ginger (Zingiber off.), angelica (Angelica archangelica) and if all else fails cayenne (Capsicum minimum) encourage heat in the body.

When managing a fever, these are the danger signs:
- Severe headache
- Nausea and vomiting
- Diarrhea
- Coughing
- Pain and spasms
- A pulse that does not rise with temperature (meningitis)

If the fever begins to burn out of control, apply a cold wet face cloth to the forehead or wash the body with tepid water, either in the tub or as a sponge bath. If you feel really uncomfortable, ibuprofen brings fever's temperature down. It will also shut down the immune response.

An Immune System Interrupted

The health challenge modern herbalists frequently treat is a confused immune system, and a viral or bacterial infection that has penetrated deeply into the body.

Think of the immune system as having layers. The first layer is physical boundaries. If the pathogen penetrates the physical boundaries, it encounters the nonspecific defences: macrophages, T-killer cells, inflammation and fever. If the pathogen hangs in a little longer plasma cells develop antibodies specific to the pathogen. Antibodies engage in vigorous battle with the germs.

Let's return to the example of a cold. The first sign of a cold is a runny nose. In allopathic medicine, nasal decongestants are the first line of defence against the sniffles. Decongestants contain antihistamines. Histamines are the early messengers the immune system uses to announce a pathogens' penetration of initial defences. Histamines initiate an inflammatory response used to seal off the infection. Interfering with the histamine response to infection is like killing the messenger and thinking the problem is resolved.

Antihistamines shut down the runny nose. Antihistamines dry up snot and all its IgA antibodies while impounding the vehicle used to remove germs, limit inflammation and the delivery of white blood cells to the area of infection. This make the cold more socially convenient but opens one up to further health risks. With the dry sinus full of unchecked multiplying viruses, there is a very good chance that the underlying tissues will become irritated. Once the cold virus has run its natural course, the site of irritation become a breeding ground for bacteria. This leads to a sinus infection.

The next step in allopathic medicine is antibiotic therapy. The antibiotics can be compared to bombs in a war zone. They kill without discretion. Friendly bacteria that are helpful in restoring order are destroyed. This leaves further room for the infections to spread. A month or two following the initial infection an ear infection develops, or tonsillitis, or perhaps strep throat, bronchitis and then pneumonia. And so it goes....

Traditional herbalists believe that when the immune system and all its agents are hampered by drugs, pathogens moves deeper into the body. The germ moves underground and conserves it resources until stress weakens the body. At the perfect moment the pathogen reasserts itself. Once or twice a year it comes out of hiding and launches a full-scale attack on the respiratory tract, the digestive tract, or will perhaps results in swollen lymph nodes. Again, allopathic treatments are used, clearing up symptoms caused by the immune response. Eventually the immune system no longer has the mustard to take an aggressive stand. Instead the body/mind is left feeling tired, depressed, and achy with no appetite. Clients with this kind of challenge say, "I never feel like I quite shake it."

In this case, the acute condition has become chronic and there may be lasting side effects due to the conventional treatment like candida infections or inflamed respiratory pathways or bladder. Even conditions like chronic heartburn can be the

Sinus Rub for Chronic Sinusitis

This formula has rescued many people from the pain of secondary sinus infections. It is a combination of tinctures.
10 mls Myrrh (*Commiphora molmol*)
10 mls Lobelia (*Lobelia inflata*)
10 mls Cayenne (*Capsicum minimum*)
10 mls Oregon Grape Root (*Mahonia aquafolium*)
10 mls Bayberry Bark (*Myrica cerifera*)
Rub over the sinus area several times a day until infection clears up. Then for one more week, continue to apply just before bed..

result of allopathic treatment of viral infections.

NSAID (Non-Steroidal anti-inflammatory drugs) also push illness deeper into the body. To understand the effects of NSAID on the body we need to begin with another class of inflammatory mediator (like histamine): prostaglandins.

There are three general classes of prostaglandins: series 1, 2 and 3. Each series has a slightly different role in inflammation.

- Series 1 and 3 are involved in the clean up of inflammation or its resolution.
- Series 2 participate in the initiation of inflammation. One of the main actions of series 2 prostaglandins is the stimulation of the pain response. Pain, being extremely unpleasant, alerts us that there is something very wrong and depending on its severity, demands attention.

NSAID inhibit production of all three series of prostaglandins. These drugs ease pain caused by series 2 prostaglandins, but also interfere with the resolution of the inflammation by impeding the actions of series 1 and 3. Studies have shown that NSAID use causes an initial sense of improvement but over the long-term delays healing.

Prostaglandins also initiate fever in the body. When suffering with a cold, taking a NSAID for body aches limits the febrile response. These drugs impede both the killing of the virus and the healing of any tissue damage caused by the inflammation process. Approximately 30 billion doses of non-steroidal anti-inflammatories are taken a year in the United States. NSAIDs are not anti-inflammatory; they are pro-inflammatory when one takes a closer look at their actions.

Chronic low-grade inflammatory conditions can go on for years before the client gives up the struggle against the immune systems efforts and arrives at the herbalist's door.

When working with long-standing infections or inflammation, it is important to know that the condition will go through a variety of stages before resolution. In homeopathic medicine, this is called The Law of Cure or Hering's Law. Hering was the homeopathic doctor who initially recorded the following observation:

...the cure takes place from top of the body downwards, from inside outward, and from the most important organ to the least important. Cure takes place in reverse order to the onset of symptoms. Therefore, for example, an ill person will start feeling better emotionally before the physical symptoms disappear and a long-standing complaint will take longer to disappear than a recent one. The Family Guide to Homeopathy Dr. A Lockie

I find it important to explain this process to my clients. This allows them the opportunity to monitor the progress of their recovery as well as not become disheartened when "setbacks" occur.

When the client religiously follows the protocol, you can expect to offer one week of treatment for every month the chronic condition has lingered.

Consider this statement by herbalist Paul Bergner:

Immune system weakness invariably arises from the first two areas (lifestyle and diet and spiritual vitality), not from herbal deficiency. If you eat a diet rich in heavy, poor-quality, or incompatible food;

Salicylates

Bitter salicylates are made by plants to discourage foragers. In the body they ease the pain of inflammation. These plant constituents are the pre-cursers to NSAIDs.

When using plants that contain salicylates to quiet inflammatory pain, it is important to offer other herbs that help bring the inflammation to completion.

suffer from chronic stress; take drugs for every ache, pain, and discomfort; indulge in addictions to destructive substances; feel a lack of connectedness to life and nature; take a self-centered approach to your fellows; feel no sense of creativity and purpose in life; and hold no feeling of the sacredness of the Creator and creation, it would be foolhardy to expect echinacea or any other herb to make up for these irregularities. It is wiser and saner to view herbs as allies – as helping gifts of nature – while you seek to grow in understanding and mastery of your life and health.   The Healing Powers of Echinacea and Goldenseal and Other Immune System Herbs

It is important to encourage your client to eat nutritious, simple foods, sleep and rest, have fun and stay off the over-counter-drugs.

Chronic Illness vs Acute Illness: Cold Vs Hot

Generally, chronic illness results in a weak fire element while acute illness burns hot. The deeper and more chronic the illness the weaker the fire element is in the body.

The fire element, centered in the heart, sparks our passion for life. Chronic illness steals passion.

Herbal treatment for chronic and acute conditions differs.

When a body has the strength to fight off an acute illness, as already stated, the herbalist follows the body's lead. For example: if the cough is wet, stimulating expectorants are offered. Thyme (Thymus vulgaris) is a stimulating expectorant. If the cough is dry and harsh, relaxing, demulsifying expectorants are used, like marshmallow leaf (Althea officinalis folia). During acute illness medicine is offered frequently and in high doses.

For example, when a client wakes up with a productive cough, swollen lymph nodes and a mild fever, recommend a tea of:

1 part thyme	Stimulating expectorant
1 part red clover flowers	Lymphatics
2 parts catnip	Diaphoretic, relaxant, bitter

Take 6 cups throughout the day, hot, with a teaspoon of honey.

When treating chronic disease, the herbalist needs to slow down and support the body on a much deeper level. Remember the illness has insinuated itself into the client's body/mind.

When a client is chronically sick, he has little energy and motivation to go out and buy nutritious food and cook it. Therefore I like to begin with nutrient rich herbal teas that are high in vitamins, minerals and chlorophyll.

Nutritious tea:

1 part nettles	- high in protein, anti-inflammatory, balances blood sugars.
1 part alfalfa	- high in minerals
1 part oat straw	- high in minerals
3 parts rose hips	- high in flavonoids, help the body absorb minerals

Take warm, 3 cups per day between meals. Add a teaspoon of honey. (The sugar in the honey will improve the absorption of the flavonoids.)

The next step is to rebuild the immune system. Herbal medicine is rich in deep immune tonics. Many of these plants are classed as adaptogens. Adaptogens help the body adapt to stress. Most moderate the immune system by interacting with the adrenal glands. However, each adaptogen has a special gift for the fatigued body. They must be studied carefully to fully understand each individual plant's nature.

Astragalus (Astragalus membranaceuss) root carries a sweet mild taste. Recall that the sweet taste "builds up" bodies. Astragalus rebuilds blood. I have successfully used astragalus to increase white and red blood cell counts during extended chemotherapy treatment.

Besides building blood, astragalus calms hypersensitive inflammation in the respiratory tract. It is my favoured herb to quiet down hay fever and allergies to animals. I find it needs to be taken a couple of weeks before allergy season and throughout the entire season for best effects.

I also use astragalus to boost a weak immune system during the early fall, preparing the body/mind for the many viruses that surface during the change of season and throughout the winter. In this case, I dose low for two months.

Although I find astragalus fast acting (I have seen it produce significant changes in the number of white and red blood cells within a couple of weeks) it is a long-term herb. Astragalus' medicine is mostly water-soluble. Traditionally it was taken in a soup based on a bone broth. This is my favoured way of having clients take the herb. However, not everyone is able to do this, so I also use a tincture of astragalus.

At times I have offered

From the Inside Out

The most inner part of our body/mind is our deeply held beliefs. Therefore it is important, according to Herring's Law to understand a client's belief about their illness to truly cure it. By discussing a client's beliefs around an illness, an astute herbalist will uncover thoughts and emotions associated with the illness. It may be necessary to offer the client new ways of approaching difficult emotions and thoughts before any real physical healing can establish itself.

a tea of astragalus, but found I have had poor compliance with it. Astragalus is a bland tasting herb and clients seem to think that herbal medicine needs a strong flavour. They typically quickly lose interest in astragulus' weak flavour.

Rhodiola (Rhodiola roscea) When anxiety accompanies chronic illness, rhodiola (Rhodiola roscea) is a good choice. Rhodiola flourishes in my garden. It has its own corner it shares with California poppy. They seem like strange bed fellows with rhodiola originally from Siberia and the poppy that loves hot, dry climates, but they like each other's company. Like California poppy, rhodiola calms an anxious mind. Unlike California poppy, rhodiola penetrates deep into the body and rebuild the immune system.

Adaptogens like rhodiola are essential in rebuilding the body and in particular the immune system. Chronic stress, an underlying cause of chronic illness, leads to atrophy of the spleen, thymus and lymphoid tissue. Each of these organs is responsible for the manufacture and storage of the white blood cells which are the soldiers of the immune system. Studies have shown that rhodiola encourages the thymus to grow and reduces the size of the adrenal glands.

I prefer fresh plant tincture of rhodiola to dry root tinctures. Rhodiola's ability to open up the mind (stress closes minds) is immediately felt with the fresh plant tincture. Rhodiola is a stimulating plant. I advise clients to take the plant in the

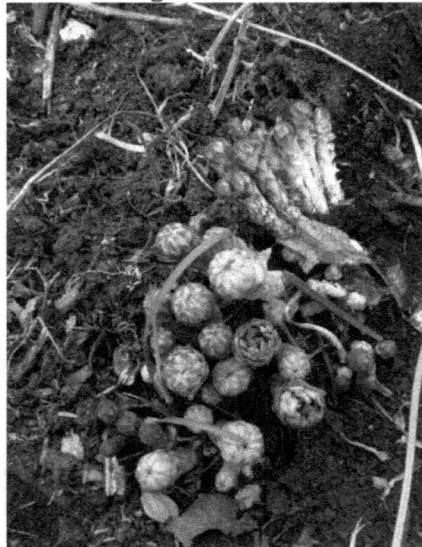

Rhodila   Abrah Arneson

190

morning. If it is taken in the evening it can cause wakefulness.

Ashwagandha When insomnia plagues a client with a weak body and agitated mind I choose an adaptogenic herb from India called ashwagandha (Withania somnifera). Some people call it Indian Ginseng. I prefer to leave the word ginseng out. Ginseng is a misunderstood plant, and I will discuss that later.

Ashwagandha helps those suffering with chronic illness put weight back on. It bestows the gift of sleep. I have one client that says, "Oh with that herb, I sleep like a baby." Ashwagandha also rebuilds blood and improves one's overall sense of well-being.

I like to offer ashwagandha in its traditional form. In India it is decocted in 1 part milk and 2 parts water for 20-30 minutes and then drank before bed. Because some of ashwagandha medicine is fat soluble, the fat in the milk draws out the medicine. The ritual of making ashwagandha medicine before bed helps the client connect with their medicine. I often suggest they think about what they want the plant medicine to do for their mind/body as they prepare the decoction. Sometimes when I have a client who is extremely preoccupied in life I offer ashwagandha in tincture form.

Adaptogens are tonic herbs that are best taken over an extended period of time, sometimes up to 6 to 8 months. They are dosed much lower than herbs used during acute illness. Generally, although I do alter dosing according to the client and her needs, I will ask the client to take 1 - 2 teaspoons of tincture or one cup of tea (5 mls) a day.

It is beneficial to combine adaptogens with gentle nervines such as oat seed (Avena sativa) and a mild liver cleansing herb such as Dandelion root (Taraxacum off. rad.). Adding a little echinacea to the formula offers the immune system an extra boost.

This is an example of a formula designed to rebuild the body. These are all tinctures.

30 mls Astragalus membranaceus   Rebuilds blood

30 mls Rhodiola roscea   Rebuilds immune organs

20 mls Taraxacum off. rad.   Cleanses liver

20 mls Echinacea angustifolia   Helps the body fight deep-seated infection

Chaga (Inonotus obliquus) is my second favourite rebuilding herb. Chaga is a mushroom and therefore theoretically not a plant. Chaga helps put weight on when a client is too thin and helps take weight off when a client is too fat. Chaga deepens sleep and improves energy levels during the day. Chaga improves the mood. Chronic illness is depressing. It steals life's optimism. Chaga brings hope back into life. Remember to cure chronic illness an herbalist often needs to offer medicine that renews the client's spirit. Chaga does this.

One of the most distressing books I have read is Cancer Ward by Alexander Solzhenitsyn. It is a grim story of the hopelessness the Russian people suffered under Stalin's brutal reign. The merciless disease cancer is used as a metaphor for the ravages of the brutal dictator. In the Cancer Ward, Solzhenitsyn dreams of the boreal forest that spreads itself across most of Russia. "He could imagine no greater joy than to go away into the woods for months on end, to break off this chaga, crumble it, boil it up on the campfire, drink it and get well like an animal. To walk through the forest for months, to know no other care than to get better."

Chaga is a famous cancer remedy in Eastern Europe. There are many stories of chaga miraculously curing cancer. It is specific to bowel and stomach cancers as well as cervical and breast cancer. In Russia, it is used for most cancers.

As with most healing herbs, its chemistry is complex, and there is no single constituent responsible for its healing activity. Listed below are a few of the beneficial constituents of chaga.

Polysaccharides

Polysaccharides are immune-modulators. Cancer is in many ways an illness that takes over when the immune system loses its vigilance. It is the immune system's job to destroy renegade cells. If the immune system is ineffective, renegade cells multiply and cancer is the result. The polysaccharides in chaga and other mushrooms stimulate the immune system and strengthen it. A strong immune system is needed to overcome cancer.

Betulin

The chaga fungus receives this constituent from the birch tree. Birch trees make betulin as protection from the sun's radiation. Without betulin, the birch tree would come down with a tree version of skin cancer. In human beings betulin has several actions, including anti-viral, anti-inflammatory, and anti-cancer properties.

Antioxidants

Free radical damage is to blame for the formation of many cancers. Antioxidants bind free radicals. When a free radical is bound, it no longer has the power to damage a cell. Studies have shown chaga to possess more antioxidants than reishi, vitamin C, or blueberries.

Chaga also makes an

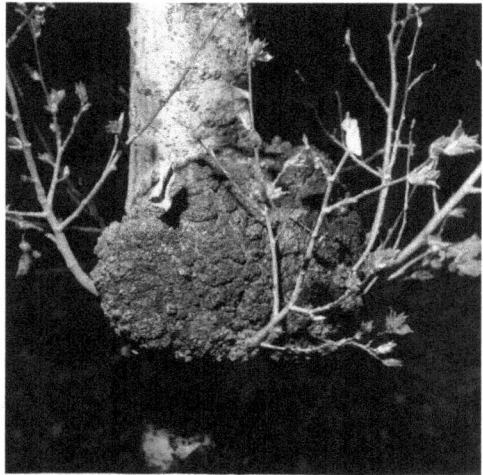

Chaga   Mark Arneson

excellent adjunct to conventional cancer treatment. It both protects against and removes radiation poisoning.

Chaga's medicine has become so popular these days that some herbalists are concerned about the over-harvesting of this slow growing wild fungus. I remember hearing a woman once say she puts chaga in all the soups she makes. It is important to remember that medicine like chaga is special. It is for those times when the body/mind is depleted by illness. Chaga needs to be respected for this purpose. Do not use it like a rose hip tea high in vitamin C to keep colds at bay all winter. Save this special medicine for the weak and sick.

This is a formula using chaga to help rebuild depleted resources:

40 mls Inonotus obliquus   Helps the body re-establish homeostasis

40 mls Avena sativa   Acts as a tonic to a frazzled nervous system

20 mls Rumex crispus   Regulates bowels and high in iron

Be aware that during acute illness deep immune tonics are not used. Their medicine is not for the initial fight. Many immune tonics rebuild the fire in the body. A vigorous immune system has enough fire to overcome acute illness. To add more fuel to the fire with a deep immune tonic could harm your client as opposed to help him.

Friend or Foe: Our Relationship with Bacteria

Our immune system happily coexists with bacteria. Remember that there are approximately 10 bacteria for every cell of your body. Our friendly bacteria play a role in protecting our body from infection. One could say that without the friendly bacteria's support, the immune system would be overrun with germs.

Our modern age just does not understand bacteria and our relationship to it. Consider this example:

What possible role can a pathogenic organism have? One image used by naturopathic practitioners is the fungus on the forest floor. As trees die and fall they leave large carcasses of relatively tough wood that would potentially litter the forest floor: the mineral and other nutrients that they contain would be locked up and unobtainable for other plants; life would be choked off. It is thus essential that organisms exist that act to rot hard wooden logs. Fungi and wood-boring insects between them can recirculate the material in a dead tree and bring it back into the ecocycle. They may marginally affect, but they do not damage, healthy living trees. Their survival depends on finding dead wood; the forest's survival also depends on them doing so. - The Essential Book of Herbal Medicine - Simon Mills

Within and on the body, bacteria exploit little tears in its tissue. Bacteria feed on dying tissue. I know this is very unpleasant to think about, but the question needs to be raised: - if 60 billion cells within your body die every day, what is taking care of the decomposing cells and recycling their valued nutrients? The answer is bacteria.

Bacteria are more friends than foe. The key to maintaining good bacterial balance within the body is nutritious food, restful sleep, moderate stress and fun.

Can herbal medicine help when an infection takes up residence in the body? Can herbal medicine help rebalance the friendly flora while destroying germs? Yes: there are many anti-microbial herbs used to destroy infecting organisms while other plants improve the overall integrity of the body.

Herbal anti-microbial

Most medicinal plants create; they make for themselves. For example: the scent of a plant is a complex blend of volatile oils designed to serve the plant in two ways. The first is to seduce pollinators such as bats, bees, and butterflies, etc. Pollinators are a essential to a plant's sex life.

Second, volatile oils kill bacteria, viruses, and fungi that threaten the plant's well-being. Volatile oils are part of the plant's immune system.

Curiously, human beings use the same plant volatile oils in perfumes and aftershave to lure mates. Humans also use volatile oils as disinfectants, such as tea tree oil, eucalyptus and oregano essential oils.

Herbalists understand that there is a relationship between humans, plants, and disease in a specific geographic area. Herbalists know these three separate entities are more entwined than can be conceived of by the limited human perception of interconnecting events. It was probably an herbalist who came up with the idea of the Christmas tree six hundred years ago.

Why is the Christmas tree a fir or pine? About six hundred years ago in a place we call Germany, the first fir tree was brought home at winter solstice. Ever since that time, during the darkest days of the year, families bundled up and ventured

Sandor Katz on Fermentation

By eating a variety of live fermented foods, you promote diversity among microbial cultures in your body. Biodiversity, increasingly recognized as critical to the survival of larger-scale ecosystems, is just as important at the micro level.: call it microbiodiversity. Your body is an ecosystem that can function most effectively when populated by diverse species of microorganisms. By fermenting foods and drinks with wild microorganisms present in your home environment, you become more interconnected with the life forces of the world around you. Your environment becomes you, as you invite the microbial populations you share the earth with to enter your diet and your intestinal ecology.

into the forest in search of a small fir tree. Once found, a tree was chopped down and dragged home through knee-deep snow. After shaking snow from its boughs, the tree was brought it into the home and covered with lit candles.

The most wonderful memory I have of the Christmas trees from my childhood are their scent. The fresh green fragrance of the fir tree filled the house and planted a forest of squirrels, rabbits, chickadees, sparkling snow, and starlight in my mind. I am sure it was the fir tree's scent that the good folks were after when they cut down the first Christmas tree.

"Have you ever wondered why the tree chosen for Christmas and Solstice celebrations is typically a fir or a pine? " The fir tree's scent is created by volatile oils found in its needles and twigs. The fir's volatile oils are antiseptic. When heated, by the candles, the volatile oils are released into the air and mingle with airborne germs. Volatile oils penetrate the cells membranes of both viruses and bacteria. Once in the cell, the oils inhibit the germ's ability to replicate.

Six hundred years ago, the Christmas tree was a midwinter flu shot without the pain in the arm or side effects.

Garlic (Allium sativum) If there was a magic bullet in herbal medicine, it is definitely garlic. Here's a short history of the herb.

Remains of garlic have been found in caves inhabited by human beings over 10,000 years ago. The first recorded use of garlic as medicine is found on a 3000-year-old Sumerian tablet. There are over 22 uses of garlic recorded in ancient Egyptian medical texts dating from 1500 B.C. The early Olympian athletes munch on garlic before a big race to enhance their strength and stamina. The ancient Ayurvedic medicine of India rubbed garlic salves over the putrefying wounds of leprosy.

What does modern clinical research say about this ancient What does clinical research say about this herb? In laboratories, it has been found that six medium size cloves of garlic pack the same antibacterial punch as 600,000 units of penicillin. The ancient Egyptians ate at least six cloves a day to maintain good health. It is not without cause that ancient Greeks called them "The Stinking Ones".

That is the problem with garlic: its medicine stinks. Garlic's amazing anti-bacterial properties are attributed to a volatile oil called allicin. A whole clove of garlic however does not contain any allicin. It is not until the clove is crushed, chewed, bruised or chopped that the medicinal allicin materializes due to the interaction between a volatile oil called alliin and enzymes called allinase. Allicin stinks.

The other important fact about the garlic is, if sautéed, the medicine is lost. Volatile oils are called volatile because when they encounter heat, they vaporize. In other words, supper smells good, but garlic's medicine has vanished into thin air.

To get the medicinal benefit of garlic, I recommend stirring it into the pot of spaghetti sauce or stew just before serving the meal. This way, most of the garlic's medicine mingles with the other flavours in the pot and the biting pungency of raw garlic is diminished. Or, crush a couple of cloves into a blend of oil and vinegar and sprinkle it on salads. Both methods of taking fresh garlic fall short of the prescribed six cloves, but it will act as preventive medicine.

A garlic salad dressing is reminiscent of a traditional anti-plague formula from the 1700's. A garlic salad dressing is reminiscent of a traditional anti-plague formula from the 1700's. When the plague struck French cities, criminals waiting execution were sent to bury the bodies of the fallen. The story goes that before going out into the plague-ridden city, the criminals drank a vile concoction of apple cider vinegar and garlic to avoid succumbing to the Black Death. The formula became known as the Four Thieves. The criminals became folk heros, for not only did they bury the dead, they also robbed them, became rich and survived to tell the story. Doctor Christopher enhanced the formula by adding cayenne pepper (Capsicum minimum).

Eating garlic daily does not only prevent bacterial infections but it also decreases one's chances of developing some types of cancer. Studies in China, the Netherlands and U.S. involving more than160,000 people have shown that being a garlic lover can significantly reduce the risk of developing stomach and colon cancer. The researchers suggest it is due to allicin's potent antioxidant effect.

Hand Washing and the Immune System

On the surface of the skin, commensal bacteria wages territorial wars with opportunistic invaders that threaten the integrity of the skin. Without the friendly bacteria fighting off the invaders, our skin would be in a constant inflammatory response struggling with fungal and bacterial infections.

When I worked in a long-term care facility, it seemed like I was washing my hands every ten minutes . We were encouraged to sing a full round of "Michael Row Your Boat a Shore" while washing our hands and were frequently reminded that the friction created by rubbing hands together loosened the infecting germs grip on our skin while running water washed them away.

On any nursing unit, someone is always allergic to soap. In this case, the person is old that soap is not really part of the disinfecting process. "Focus on rubbing your hands together and keeping them under the water," she is advised. The nurse allergic to soap always has the nicest hands on the unit.

Those who were not allergic to soap have dried, red hands. The nurses who regularly used the alcohol based hand sanitizers have deep, raw cracks i their skin that stretch across their hands. The cracks are a breeding ground for infection.

A Post Antibiotic Era?
"The dangers of hubris on human health - the rapid emergence of antimicrobial drug resistance" is about the global heath security emergency that is arising due to emergence of microorganisms that are no longer treatable because of their resistance to virtually all available antimicrobial treatment options. - Dr Keiji Fukuda, WHO Assistant Director General, World Economic Forum's Global Risk Report 2013
There are a number bacteria resisting antibiotic therapy. Resistance to an antibiotic occurs when a bacteria mutates and renders the drug ineffective.

The following are just a two of nasty bacteria developing resistance:
MSRA - Methicillin-resistant Staphylococcus aureus. This is an epidemic infection in some hospitals
In 1999, there were 2 cases of MSRA per 1000 hospital admissions.
In 2005, there were 5.2 cases per 1000 admissions.
In 2006, 893 Canadians contracted a MSRA infection outside of the hospital.
In 2007, the number of cases contracted outside of hospital increased by 50%.
In 2008, 18,650 Americans died of MSRA infections-- more than those who died of AIDS that year.
Can herbal medicine presents some solutions?
In the burn unit at the Wythenshawe Hospital in Manchester, England, an essential oil blend of lemon grass (*Cymbopogon flexuosus*) and geranium (*Pelargonium graveolens)* was diffused into the air in hopes of limiting airborne bacteria, including MSRA. After burning the essential oils for 15 hours, there was an 89% reduction of air born bacteria. After 9 months of diffusing the oils, MSRA infections disappeared and there was a dramatic decrease in other infections. Following the removal of the diffuser, there was an MSRA outbreak.

Our skin has two levels of bacteria and oil for protection. Constant hand washing is a necessity in a care facility. However, one really has to question using a substance like alcohol that kills all bacteria living on the skin. The friendly bacteria dwelling on skin is part of our first line of defence against infection. Oils secreted by the tissue living just under our skin keep it elastic and malleable. The oils hold the skin together. Without them cracks develop. Soap strips oil from skin. Replacing the skin's oils with cheap hand creams is not a solution.

Physiology of Elimination - Letting Go

Floating on the murky surface of the lazy river are lovely, white water lilies. The water lily's petals are not stained with dirt or collapsing under the weight of mud stirred up by the river's slow moving current. The white petals are brilliant in the sun. Even the lily's leaves lying flat on the water's surface are pristine green. The water lily is a perfect example of nature's self-cleaning abilities. The water lily's leaves have a waxy surface that repels water. Most plants are self-cleaning. Other than after a heavy rain or flooding, it is rare to find dirty plants in nature. Like the plants, nature has provided the human body with efficient self-cleaning processes.

Before the study of physiology and anatomy took on a reductionist precision, people were in awe of the body's power

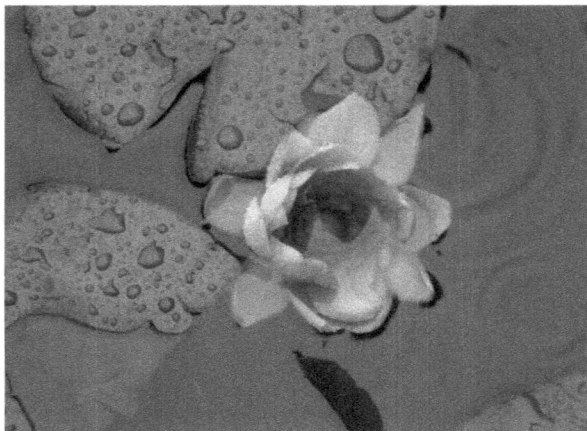

Water lily   Abrah Arneson

to transform one substance into another. The carrot eaten does not leave the body as a carrot. The air on the "in" breath contains more oxygen than the exhalation. A fresh sip of water is expelled as a yellowish liquid with a sour smell if left exposed too long.

Today, modern physiologists can describe these processes to a certain degree. There is all sorts of information on how the kidneys continually monitor and adjust hydrogen ions to regulate the acid/alkaline balance in the body. We know that bacteria in the gut have a similar role in breaking down dead vegetable matter just as it does on the forest floor. The exchange of oxygen and carbon dioxide in the lung's alveoli can be described in a complex diagram of arrows, numbers and letters. But the very essence of the transformation of matter within the body from one substance to another remains a mystery. It is just too complex to be defined through reductionist methods. Unfortunately, because the body transcends reductionist reasoning, it is viewed as suspicious and untrustworthy. This leads to many, many conflicting and subjective points of view, including the belief that the body is dirty.

The reductionist thinker sometimes considers spinach a healthy food containing iron and other minerals. Other times spinach is a food to be avoided, because it contains oxalic acids that interfere with the absorption of iron and can be hard on weak kidneys. Beets in Ayurvedic medicine are considered superior medicine for a congested liver. Western medicine cautions diabetics from eating too many beets because of their high sugar content. (Most diabetics have challenges with liver function, particularly Types II's). The latest demon food is the banana, because of its sugar molecule. But what about the banana's high potassium content that is essential for smooth heart contractions?

It is my experience that the reductionist expert confuses and bewilders to the point that the lay person no longer trusts her own body's power of transformation. Or perhaps it would be more accurate to say that many people no longer notice their body's transformative powers.

When was the last time you had a really good bowel movement and thought, "Wow, I wonder how last night's crispy green salad, yummy sweet potato fries and lemon ginger chicken became that long, brown thing floating in the toilet?"

When body's powers of transformation stall (usually on the elimination side of things) we notice something awry. Unfortunately most people have little experience with interpreting the body's signals and doubt their intuitive understanding of the body.

In clinic, one of the most common questions an herbalist asks a client is: what triggers your condition? "Do you know what aggravates your skin rash?" I might ask. "I am not really sure," is the answer, "but dry weather seems to irritate it." Or, "What makes the cough worse?" "I am not sure, but it is always bad in the summer, when the air conditioning comes on."

Most people have an intuitive understanding that weather, the change of seasons, food consumed and certain times of day affect a health condition. But because people are often trained as reductionist thinkers, these generalized observations are discredited as too simple. Very basic truths about their health are discarded in exchange for something more complex and just beyond understanding. This opens the door for the expert in health matters to come in and tell us what is wrong and how they will fix it.

The remedy to this lack of faith in understanding one's physiological and psychological process is the language of elements. When the processes of elimination fail or become erratic, think in terms of the elements and you will have a language to define the condition and know which plants will help.

In this chapter we will study the elements through the processes of elimination, beginning with the question: What is elimination?

Then we will move on to:

- The Liver: The Stay at Home Mom
- The Earth Element: The Bowel
- The Water Element: The Kidney
- The Air Element: The Lungs
- The Fire Element: The Skin
- The Space Element: The Mind

What is Elimination?

The body is not really a living thing; it is a living process. It is a process in a constant state of change or adaptation. The body/mind is adapting to the weather, the veggie somas you had for lunch, the quality of your sleep the night before, the amount of sunlight you received during the day, the minerals in the water you drink, and on and on and on. Mostly we do not notice the shifts in balance the body makes except when it needs our participation. For example, when the body is hungry it needs you to open the fridge and take out the apple, wash it and eat it.

What is the body adapting to? Perhaps it is helpful to think of adaptation as the process of homeostasis The body is constantly working to achieve the most comfortable state of balance it can in any given moment as you move though different environments , eat lunch, wake to an alarm clock, or express sadness with a friend's parting. The body is continue adjusting and adapting to myriad unseen influences.

It is important to think of balance as an ever-changing state of being. For example, when you are sitting calmly and sipping a cup of tea, your breath is quiet and calm. However, after chasing the garbage man down the street because you slept in and forgot to put the garbage out the night before, your breathing becomes rapid and shallow. Running requires more oxygen so the body turns to chest breathing. Neither breath is the "right" breath. They are both appropriate to the situation the body finds itself in at the moment.

Symptoms of ill health generally manifest when the body/mind is unable to maintain balance. For example, shortness of breath when resting suggests insufficient levels of oxygen in the body. A variety of health challenges can produce this symptom, such as anxiety, asthma, pneumonia, congestive heart failure, lung cancer, etc.

The medical term used to express this balancing principal in health is Homeostasis.

Homeostasis n. The ability or tendency of an organism or cell to maintain internal equilibrium by adjusting its physiological processes.

Elimination processes are essential for maintaining balance. It is usually processes of elimination that we first notice to be out of balance.

But before exploring the process of elimination, what does the body eliminate? The answer is toxins.

What is a Toxin?

According to the Merriam Webster Dictionary a toxin is: a poisonous substance that is a specific product of the metabolic activities of a living organism and is usually very unstable, notably *toxic* when introduced into the tissues, and typically capable of inducing antibody formation.

According to this definition, there are two different types of toxins that bodies need to eliminate. The first are waste products of metabolism such as the free radical. The second types of toxins are bits and pieces of used cell parts and bacteria. These bits and pieces are proteins, and some of these proteins are recycled and used again, such as for the production of hormones. Other bits and pieces the liver dismantles and ships to the kidneys for elimination. Bacterial wastes are flushed through the bowel.

Bodies have eliminated protein through the kidneys, dead bacteria with bowel movements, and carbon dioxide with each exhalation for a very long time. The body can achieve balance through elimination of these toxins without you even thinking about it.

Detoxifying Plants

Plants help clean up toxic land sites. Yellow dock's deep taproot (*Rumex crispus*) pulls heavy metals out of the earth where gas stations or industrial developments stood. Cat tails (*Typha latifolia*) cleans water. Cat tails absorb arsenic, mercury, nitrates and ammonia. Cilantro (*Coriandrum sativum*) limits the absorption of lead into human tissues.

Cruciferous vegetables such as cabbage, kale, and broccoli support detoxifying processes in all the body's cells. They are particularly adept at supporting the removal of carcinogenic toxins from the body. White birch (*Betula spp*) helps the body remove cadmium, a heavy metal absorbed through cigarette smoke and gas fumes.

Today the body is coping with chemicals it has never before known. We are living in a chemical age that requires a new definition for the word toxin. Environmental toxins have become part of our nomenclature. Environmental toxins are found in supermarkets, furniture, water, hair salons, hospitals, and toy boxes--literally everywhere.

Free radicals are toxins that result from metabolic processes. A free radical is an oxygen molecule with an odd number of electrons. Electrons like to travel in pairs. When single, electrons steal from other molecules and oxygen molecules with an unpaired electron prey on the molecules that make up fatty acids responsible for maintaining cell membranes. When there is an abundance of free radicals circulating in the body, cell membranes are harvested for electrons. This weakens them and makes them porous, allowing toxins to pass into cells and disrupt DNA. Cancer may result.

The challenge many modern humans have is they do not understand that they are the environment they live in. Our body/mind is the same environment where fish swim, sunflowers sprout, deer forage, cattle graze and chickens lay eggs. We are all part of this earth and our environment. Just as environmental toxins affect seagulls, maple trees and marine algae, human bodies and minds are also affected. As the rest of nature struggles to understand the nature of these new chemicals, so do our bodies. Nature has little experience with their elimination.

In previous generations, herbalists considered elimination to be of primary importance for health. In today's chemical age it cannot be ignored.

Plant medicine offers tonic herbs to support the body and limit the influence of toxins on the body. Use plants high in flavonoids like rose hips (Roscea spp.) or hawthorn (Crateagus spp) to support the removal of chemical toxins. To support the absorption of flavonoids in the body, add a bit of unpasteurized honey to the medicine. Polyunsaturated fatty acids such as those found in sunflower seeds protect cell membranes from damage by chemical toxins. Sunflower oil also pulls heavy metals from the body. Put a teaspoon of the sunflower in your mouth and hold it under your tongue. When the oil starts to burn, spit it out. Do this several times a day, until the oil no longer burns.

The Spring Cleanse

Consider a time before every home had a refrigerator. Green vegetables were as scarce in January as a robin's song. Salted meat was chewed on through short days and long dark nights. By February the root veggies in the cellar were limp and spongy. Pickled eggs and fish were a treat.

Imagine nibbling the first green fiddlehead spirals and the first tender shoots of nettle and bitter dandelion leaves. Their green |spring-ness" awakened the mind and body from the monotonous white landscape of winter.

The burst of minerals in the mouth, fresh from the moist earth and filled with the promise of warmth, sunlight and summer was the traditional spring cleanse. The spring cleanse unburdened the body of the "phlegm" humour produced by winter's diet heavy in protein and fatty foods. The spring cleanse was a time of both elimination and renewal.

Recall that my friend and Cree elder Corky advises, "Look to the trees to know what to do." Compare the spring cleanse to the tree's

Other Toxins

Today the word *toxin* has even broader meaning than metabolic wastes or chemical poisons. We commonly talk about toxic relationships, toxic emotions, toxic beliefs, toxic jobs, toxic homes and toxic bosses. Some people even talk about toxic politicians. Anything that is not in the best interest of the mind/body is considered toxic. When assessing an individual health plan/protocol, a holistic practitioner needs to be aware of these toxic events and people in their clients' lives.

activity during April. The tree's roots thaw as the sun warms the soil. The sugars and minerals stored in the roots deep under the earth soften; sap is formed and begins to flow up the tree's trunk to the highest branch. The sap delivers minerals from the soil to nourish new green growth.

Today, most think of the spring cleanse as a time to eliminate toxins. They forget that the spring cleanse is about regrowth and renewal. This is erroneous and dangerous in today's toxic landscape. Strengthening the body mind with nutritive cleansing plants is more important than purging the bowels with laxatives and pushing toxins from the tissues with fasting.

Cleansing Tincture

2 part *Articum lappa* (moistens winter's dryness)

2 part *Taraxacum off radix* (cleanses liver)

1 part *Xanthoxylum americanum* (opens circulation)

1 part *Echinacea angustifolia* (removes lymph stagnation)

1 part *Rumex crispus* (opens up the flow of bile)

Dosage: 1 tsp. twice a day for 1 month.

Cleansing Tea

1 part Alfalfa (high in minerals)

1 part Nettles (high in minerals)

1 part Red Clover Flowers (flavonoids)

1 part Mullein leaf (cleansing to lungs)

Dosage: 1 cup three times a day.

Think of a cleanse as a new beginning. A spring cleanse is about learning a new way of being. Every beginning is defined with intention. Intentions are seeds and the seeds planted in the spring determine the harvest in the fall.

To begin a cleanse start with considering these questions from the perspective of your mind, body and spirit: Why do I want to do this cleanse? What is its purpose?

Actions (such as what you eat) are rooted in thoughts. Thoughts are rooted in emotions. Emotions are driven by intentions, both conscious and unconscious. If there are any toxins we really need to concern ourselves with, it is toxic intentions, particularly the ones rooted in greed, hatred and denial. It is important that cleansing is not based on fearful or hateful intentions towards our body/mind or environment. Cleansing needs to be founded on the desire to live a fuller life. Remember, cleansing is not just about releasing toxins; it's about replacing them with nutrients.

The word 'nutrient' is being used broadly here to include everything that nourishes your body, spirit and mind. During a cleanse, it is as important to keep your awareness focused on what nourishes you as it is letting go of toxins.

A Cleansing Meditation
Breathing Rainbows (Somewhere Over the Rainbow)
This meditation cleanses the emotional body and opens up new possibilities.

Breathing in rainbows...have fun with this.
Face the sun; you can be standing or sitting outside, or sitting in a sunny spot inside.

Image the spectrum of light from the sun coming into your body.
Breathe in deeply the colour violet and feel it move through your body.
Then breathe the violet colour out, imagining that it carries away any toxins or unhappiness in a sooty grey shade to the violet.
Repeat with:
Red
Orange
Yellow
Green
Blue
Repeat this entire sequence three times.

The Liver: The Stay at Home Mom

...the Liver official referred to in the classics "the Military Leader who Excels in Strategic Planning." We can see why this minister belongs in the Wood element, as qualities of discipline, focus, structure, and vision that are required for running an army are also needed to make growth possible. - Archetypal Acupuncture, Gary Dolowich

However much I respect Traditional Chinese Medicine, at times the hierarchal and imagery of war used to describe the nature of the body and its functions seem to me to impede our ability to see the body as a peaceful organism seeking to live in harmony with its environment. This is particularly true for the liver.

Dissect the word liver and one finds the word LIVE. Add 'er' to the end of the LIVE and one has liver: someone who lives. There was a time in the middle ages when the liver rivalled the heart as being the home of love and passion in the body. In medical astrology the planet Jupiter is aligned with the liver. Jupiter is the planet of abundance, expansion and good fortune. These ideas of the large organ suggest something very different from a

Maple Syrup

When I lived in Ontario, every Easter we would take t a trip to the maple syrup farms. We would taste fresh sap dripping from taps in the trees right out of the buckets. I remember the taste of minerals tingling on our tongues. We always left with several gallons of syrup to last us for the year.

Maple syrup is high in antioxidants and minerals. I often substitute it for honey in syrups, particularly for small children who cannot take honey. I also encourage a small dollop of it in herbal teas. It is a great addition to any spring cleanse.

general conducting a war. Western descriptions paint the liver as an organ that nourishes life. The liver encourages life to grow to its highest potential.

I suggest a kinder and more nourishing metaphor for the liver: the stay at home mom.

When a woman stays home to look after children, she spends much time in the kitchen. She implements systems to ensure that what needs to be recycled is recycled and what should be thrown out gets thrown out. She knows when the apples bought last week need to be made into apple sauce, which containers of leftovers need to be eaten first and what the expiry date is on the yogurt. The kitchen is the hearth of the home where children are nourished. Under loving care, ,the kitchen is a warm and fragrant place where the sensual delights of nutritious food builds strong bones and blood, smart brains, and gentle souls.

But when the stay at home mom decides to get a full time job, the kitchen can fall into chaos. The recycling piles up, the garbage always needs to be emptied, the leftovers slowly make their way to the back of the fridge where they become forgotten and there always seems to be more yogurt in the fridge than

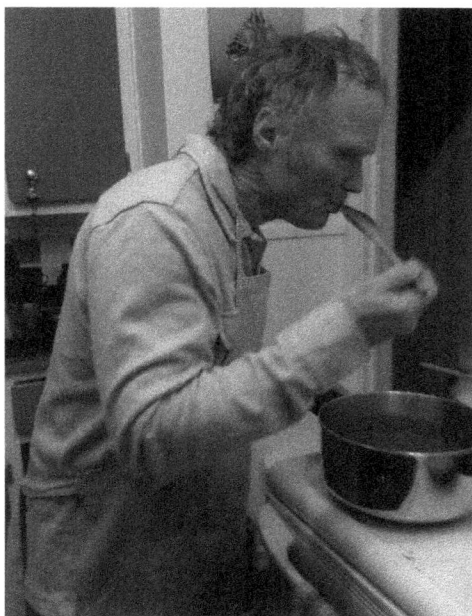

I don't want to appear discriminatory here. Many men are wonderful, nourishing cooks as well as take the garbage out! But I like the metaphor of a mother.

can be eaten in a week. The smooth flow of a nourishing kitchen becomes fragmented as Mom's time becomes burdened with demands beyond the kitchen.

This analogy fits the liver in our day and age. Like the stay at home Mom ,the liver carefully discriminates between what is nourishing to the body, what needs to be recycled, and what is trash. If the liver is burdened with pharmaceutical drugs, alcohol, pesticides, an abundance of hormones, food additives and all the other toxins of modern life, it has little time left to make nutritive substances to feed the body. When the liver is stressed, disharmony within the body and its relationship to the environment prevails.

Like a hurried mom, when the liver's natural flow is disrupted it begins to store wastes to be processed later. Body fat becomes the broom cupboard bursting with plastic bags to be dealt with or the disorganized junk drawer crammed full of twist ties, rubber bands, finishing nails, hard dried up glue, rubber gloves, etc.

Liver Facts

The liver is the largest internal and most metabolically complex organ in humans.

The liver is about 8 inches (20 cm) wide, 6.5 inches (17 cm) long and 4.5 inches (12 cm) thick and weighs approximately 3.5 pounds (1.6 kilograms).

It has two large lobes: a large right lobe and a smaller left lobe.

Your liver is located under your ribs in the upper right part of your abdomen just below your diaphragm.

The liver is the only organ that regenerates itself.

No matter the challenge in the body, whether depression, PMS, constipation, autoimmune disease, arthritis, cancer, etc., the liver's role as the organ that sorts through the recycling and the trash is always needs supports. It is in many ways the primary organ of elimination. The number one herb for this task is the bright and sunny dandelion (Taraxacum officinalis).

The Dandelion: A Plant for our times.

The Cherokee people have a beautiful saying that goes like this:

Each tree, shrub and herb, down to the very grasses and mosses, agreed to furnish a remedy for someone of the diseases named, and each said: I shall appear to help man when he calls upon me in his need. - Herbal Medicine, Healing and Cancer, Donald Yance

I often think of the dandelion as the plant for our times. But let's begin by exploring dandelion's traditional uses.

In western herbalism, the dandelion leaf is classed as a diuretic and dandelion root is offered to improve bile flow through the liver to support cleansing. Generally western herbalists offer the root and leaf separately. In TCM the root and leaf are taken together for cleansing the liver.

Let's begin with a look at pathways of detoxification in the liver.

Detoxification in the human body involves Phase I and Phase II enzymatic reactions that occur in virtually all cells. Phase I reactions change non-polar, water-soluble chemicals into polar, water-soluble compounds. Phase II reactions involve the addition of chemical groups to the toxic intermediates to make them water soluble and thus easily excretable from the body in urine and/or feces. Many of the Phase II enzymes detoxify carcinogenic compounds in the body reducing the susceptibility of cells to these substances. - American Botanical Council: Herb Clips. Phytochemicals in Vegetables Can Assist Detoxification, Brenda Milot, ELS

Although every cell in the body is involved in this detoxification process, the liver is the mother of detoxification, and if she is not happy, nobody is happy. Now let's revisit the humble dandelion.

Research demonstrates dandelion root is very active during Phase 1 detoxification in the liver. In Phase 2 the leaf's medicine is active. Taking the root and leaf together is the most effective support for the body's detoxifying work. Dandelion's ability to enhance the detoxification process conserves the liver's resources. It simply has more time for all its other functions, including formation of antioxidants. Dandelion's quiet support for the liver is one of the reasons it is frequently used in cancer protocols.

Why do I think Dandelion is the plant for our time? Dandelion's bright yellow flowers bloom abundantly every spring. Are the dandelions colonizing our lawns and parks because they are responding to our call for help to relieve illnesses caused by environmental toxins, just as the Cherokee prayer stated? No matter what herbicides we throw at it, it not only survives, but it thrives. Is dandelion trying to tell us something? Listen.

The Earth Element: The Bowel (Also referred to as the Colon)

Earth Element: Stool is strongly associated with the earth element; It is after all one of the main components of soil.

My friend Grant once told me that if you let any group of people roam freely in conversation long enough they eventually share the secrets of their bowels. He claimed this is because bowel movements are one habit shared by all humans. I am not so sure about the truth of this statement but I do know herbalists spend a lot of time talking about bowel movements while gathering essential information about a client's health.

Talking about bowels is not always comfortable for either the herbalist or the client. I find using a professional language to discuss a client's bowels softens any discomfort. Remember that if the client's bowels are not functioning with regularity, he will want to talk about them. You may need to supply the client with a vocabulary to describe their bowel movements accurately.

The Vocabulary of Bowel Movements

Frequency: How often does he go to the bathroom? Get specifics here. People with a history of constipation may consider a bowel movement every three days normal.

Formed stools: Stools do not fall apart in the toilet, have length and are passed easily. These are well-balanced stools.

Loose stools: Stools fall apart in the toilet and are part watery and formed.

Diarrhea: Watery stools with little form if any at all.

Another way of approaching a description of the bowels is to ask about the stools consistency. Are they hard and dry? Soft and wet? Mixed?

Other Useful Descriptions

Colour: The colour of stools tells the herbalist about the body's ability to absorb nutrients and discern how deeply the imbalance has penetrated the body. A healthy stool is golden brown in colour. This colour is caused by the breakdown of bile salts in colon. A healthy liver releases enough bile to facilitate the absorption of fat and stimulate peristalsis.

The traditional system of medicine from the Middle East called Tibb assesses the colour of stools in the following manner:

Whitish stools are caused by a lack of bile secretion from the liver or a blockage in the gallbladder or bile duct. The clients with white stools will have difficulty digesting fats and probably be in pain.

Colon Facts

- The Colon is about 1.5 meters long and 6.5 cm in diameter
- It has five principal sections: the ascending colon, transverse colon, descending colon, sigmoid, colon and anal canal which includes the rectum
- Chyme (the processed food stuff from the small intestine) moves into the colon through the ileosecal valve
- The appendix (a lymph organ) is just below the ileosecal valve
- The colon is divided into pouches called haustra by circular muscles
- It is lined with bacteria and a mucosa

Very red stools indicate the imbalance has reached its peak. Red stools are associated with a healing crisis. Note that eating beets also causes red stools.

Black stools as we previously learned are associated with internal bleeding. In traditional medicine, black stools were considered a grave sign of excessive black bile humour and impeding death. In either case, if a client reports black sticky stools, consider it a medical emergency.

Green stools suggest heat deficiency in the digestive tract.

Intensely yellow stools are classed according to when they occur in the disease process. At the beginning of a disease yellow stools are a good sign. Tibb herbalists say an excess of yellow bile humour causes the bright yellow stools. Recall the yellow bile humour is related to the fire element. The fire element is acutely active during the early stages of infection. The stools' yellow colour is a result of the extra work the liver does during infection when processing wastes created by the immune system's battle with the pathogen. The wastes are eliminated through bile.

When bright yellow stools occur during chronic illness, they suggest the imbalance is resolving itself. Chronic disease wears out the body's defence mechanisms and creates coldness. The return of heat to the alimentary tract and increased bile from the liver is a sign the body is regaining its ability to fight.

Multi-coloured stools with pus signal a deeply penetrating illness and damage to internal organs.

Urgency: The bowel movement comes on quickly.

Odour: Healthy stools have a mild smell unless left exposed to air for a period of time. If stools have an unpleasant smell, this suggests infection or fermentation.

Mucous: Mucous in the stool is caused by irritation on the bowel's lining. Mucous soothes and protects abrasions on the

Physiological Facts about the Colon
Chyme moves from haustra to haustra as the pouches fill up and pressure is experienced on its walls. This moves the chyme from pouch to pouch.

Approximately every 8 hours a grand movement of peristalsis pushes the chyme against the wall of the rectum. This becomes a conscious sign that a bowel movement is imminent.

Absorption continues in the large intestine (this is the balancing principal at work).

Of the ½ litre to 1 litre of water that enters the colon, all is absorbed but 100 to 200 milliliters

Electrolytes, primarily sodium and chloride are absorbed

Vitamins K and biotin are the principal vitamins absorbed in the large intestine due to interactions with bacteria

Some water-soluble vitamins are also absorbed

Carbohydrates are further synthesized and absorbed as fatty acids

Once bulked up through loss of water,chyme becomes feces

Feces consist of:
- Water
- Slough of cells from the GI tract
- Bacteria and dead bacteria parts

bowel wall. .

Blood: I am always surprised at clients who do not initially divulge blood in their stools. This is an important symptom that suggests a serious underlying condition. There are three basic appearances of blood in the stool:

- When blood is on the surface of the stool, there is bleeding in the rectum. Hemorrhoids frequently cause this.
- Blood mixed in with the stool suggests bleeding in the colon. This type of bleeding is often caused by inflammatory bowel disease, as well as bowel cancer.
- The stool resembles sticky, black tar. In this case there is bleeding higher in the alimentary tract, possibly an ulcer within the alimentary canal, liver disease or internal bleeding.

Pain: Abdominal pain is one of the most frequent concerns an herbalist sees. Ask the seven essential questions needed to understand the pain:

Castor Oil Packs clear toxins from the bowel as well as initiate bowel movements. They are a gentle relaxing way to encourage sluggish bowels.

How to do a Castor Oil Pack:

On a piece of flannel or a cotton dish towel, pour castor oil until it is soaked into the cloth.

Fill a hot water bottle with hot water or heat up a barley bag. Place the cloth soaked in castor oil over your abdomen and cover with a plastic bag. Place the hot water bottle over the plastic bag and relax for 20 minutes.

When you are finished, fold the flannel and place it in a plastic bag, store in a cool place, and reuse next time.

Repeat this for three days, take a rest for two days and then do it again for three more days.

- Timing of the pain. When does it occur?
- History of pain. When did it start?
- Description of the pain. How does it feel?
- Quantity of the pain. On a scale of 1-10 (10 being you are ready to die to relieve the pain) how do you rate the pain?
- Aggravating factors. What makes it worse?
- Relieving factors. What makes it better?
- Associated symptoms. Are there any other symptoms that accompany the pain, such as blood in the stools?

Undigested food: Undigested food suggests a problem within the stomach and small intestine.

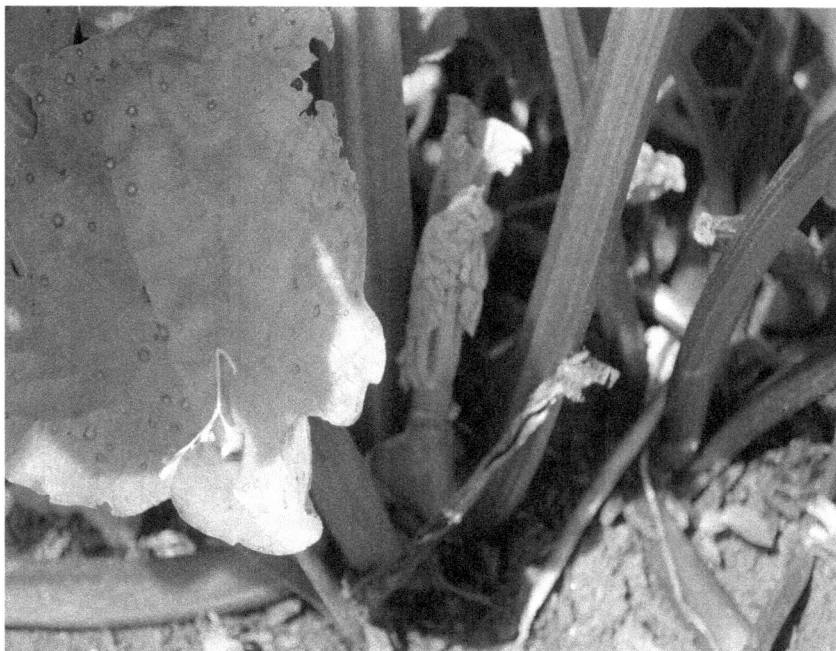

Rhubarb   Mark Arneson

Herbs for Healthy Bowel Movements

Form of stool	Description	Appropriate herb
Loose	Formed bits that fall apart easily Check for food allergies and sensitivities.	Herbs containing tannins: aAgrimony, blackberry leaf, meadowsweet Herbs with mucilage: marshmallow, slippery elm
Constipation	Hard, small stools Explore diet for amount of fruits and veggies as well as water: diuretic intake.	Mild laxatives: yellow dock, turkey rhubarb Chologogues oregon grape root, wild yam
Constipation	Formed stools every few days Check to see how much they are eating and beliefs around food.	Mild laxatives: Turkey rhubarb, licorice
Alternating stools	Some days stools are loose and others they are constipated. Explore their mood and its relationship to their bowels as well as food sensitivities and allergies.	Herbs containing both tannins and anthraquinones such as yellow dock Carminatives to calm the nervous system in the gut: peppermint or lemon balm.

Note about laxatives: The plant constituents in most herbal and pharmaceutical laxatives are anthraquinones. such as: aloe-emodin, sennosides, and cascarosides. These plant constituents irritate the bowel's lining, forcing peristalsis. A plant that irritates the body and provokes activity from any organ is classed as a stimulating herb. Laxatives are stimulating herbs.

Anthroquinones taunt the bowel. The bowel's gut reaction is to expel the irritant as quickly as possible. Painful cramping ensues. Plants containing anthraquinones are often paired with carminative herbs to ease cramping.

A skillful herbalist avoids using anthroquinones to relieve constipation. Regular use of anthroquinones causes the bowel to become desensitized to endogenous stimulation of peristalsis. The bowel develops dependency on anthroquione's harsh commands. I frequently witnessed laxative dependency when I worked in a long-term care facility. The pain associated with this form of over medication determined how I work with laxatives in my practice.

I have never had to use the stronger laxative plants such as senna (Senna alexandria) and cascara (Rhamnus purshiana). My first choice for a laxative herb is yellow dock (Rumex crispus) and if the constipation is stubborn I use turkey rhubarb (Rhuem palamata). I strongly encourage clients struggling with constipation (and there are many) to eat an apple a day, go for a good walk, drink water and take ground flax seeds. It is always better to teach a client simple ways to keep bowels regular than to use harsh, purging laxatives.

When a child is chronically constipated, I recommend apple crisp made with rhubarb for breakfast. This breakfast will regulate the bowels.

The Colon and The Lungs

TCM pairs organs as a husband and wife. Each pair complements the action of each other. The colon is paired with the lung. TCM physiology describes the lungs as grasping what the body needs: air. The colon lets go of what is no longer needed: soil. In other words, the two reflect how we hold onto what we need and how we let go of what no longer has value.

It is my experience in clinic that there is generally a relationship between the health of colon and the respiratory tract. It is rare that I see someone who has chronic issues with their sinuses and does not struggle with constipation.

I have never worked with an individual who did not suffer with both asthma and irregular stools. Asthma's primary symptom is a wheeze caused by narrowing bronchi trapping spent air in the lungs. When stale air cannot get out, fresh air cannot get in. The bowel of an asthmatic tends to be loose. In TCM one would say the bowel compensates for the lungs inability to let go and release what is exhausted.

Asthma Protocol
Tincture of:

Glyzzhiriza glabra	resolves inflammation, heals to damage mucous membranes
Astragulus membranous	moderates the immune system, mucous membrane tonic
Curcuma longa	Resolves inflammation
Schizandra chinosis	A liver and lung tonic.
Lobelia inflata	relaxes the bronchi

Tea of:

Nettles	Anti-histamine effect
Hyssop	Relaxes the bronchi as well as helps move mucous from the bronchi
Mullein	Anti-histamine effect as well as helps move mucous from the bronchi
Peppermint	Carminative effect

The real concern for the asthmatic is being able to get a breath, or in other words, grab hold of fresh air and let fresh air into her life.

In TCM, liver and bowel herbs are used to relieve asthma. I find a blend of TCM and Western herbal practices most effective in relieving frightening asthma attacks. I also recommend significant dietary changes to heal the bowel.

The Golden Rule

Be aware of the golden rule when treating inflammatory conditions. (Asthma is an inflammatory response.) No matter whether the condition is asthma, fibromyalgia, or bloating, if is there is either a substance being taken in or in the surrounding environment that is triggering the immune response, the condition will not resolve until the irritant is removed.

Cleanse as much as one wants, but if the aggravating factor is continually introduced, the cleanse will simply deplete the body's resources and cause a deeper illness.

The Water Element: The Kidney

Water Element

Whenever we treat a disease, we must approach it at the base. Base here means root or source. Every stream on earth has a source, and every plant has a root. If all murky sediments settle at the source, the downstream waters will naturally be clear and fresh, and if we water a root, it will grow and branches will sprout; these are the laws of nature. The experienced physician, therefore, will always consider the source. - From Li Zhongzi, A Primer of Medical Objectives (Yizong Bidu), 1637

Jing

Traditional Chinese Medicine teaches that the kidney houses jing. Jing is defined as congenital chi or the life essence we inherit from our parents. Sometime jing is called the body's original water. Your jing's strength is measured by your ability to choose your response to life's blessings and challenges. Jing is your capacity to pause and consider your reactions to life's circumstance. In the West, jing is equated with will power.

In the West will power is defined as the ability to withstand outside forces or impose your will on others. Consider Nike's formula for a good life: get out there and "just do it". Nike promotes a will that is forceful, active, competitive and hot and yang in nature. The athletic shoe company's recommendation lacks the thoughtfulness and careful timing of a will power influenced by the energy of yin.

Taoists (eastern mystics) have a more yin view of will power. Eastern philosophy considers will power to be the ability to control your mind. Taoists train their body-mind to choose harmonious, peaceful thoughts and emotions. The power of your jing or will is used to calm thoughts that lead to discord and strife. Disharmonious thinking and emotions are called ill will. Thinking harmful thought, whether directed at yourself or others, is a symptom of a will that is ill. Or more simply put, ill will is a weakness in will power and low functioning jing.

TCM teaches jing is the original source of yin. Let's do a quick review of the concept of yin.

Yin is essentially the receptive side of life. Yin is the ability to receive and be in the moment. Its qualities are cool and moist. The moon and the quality of darkness are yin in nature.

Water is the element associated with jing. Water is able to take the shape of any container. For the most part, water flows harmoniously through landscapes carrying moisture and nutrients to plants, animals and humans.

Each element interacts with all life in an indiscriminate manner. Water quenches thirst whether you are a saint or a mass murder. Altruistic actions, like water, are able quench the human thirst for meaning. The ultimate expression of the will is altruism: the desire to create happiness for others. Understanding that your own personal happiness is dependent on the happiness of others carries power to your will and heals ill will.

To express this truth, first be still, quiet and open and rest in the energy of yin. Only in a calm, easeful state of mind can you drink deeply from the well of wisdom: the understanding of interdependence of life.

In TCM the kidney's essence is quality of yin that contains yang. When your actions are created by a mind endowed with calm surrender, the kidney's yin and yang are in balance. Your actions are contained in the reserved thoughtfulness of yin.

The adrenal junkie who Nike ads appeal to does not act from within a state of yin. Their adrenal glands (which sit directly on the top of the kidneys) are too hot for them to rest and receive life. These people require yin tonics. Yin tonics are sweet and cooling plants. The roots of solomon's seal (Polygonum multifolium) are a yin tonic. It cools heat throughout the body and moistens dry hot tissues. Solomon's seal is used for any part of the body that is dry from heat. It moistens cracking joints and creaking ligaments. It soothes hot digestive tracts and lungs. Chinese herbalists use solomon's seal specific to nourish deficient kidney yin.

The other extreme is yin without yang. Too much yin is cooling and the water element freezes. When the water element freezes life is governed by fear. TCM teaches the emotion associated with the kidney is fear.

A Case History of Fear Creating Illness

Susan's job is making her sick. By the end of every workweek, Susan suffers with debilitating headaches. She spends the weekends recovering. Her friends are abandoning her because they can no longer tolerate her constant bitter and angry whining about her job and how it is making her sick. Unfortunately Susan worries leaving her job will lead to a loss of income. She is committed to her current lifestyle even though it is meagre due to her poor physical and mental health. She believes loss of income will be too difficult for her to cope with. The fear of loss has frozen Susan in place. As she becomes sicker, she has less energy (will power) to seek better

Sick Building Syndrome (SBS)

SBS occurs with when there is poor or little air ventilation in a building. This is often the case with the closed air systems that are commonly used in office type workplaces. Sufferers of SBS will note that symptoms are at their worst when either the air conditioning or the central heating comes on. Unable to open windows, stale air is continually recirculated and if it carries toxins such as molds, off gassing building materials or organic volatile chemicals such as those found in industrial (industrial what??), those breathing the air become sick.

SBS cause a wide range of symptoms:

* Headaches
* Muscle aches
* Depression
* Foggy thinking
* Ringing in the ears
* Runny nose and eyes
* Skin rashes
* Unpleasant taste and smell sensations

Herbal medicine can be used to rebuild the body after exposure to a sick building, but the real cure is a change in workplace.

employment and her life force wastes away. Her thoughts spin endlessly around in her mind alternating between blaming others for her misfortune and wondering what she did to deserve such a fate. It is a sad, tragic story.

This is a common condition seen in the herbalist clinic. The will to change for the better is weak due to life circumstances and poor mental and physical health. When jing is weak there is little acknowledgement of self-responsibility and an impoverished understanding that one's own personal happiness is dependent on the happiness of others. It requires great patience to heal from this desperate situation.

Susan needs to strengthen the kidneys while cleansing her fears. Many fears are tangled up in the past. Unfortunately we tend to project unhappy moments from the past into our futures and recreate fearful events again and again and again.

Relaxing and Stimulating Diuretics

Most cleansing herbs, laxative, expectorants and diuretics can be classed as relaxing (yin) or stimulating (yang) in their effect. Demulcents are yin in nature. They soothe, moisten and nourish. Plants like marshmallow and solomon's seal are relaxing diuretics.

Stimulating diuretics are plants that carry the strong scent of volatile oils or resins. Plants with volatile oils are irritating to the kidneys and carry anti-microbial actions. Energetically these plants are hot and dry. They are yang in nature.

Cornsilk (*Zea mays)* is a relaxing diuretic. When reading a plant's medicine there is a number of ways to discern whether a plant is predominately yin or yang. To class a plant as yin or yang consider the plants preferred landscape, appearance, texture and taste.

Cornsilk's yin signatures:

- Flowers are yin in nature. Cornsilk is the corn flower's long stamens.

- Swaying, drooping flowers are particularly yin in nature. Cornsilk does both.
- Plants containing yin medicine are soft and silky to the touch. Corn silk is soft and silky.
- A mild sweet flavour is characteristic of yin medicine. Corn silk tea has almost no taste.
- Yin plants act as demulcents, soothing and moistening irritated tissues. Corn silk is a demulcent specific to urinary tract.
- Drinking corn silk tea helps the kidneys return to a yin state.

A Case History using Corn Silk

Lisa was 7 months pregnant when she developed intolerable heartburn and a burning sensation in the bladder. The doctor tested Lisa for a urinary tract infection. The test came back negative. In my interview with Lisa I learned that there was considerable tension in Lisa's household because of her husband's desire to move across the country. Lisa did not want to move.

Lisa had two boys, both school age, and when she learned she was pregnant again, she had to put plans to return to school on hold. She felt being pregnant again was like having her future denied. At seven months, she had made peace with her pregnancy but was still struggling with the idea of a

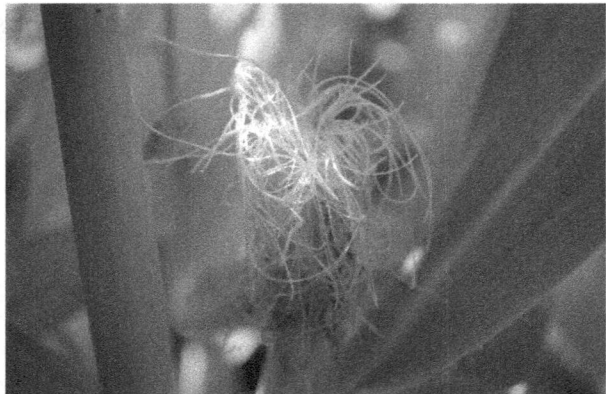

Corn silk   Mark Arneson

major move. She was insecure about of leaving everything familiar. The heartburn and bladder irritation were making matters worse as she was getting very little sleep.

I offered Lisa the following tea:

1 part lemon balm Cools both the heat in the stomach and mind.

1 part corn silk   To calm the irritation, spasms and burning in the bladder

I asked Lisa to drink 3 cups a day. Within a day or two, both the heartburn and the burning sensation in her bladder resolved. Lisa continued to drink the tea throughout her pregnancy and had no further heartburn or bladder irritation.

To help Lisa make the transition into a mother of three children and through a move, I offered her Bach's walnut flower essence. Her little girl is now three. Lisa has made many new friends in her new home and has returned to school.

Juniper Berry (*Juniperus spp.*) is a stimulating diuretic.

Juniper, particularly the prickly version of this coniferous shrub, is considered to be a female plant in Cheyenne medicine. The Cheyenne people compare juniper's prickly nature with a woman who is pissed off.

From a Taoist point of view, juniper is a yin in nature, although not as yin as cornsilk. The following are juniper's yin characteristics:

- Yin plants like to stay close to the ground. Juniper is low growing with drooping branches.
- Cool colours signify yin. Juniper's boughs are dull green and its berries are blue.
- Juniper also has the following yang characteristics:
- Sunny hot, dry landscapes are yang. Juniper prefers dry soil, and lots of sun.
- Pungent tastes are characteristic of yang. Juniper's berries have a pungent taste due to their high

volatile oil content. Juniper's volatile oils have a diuretic effect on the kidneys because they aggravate the kidney's delicate nephrons. When aggravated, the kidneys react by trying to expel the irritant. This increases urination.

- Yang carries the energy of warming and drying. Juniper berry's pungent taste is warm and drying.

The juniper plant is similar to the kidney: it is a yin-containing yang. The plant itself is yin in nature, while the medicine contained in the plant is yang.

Juniper berries are offered during persistent urinary tract infections with thick and cloudy urine that passes painfully in small amounts. These are the symptoms of a boggy urinary tract. The urinary tract is damp and sluggish. Juniper berries warm the tissue and dry up the excess moisture. One could say the yang quality of juniper berry restores balance when yin has overwhelmed yang within the kidney.

From a physiomedical viewpoint, juniper's volatile oils are able to penetrate the cell membranes of infecting organisms and disrupt their replication. The irritating effect of volatile oils

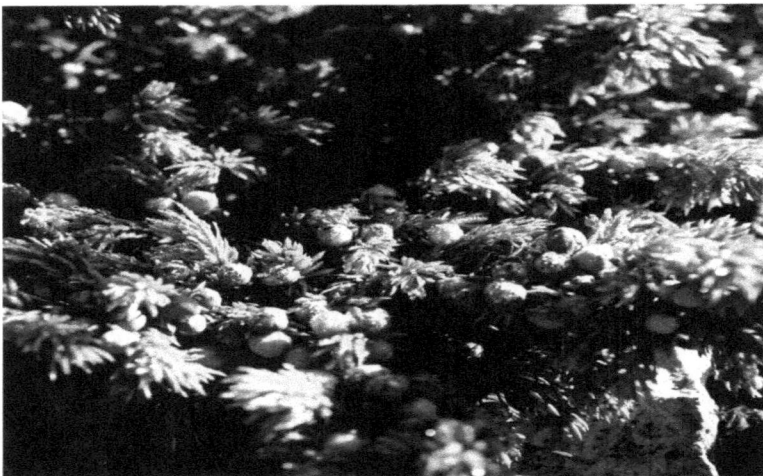

Juniper   Mark Arneson

on the nephrons attracts more white blood cells to the urinary tract, invigorating the battle with the pathogen.

Please note that the irritating effect of juniper berries on the kidneys make it contra-indicted in kidney disease and pregnancy.

Breathing: The Air Element

And the Lord God formed man of the dust of the ground, and breathed into his nostrils the breath of life; and man became a living soul. Gen. ii, 7

spirit (n.) mid-13c., "animating or vital principle in man and animals," from Anglo-French spirit, Old French espirit "spirit, soul" (12c., Modern French esprit) and directly from Latin spiritus "a breathing (respiration, and of the wind), breath; breath of a god," hence "inspiration; breath of life," hence "life;" Meaning "supernatural immaterial creature; angel, demon; an apparition, invisible corporeal being of an airy nature" is attested from mid-14c.; from late 14c. as "a ghost". www.etymonline.com/index.php

Clearing the Air

It was a difficult summer. The bears were hungry and on the prowl. Waking to bright daylight at 5 am, most mornings we'd find a bear sprawled across the cabin's front window. The hairy beast gnawed on the wooden bear bars nailed to the window frames intended to keep him out. It was the rainiest summer in the memory of most Yukoners and the mosquitoes were as thick as molasses. Mark and I longed for the cold, quiet days of winter when the bears slept and the incessant buzzing was silent.

When a couple from the small Dene village that was about an hour and a half hike from our cabin asked if we would like to house sit for a couple weeks, we welcomed the opportunity.

During the first few hours in the house, we thoroughly enjoyed the electricity, indoor plumbing and a real stove. (I made a turkey supper on that very first day.) For almost a year we had lived without these luxuries. Mostly we were relieved to be away from the bears. Our contentment was short lived.

At 2:45am, Mark and I both sat bolt upright in bed, a chill creeping across our skin, our hearts pounding. The next day, walking down the hall toward the bathroom, a breeze prickled my skin and suddenly I felt ice cold. A couple of steps further, heat licked my skin and every hair on my body stood upright. Turning quickly, out of the corner of my eye, I saw blood running down the wall. When I looked again it was gone. We had traded bears for ghosts. The tiny house was haunted.

Undaunted, Mark and I hiked back to the meadow where our cabin sat calm and quiet and picked a large bundle of sage (Artemesia frigida). Back in the small house, we tied the sage into bundles and hung them throughout the house. Then we prayed that the spirits lingering there find happiness and contentment.

For three days we preformed these rituals. Each morning we replaced the bundles of sage. As we gathered sage bundles from the many corners of the house, it was easy to feel the dark energies the soft leaves had pulled from the air. Before replacing the bundles, we tossed the spent ones in the river running alongside the small village. We asked the river to wash away any unhappiness the sage had absorbed.

On the forth night we slept straight through. As we continued our rituals of hanging sage and performing prayers the house became calmer. The erratic temperatures evened out and a sense of peace entered the house. At the end of two weeks, the owners of the house returned and we returned to the meadow with a sense of accomplishment.

Plants have a long history of cleaning the air. Here are just a few:

- Members of the sage family were laid on the floor in sick rooms to clean the air.
- In medieval Europe, posies made with lavender, rose and rosemary were carried to purify the air one walked through. It was hoped that the sweet scents offered protection from the plague. (It did not always work as the pathogen was carried in fleas and was not an airborne bacterium.)
- First Nations peoples burn a number of plants: cedar, sweet grass, sage and juniper, to cleanse both the spiritual and physical realms of disturbance. This plant ritual is called smudging.
- In TCM mugwort (Artemesia vulgaris) is burned over areas of disease in the body to improve the movement of chi. This type of treatment is called moxibustion and can be used in place of acupuncture needles.
- Many workplaces grow plants indoors to remove toxins and increase oxygen levels in stale air. Nasa has compiled a list of 10 plants that remove toxins such as formaldehyde, benzene and ammonia from the air. See: http://en.wikipedia.org/wiki.NASA_Clean_Air_Study

Breathing

My lungs have had a hard time in this life. I recklessly started smoking cigarettes when I was 15. At 24, I became deathly ill with a malarial parasite. The parasite ravaged my lungs. My heroic doctor (and I mean that in the positive sense) used a metaphor of bubble gum to describe them, saying "They are stuck together just like bubble gum after blowing a bubble too big".

I spent six weeks with a tube in my trachea and a machine pushing air into my lungs. A tube in each side of my chest drained fluid from my pleura. Strange as it may seem, when I realized that I was breathing through a machine, my first thought was I would never be able to meditate on my breath again.

While breathing through the machine, I longed for the sweet bliss of riding the breath to the still pool where calm and clarity pervades the mind and the breath becomes a fine silk thread weaving me into life. The machine's hissing and sighing was crude compared to the soft, subtle featherlike breath of bliss.

Two years before I became ill, I had done my first mediation retreat. I remember one day after meditating watching my teacher, Cecilie, clean paint from a brush in a bucket of water. Clear water from a hose ran over the red paint, washing it from the brush. At first I could see the water separate from the paint. The paint swirled in the water like red ribbons. Slowly the paint and water merged, blending, and water became pink. "It is like the breath and the mind," Cecilie said giving me a generous smile. Being in a quiet state of mind, I said nothing and just watched.

In traditional forms of meditation, the breath reflects the emotional body and weaves the mind and the body together. Many meditative traditions use the breath to cleanse the body, emotions and mind.

Let's look at some ways the breath cleanses the body.

Deep breathing improves lymphatic drainage.

Lymph, containing metabolic toxins and inflammation's debris, flows up hill in the body to drain into the circulatory system through two ducts at the base of the neck, the thoracic duct and the right lymphatic duct. Once back in circulation, lymph is filtered by the liver and kidneys where toxins are processed for elimination.

This is a tricky feat for the lymph. Unlike the circulatory system, the lymphatic system has no pump and is reliant on the movement of muscles to flow. Particularly important are the chest muscles and the diaphragm that expand and contract with deep breathing. Deep breathing enhances lymphatic drainage.

Deep breathing stimulates the parasympathetic system.

As the diaphragm rises and falls with each breath, the vagus nerve is massaged. Recall that the bitter taste triggers the vagus nerve which prepares the digestive system to receive the goodness of a home cooked meal. Remember the phrase "rest and digest." Stimulation of the vagus nerve triggers the release

Respiratory System Facts :A Tree in the Body
The Trunk:
Nose connects to pharynx
Pharynx connects to larynx
Larynx connects to trachea
The Branches
Trachea connects to bronchus (2 branches)
The bronchus connects to further bronchus
The bronchus connects to bronchioles
The leaves
The bronchioles connecs to the alveoli
Physiology
Air is breathed in through the nose (lined with hairs) and swirls around in the sinus (warm and moist). In the sinus thre mucous membrane begins. The air travels in a spiral to the bronchus where the muco-cilary escalatory ripples inhaled particles up into the trachea to trigger cough reflex or swallowed. Cleaned air travels through bronchus to alveoli where the oxygen is exchanged for carbon dioxide.

of a neurotransmitter called acetylcholine. This calming neurotransmitter turns off the stress response and relaxes the heart, the larynx and trachea, the stomach, liver and kidneys, and the small and large intestines.

Acetylcholine does not only affect our physiology; it also affects our psychology. Acetylcholine increases attention, focus and memory. Low levels of acetylcholine are linked with depression.

In a study of several depressed patients on a psychiatric ward, 45 adults were assigned to three groups. The first group was given only SKY (a yogic deep breathing technique) breath training and no medication. The second group was given 150 mg/day of an antidepressant, imipranine. The third group was treated three times a week with unipolar electroshock therapy. At the end of four weeks, the patients were retested, using the Hamilton Depression Scale and the Depression Inventory. The group given SKY breath training showed as much improvement in their depression scores as the group given imipramine. Sky and imipramine groups did almost as well as the electroshock group.
- How to Use Herbs, Nutrients and Yoga in Mental Health Care, Richard Brown MD, Patricia Gerbarg MD, Philip Muskin MD. pg 60

Deep breathing increases the release of carbon dioxide.

Stress is oxygen hungry. Stressful thoughts trigger chest breathing to supply the increase demand in oxygen. Chest breathing is short shallow breaths gulping oxygen and limiting carbon dioxides elimination. Chronic chest breathing results in high blood levels of carbon dioxide. Here are just a few symptoms of moderately high blood levels of carbon dioxide.

Headache	Dimming of eyesight
Blue fingers	Swollen ankles

Difficulty hearing	Increase heart rate and blood pressure
Flushing	Confusion
Drowsiness	Muscle tremors

If the CO2 level are really high, death

Deep breathing enhances the elimination of carbon dioxide.

Two herbs that open up airways

Hyssop (Hyssopus officinalis)

Then shall the priest command to take for him that is to be cleansed two birds alive and clean, and cedar wood, and scarlet, and hyssop: And the priest shall command that one of the birds be killed in an earthen vessel over running water: As for the living bird, he shall take it, and the cedar wood, and the scarlet, and the hyssop, and shall dip them and the living bird in the blood of the bird that was killed over the running water: And he shall sprinkle upon him that is to be cleansed from the leprosy seven times, and shall pronounce him clean, and shall let the living bird loose into the open field. (Leviticus 14:4-7 KJV)

...recent analysis has found that the mold that produces penicillin grows on the leaves of Hyssopus officinalis. So when lepers were forced to cleanse themselves ritualistically with hyssops before being

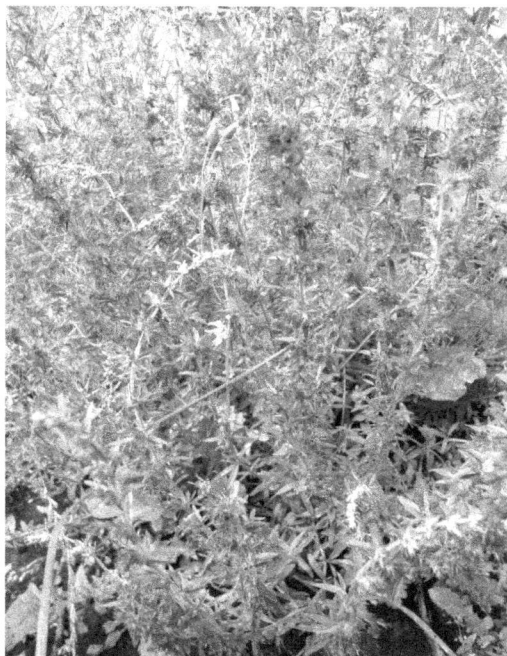

Hyssops   Abrah Arneson

allowed contact with their healthier kin, compassionate Nature provided a very suitable protection for parents and relatives, a powerful antibiotic. - The Book of Herbs by Dorothy Hall pg 127

It is not surprising hyssops was historically used against a leprosy's air bourn bacteria. Although I have never had a case of leprosy in the clinic, I frequently recommend hyssop either as a tea or tincture to open up the respiratory passages while killing off infecting pathogens. Hyssop tea also makes breathing easier for those struggling with asthma, bronchitis or congestive heart failure.

Hyssop is easy to grow in the garden. It enjoys the sun and is not too fussy about water. In the garden it has done well during rainy and dry summers. Hyssop's medicine is made up of volatile oils. During dry summer days, hyssop concentrates its volatile oils. Tasting a leaf during hot summer days leaves an intense pungent tingle on your tongue. Rain dilutes hyssop's volatile oils. If you are growing and making your medicine, it is best always to harvest your plants after a few days of dry, hot weather.

I only occasionally take advantage of Hyssop's secondary anti-microbial action particularly when I suspect parasites.

Lobelia *(Lobelia inflata)* is the number one herb to open airways and was the darling of the venerable American herbalist Doctor Christopher.

The following is one of his stories of using lobelia to cure asthma.

One night...I heard a knock at the door. There stood two young fellows carrying a wizened little gentleman between them. They asked, "Can you help Dad? We can't reach his regular doctor, who has cared for him all these years, and he needs help."
We brought him in and gave him a cup of peppermint tea. He had to sit up, because he had not been able to lie in bed for over twenty years. He had suffered severe asthma attacks for twenty-

six years, and for twenty of those years had been propped up at night and could sleep for only short spells of thirty minutes or so. He has been under heavy medication during all that time, with no hope of ever getting well. After the peppermint tea had been down for fifteen minutes or so, I gave him a teaspoonful of tincture of lobelia, followed ten minutes later with a second teaspoonful. He started to throw up phlegm from his lungs. During this time the emetic principal was working and bringing up phlegm from his lungs and bronchial cavities, he ejected over a cupful of varicolored materials, ranging from light to dark, plus other liquids. At five o'clock, we released him, and the boys took him home. Two days later, I heard the results. Instead of being propped up as usual in the chair, he said to his boys, "I'm going to lie in a bed; I can sleep tonight." For the first time in twenty years, he slept the full night in bed, and he has slept in a bed from that day on. - School of Natural Healing, Dr. John R. Christopher pg 401.

Lobelia has a complex chemistry made up of at least 14 alkaloids with divergent actions in the body. Some stimulate the central nervous system while others relax it. Whatever its contradictory chemistry indicates, lobelia relaxes spasms and is a traditional remedy for easing bronchial spasms associated with asthma. Lobelia is useful whenever the breath needs to deepen, as in congestive heart failure and chronic anxiety.

Lobelia relaxes skeletal muscles releasing tension held in the shoulders and neck. Shoulder and neck muscles are over used in chest breathing. A little lobelia eases tension from the shoulders and allows the rib cage to open and lift, deepening the breath. In a tincture formulated to encourage deep breathing I add 10mls of lobelia for every 100mls of herbs.

Lobelia's other common name is Indian Tobacco. This name refers to the First Nations practice of smoking dried lobelia mixed with mullein (mullein supplies

Puke Weed
Lobelia's alkaloids have an acrid taste that triggers the gag reflex and induces vomiting. Lobelia is such a potent emetic that it's common name is "puke weed." In high doses, Lobelia is guaranteed to induce vomiting.

the nitrogen that helps the other herbs burn) and perhaps some wild mint. Just like a tincture, lobelia's smoke opens the bronchial passages. Smoking lobelia helps to cough up phlegm. Susan Weed says smoking lobelia brings clarity to the mind.

The Cough

Coughing is the body's way of protecting the lungs from irritants in the air. Coughing clears liquids and food that find their way into the trachea as opposed to the esophagus. A cough also removes debris from chest infections: cold, bronchitis, and pneumonia. Lingering coughs can be one of the initial signs a serious illness is brewing in the respiratory passages like cancer. A cough can be a nervous response to an uncomfortable experience.

The problem with the cough: an explosion of air traveling 100 miles per hours from your chest out your mouth ranges from awkward to unbearable in its expression. Coughing intrudes upon our sense of politeness. A cough can be extremely painful. Coughing can keep you and your bed partner up all night. Coughs are messy and gooey.

For many people there is a strong desire to suppress a cough. A smart herbalist knows the cough is a cleansing mechanism the body uses and may need to be encouraged but also knows when a cough needs to be quieted down. A smart herbalist asks the following questions:

Does this cough need to be suppressed?

When a cough is interrupting sleep and the client is exhausted, an anti-spasmodic herb to calm the cough is a good idea. Sleep is deeply healing. I use valerian (Valeriana officinalis) to suppress coughs because I always have it in the apothecary. (I tend to keep herbs with many different applications on hand and valerian is one of them.) Usually 10 drops 20 minutes before bed will quiet down a cough.

Wild Cherry Bark (Prunus serotina) is another commonly used cough suppressant. Many herbalists make syrup of wild cherry bark and offer it to clients who need peace from a hacking cough in the night.

Is the cough effective?

A productive cough produces mucous. Mucous is the vehicle on which germs and debris from the infection are removed from the respiratory tract. When a cough is effective, it is shorter in duration and less harsh.

A skilled herbalist offers herbs to increase a cough's effectiveness. He does this by using a class of herbs called

Understanding Mucous

Yellow or green mucous is a sign of a bacterial infection. The greener the mucous, the more intense the battle the body is waging against the infecting organism.

Rust coloured or brownish flecks in mucous suggested the mucous membranes are several irrated and are bleeding a small amount. If the mucous is similar in colour and texture to prune juice, there is a severe bleed somewhere and should be treated as a medical emergency.

Mucous with air bubbles in it suggests fluid is accumulating in the lungs and often accompanies advanced heart disease.

Asthma produces a clear mucous with a ropey texture.

expectorants. Like laxatives and diuretics there are two classes of expectorants: stimulating expectorants and relaxing expectorants.

Stimulating Expectorants

Stimulating expectorants are also called warming expectorants. When does one use stimulating, warming expectorants? When the chest is cold and the cough wet with copious amounts of mucous. This cough is referred to as productive. Warming herbs have a slight irritating effect on the respiratory tract's mucosa triggering the cough reflex. This clears the excess mucous and any germs imbedded within it. Warming expectorants also dry up excess mucous.

There are many stimulating expectorants: poplar bud (Populus canadensis), english daisy (Bellis perennis) and horehound (Marrubium vulgare). My favourite is elecampane (Inula helenium).

Elecampane (Inula helenium) bright yellow flower bursts like sunshine. Elecampane leaves are rough with fuzz, wide and long, and deeply ribbed. Its sun like flowers suggest the plant's warming action while its leaves resemble the shape and structure of lungs. In herbal medicine, elecampane's thick, deep roots are used. The root has two chemical constituents that act on the respiratory passages stimulating a cough.

First, elecampane is rich in volatile oils that warm the lungs. Volatile oils irritate the lining of the bronchioles

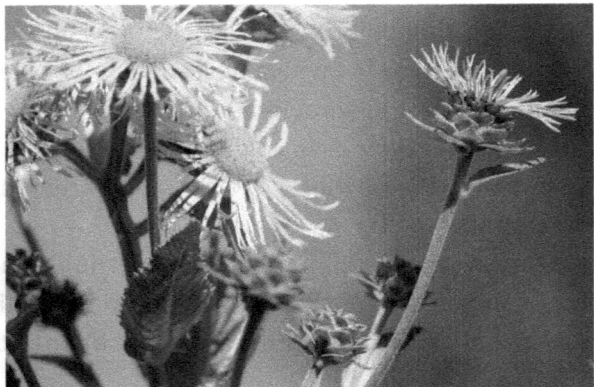

Elecampane　　　　Mark Arneson

al initiating the cough reflex. The irritation stimulates the flow of blood into the bronchiole, delivering nutrients and white blood cells designed for killing invaders in the body. The increase in circulation thins thick mucous facilitating its climb up the cilary, preparing it for expulsion.

Elecampane's second constituent that irritates the bronchioles and triggers a cough are saponins. Herbs high in saponins create foam when mixed with water. Herbalists easily spot herbs high in saponins when making tinctures. Saponins cause tinctures to foam up like a bubble bath. Saponins' action is that it is effective at thinning thick mucous.

A couple of winters ago an elderly client's wife called me to come see him. This client suffered with congestive heart failure and shortness of breath. His wife was particularly concerned about a cough that had developed and was fearful it was the beginning of a nasty respiratory flu that was making its way across the country. I asked the client if he could cough up a little mucous for me to take a look at it. The mucous was clear, thin and full of small bubbles.

I gave him a tincture of elecampane to take three times a day. Within a week the cough cleared up. Elecampane brought heat into the lungs, dried up the mucous and relieved the cough. The bubbles in the mucous suggested elecampane.

Relaxing Expectorants

Relaxing expectorants calm hot, dry "barking" coughs. Dry coughs hurt. Relaxing expectorants are cooling and moistening. These herbs are classed as demulcents and the principal active constituent is mucilage.

There are many relaxing expectorants to choose from: marshmallow (Althea officinalis), licorice (Glycyrrhiza glabra) and iceland moss (Cetraria islandica). Mucilage coats hot, dry respiratory passages and soothe irritated tissues while trapping irritants. Mucilage thins and loosens viscous mucous.

A tea made with relaxing expectorants changes a nonproductive cough into a productive cough.

Mullein *(Verbascum thapsus)* loves to grow in dry soil lacking nutrients. In my herb garden it only grows as high as my knee. Beside the railroad tracks by my home, mullein towers about the prairie grasses. Mullein's preference for dry soil reflects its medicine. Its leaves are an ideal plant for dry, harsh coughs. Matthew Wood refers to mullein's salty taste as the signature of the plants medicine. The salty taste draws water into the respiratory passages thinning hard, encrusted mucous, and creates a productive cough.

Mullein contains both mucilage and saponins. Recall that saponins irritate the bronchi and trigger coughing while mucilage thins and loosens mucous. When a plant like mullein contains two seemingly opposing actions it is called an amphoteric herb. The word amphoteric comes to herbal medicine by way of the chemistry lab. An amphoteric compound can react either as a base (alkaline) or as an acid, depending on the compound it is interacting with.

Mullein is both a relaxing expectorant because of its mucilage and a stimulating expectorant due to its saponins. (Licorice is a similar herb with both mucilage and saponins.)

In my practice, I use mullein to clean out smoker's lungs. More than once mullein has taken care of chest pain caused by

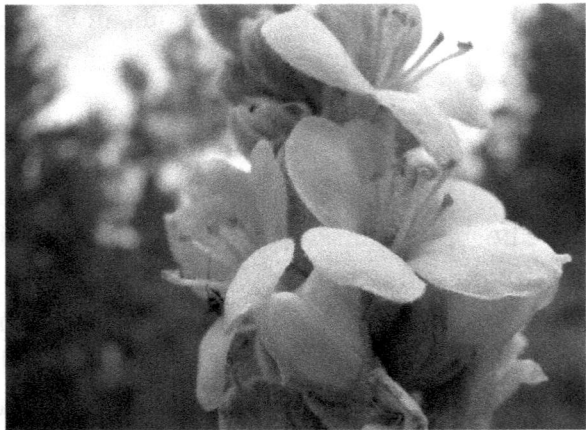

Mullein   Rosalee de la Forêt

smoking while making a chronic morning cough more productive. I encourage smokers to drink several cups of mullein tea a day.

When a client smokes cannabis, I recommend that she add a little mullein to her smoke. Although it has many medicinal effects on the body, smoking cannabis leaves tar behind in the respiratory tract. Mullein soothes the harsh cannabis smoke on the back of the throat while clearing tar from the bronchi.

Case History of a Wheeze

Sydney was 12 weeks old when she developed a wheeze. Her mother took her to the doctor and he wrote a prescription for an inhaler. Her mom was not comfortable with this suggestion. A chiropractor

Sidney's Formula
Formula for Sydney's Infusion
1 tablespoon of marshmallow root
1 cup of cold water.
Cover and infuse over night in the fridge
1 tsp of thyme leaf
1/2 cup boiled water
Steep 20 minutes.
Combine the two teas in a jar and store in the fridge for two days.

who specializes in pregnancy and infants recommended that mom bring Sydney in to see me. I made Sydney an infusion of marshmallow root and thyme (Thymus vulgaris) and asked mom to give her two drops three times a day for two days. In the afternoon on the second day, Sydney coughed up a plug of mucus and the wheeze completely resolved and never returned.

Lungs and Sorrow

TCM associates the emotion sorrow with the lungs. Sorrow's loneliness lays heavy on the chest. Sorrow's thick weight longs for connection with life. The connection with life that our first breath weaves together with our last is the remedy for sorrows solitude. Sorrow's medicine understands the interconnectedness of life. My favourite story illustrating the interconnectedness of life is told by Old Man's Beard.

Old Man's Beard (*Usnea spp.*) in the First Nation's medicine wheel usnea sits in the North, the place of wisdom. I remember my first taste of old man's beard tincture. I felt I was sipping ancient green wisdom. It filled me with the humble quiet sense of awe that I feel when standing amongst venerable trees in old growth forest, usnea dripping from the branches,the forest pregnant with the silence and mystery of life. No plant (usnea is not really a plant) gives meaning to the interdependence of life like usnea.

Usnea is a symbiotic relationship between algae and fungi. Algae forms the green/grey outer surface, and fungi, the inner the white elastic like substance. Usnea grows all over the world, and all over the world it is used to treat cancer, wounds, and lung infections. Usnea's grey green algae are strongly antibacterial. The inner fungus, the thallus, is immune-modulating.

It was once thought that Usnea was a plant parasite because it

The Breath of Interconnection
The carbon that is exhaled as CO2 originates from carbohydrates. The carbohydrates are turned into glucose. Glucose is what every cell in the body feeds on. After the glucose is turned into energy, whatis left over are lone carbon molecules that join up with 2 oxygen molecules. These are no longer of value to the body, so they are exhaled through the lungs as air.
This is the elegant relationship between green plants and animals.
Chemical formula of glucose   is: C6 H12 O6
It is made through this formula:
C6 H12 O6 + 6O2 = 6CO2 + 6H20 + 6CH12602
Glucose + Oxygen = Carbon dioxide + water + energy
Chemical formula of photosynthesis:
6CO2 + 6H20 sunlight received via chlorophyll C6H12O6 + 6O2

prefers to grow on trees where the bark is damaged. It was believed that Usnea drew nutrients from the tree. We are now wiser.

Usnea acts as medicine wherever it perches on the damaged skin of a tree. Usnea protects the tree from invading plant pathogens. Usnea takes nothing from the tree.

How does Usnea eat? The alga absorbs energy from the sun and feeds the inner fungi. The fungus, catching minerals and moisture from the air, makes its own food and feeds it to the algae. Usnea is self-sustaining. As Usnea is dependent on the air for its source of nutrients, it is very sensitive to air pollution. If the air is thick with pollution, Usnea grows slowly if it grows at all. In clean air, usnea hangs from trees like an old man's beard. In northern California Usnea is used to track levels of air pollution in old growth forests.

This strange combination of algae and fungi that care for the

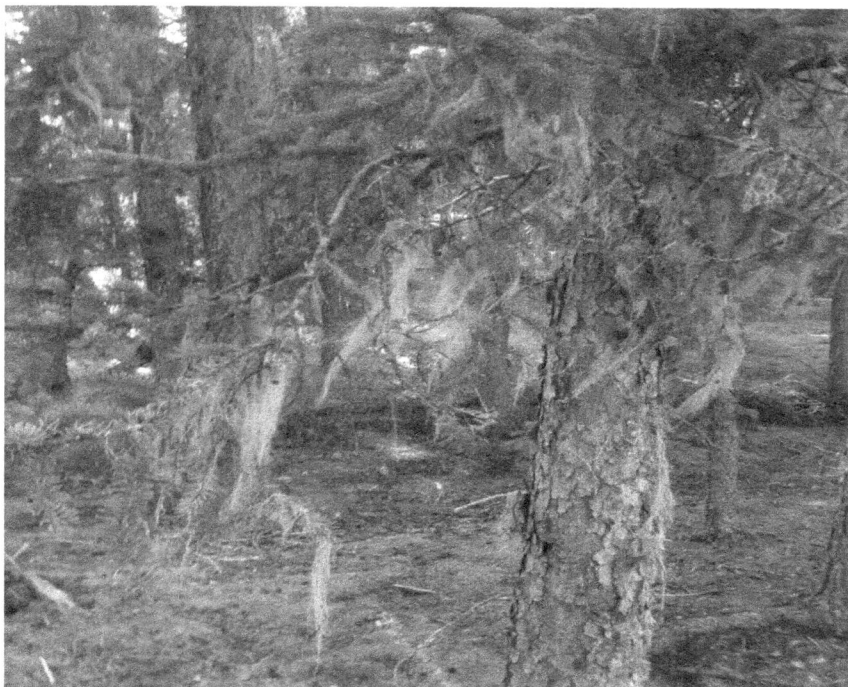

Old Man's Beard   Mark Arneson

trees-- the lungs of the planet-- informs us about the quality of the air and helps us heal our own lung deficiencies. It is a sublime dance of interdependence.

It is the lack of understanding of the interdependence between all living things and the mutually supportive relationships found in nature that is the source of the great sorrow infusing our world. Beliefs like "life is a survival of the fittest" and "it's a dog eat dog world" (although I have never seen one dog eat another) keep hearts guarded and kindness on a leash. Usnea's story inspires trust and releases sorrow's isolation.

The Skin - The Fire Element

The body uses its skin and deeper fascia and flesh to record all that goes on around it. Like the Rosette stone (for those who know how to read it) the body is a living record of life given, life taken, life hoped for and life healed. It is valued for its articulate ability to register immediate reaction, to feel profoundly, and to sense ahead.

The body is a multilingual being. It speaks through its colour and its temperature the flush of recognition, the glow of love, the ash of pain, the heat of arousal, the coldness of non-conviction. It speaks through its constant tiny dance, sometimes swaying, sometimes a-jitter, sometimes trembling. It speaks throughout the leaping of the heart, the pit at the center and rising hope.

The body remembers, the bones remember, the joints remember, even the little finger remembers. Memory is lodged in pictures and feelings in the cells themselves. Like a sponge filled with water, anywhere the flesh is pressed, wrung, even touched lightly, a memory may flow out in a stream. - Women Who Run with the Wolves, Clarissa Pinkola Estes pg 200

Skin is our most sensitive organ. Skin wraps our bony frames and contains our squishy, pulsating organs. Skin makes our bodies composed of many parts whole.

One of the purest pleasures in life is the feel of a baby's skin-- soft, free of blemishes, smooth, sweetly scented. An infant's skin does not know the burn of the sun or embarrassment, the chill of the North wind or rejection. It has not been bruised (unless the baby was birthed with intrusive methods) by the rough and tumble of life, nor has its natural glow been dulled by a reckless life style. A baby's skin bares no scars.

Life's sufferings leave tell tale signs on our skin. Skin becomes scarred by cuts, surgeries, broken bones, vaccinations, tattoos, falls, burns, birthing, and car accidents. Young scars are tender welts marking hurts. As scars age, they become dense and bloodless skin with little to no feeling.

As we age, wrinkles, creases and lines appear where skin was once smooth. Laughter and tears carve lines around our eyes and mouths. The sun and wind chisel crevices in the skin. In some cultures the appearance of wrinkles marks the transition into elder hood, a time when wise counsel can be offered to those who have yet to grown lines on their skin.

When life no longer pulls us in the many directions of middle age, skin begins to become thin. Those close to death have skin so thin, it's like the light from the other side of death's doorway shines through them, reminding those who stay behind of the journey's end we all must discover. Slowly as one slips from the body, the skin over the feet and hands darkens like bruises. At death, the light moves on and the skin becomes the colour of ash.

The Medicine in Sweat

Lying on the damp, cool earth, breathing deeply Mother Earth's eternal embrace, drenched clothing sticks to my hot skin. I prayed for patience as the woman on the other side of the sweat lodge recited the many sufferings her relatives continue to endure. Her pleas for a peaceful existence in a world that divides people by the colour of their skin made my prayers for patience seem trivial. The shame of the actions of my white ancestors pierced my heart as the shame she was made to feel for her brown skin left hatred in hers. Shame's heat passed from my burning skin into the cool earth that supported us all.

Most sweat lodges I have participated in are smallish structures made with a skeleton of aspen or willow branches (favoured for their flexibility) and covered in a hide of many, many blankets.

Inside the sweat lodge, smoke from herbs and heat from glowing red rocks and water are blended with prayer to encourage profound sweating of both a physical and spiritual nature. As sweat drips from every pore of your body, prayers are wrung from your heart. After four rounds of sizzling water on hot rocks, the pungent sweet scent of plants mingle with prayers and sweat. Your body and mind become a clean, empty vessel. The discomfort of the sweat lodge forces hearts to open and give expression to life's sorrow while finding comfort in the community.

The sweat lodge is an ancient ritual practiced by many cultures. The oldest ring of stones that suggests the use of sweat lodges is found on the steppes of southern Russia. Archaeologists date the rings of stone to 5 B.C.

Sweating is an ancient healing therapy used today by many cultures who live close to the earth. In Mayan culture the sweat lodge is referred to as the steam bath. One takes a steam bath to "warm the flesh and blood,' to expel pathogenic "cold winds" from the body and to restore vital "heat" or "warmth". It is believed sweating is necessary for a long healthy life. - Kevin P. Groat Jornal of Latin American Lore 20:1 (1997) 3-96 To Warm the Blood, to Warm the Flesh, The Role of the Steambath in Highland Mayan Ethnomedicine.

The Mayans use of sweat to heal is reminiscent of Samuel Thompson's use of sweating in the 1800's.

In all cases where the heat of the body is so far exhausted as not to be rekindled by using the medicine and being shielded from the surrounding air by a blanket, or being in bed, and chills or stupor attend the patient, then applied heat by steaming becomes indispensably necessary; and heat caused by steam in the manner that I use it, is more natural in producing perspiration, than dry heat that can be applied to the body in any other manner, which will only serve to dry the air and prevent perspiration in many cases of disease, where steam by water or vinegar would promote it and add a life and motion, which has lain silent in consequence of the cold. - Samuel Thomson - New Guide to Health, or Botanic Family Physcian pg 20

Skin Facts
Skin, made up of 1.6 trillion cells is the body's largest organ and about 16% of your body's weight. Spread out, it covers approximately 2 square meters or 22 square feet.
It is made of three layers:
1. The epidermis is several layers of protein rich cells called keratinocytes. The epidermis' superficial layers are dead cells and are referred to as the horny layer.
2. The dermis supports the epidermis and is woven with collagen and elastin giving skin its stretch. It is also home to hair follicles, sweat and sebaceous glands, blood vessels and sensory nerve receptors.
3. The deepest layer of skin is called the subcutis. It is made mostly of fat and provides insulation and cushioning for the collisions with the hard surfaces of life.

Our modern medicinal system does not recognise the value of a good sweat. Sweating is viewed as uncomfortable and should be suppressed using heat reducing drugs like aspirin. Western culture believes sweating lacks sophistication and is embarrassing (other than when in a hot yoga class or at the gym). Pharmacy shelves are lined with a colourful selection of antiperspirants and deodorants. You would be hard pressed to find a medicine cabinet in North America that did not contain these anti-sweat compounds.

Our communal dislike of sweat and its odour may in the long run not be so healthy for us as a society. Limiting sweating and its odour isolate us from each other. Sweating is a display of our common humanity and constant struggle with discomfort. Sweat's odour reveals essential information about that which we are to those we love, hate and are indifferent to.

Sweat carries the scent of illness and health. In a quiet and unconscious way it informs on us. Sweat reveals what we wish to hide.

Researchers at the Institute of Cytology and Genetics in Novosibirsk, Russia studied women's ability to identify men with gonorrhea through smell. A group of women were asked to sniff men who have never had gonorrhea, men currently carrying the infection and men who had been treated for it. The women described the scent of healthy men as floral, while the sick men smelled putrid.

The researchers suggest that the scent of gonorrhea is the result of the immune system's interaction with bacterial changes in the body due to the infection. They go on to suggest that gonorrhea's scent may be a sort of communal immune defense for our species. Untreated gonorrhea leads to infertility in women.

Sweat is good. It's healthy for our bodies to do and it's important to sniff each other's sweat. But what is it?

Sweat forms in the apocrine glands, or commonly referred to as sweat glands. Sweat glands are a tangle of tubes (resembling the kidney's glomerulus) entwined with capillaries in the skin dermis When the body's temperature rises, water, urea, creatine, salts and metabolic acids diffuse across the capillaries and into the sweat glands. As the glands fill, the sweat spills over onto the surface of the body. When sweat drips from your nose in when in downward dog, metabolic wastes are being washed away.

The composition of metabolic waste changes with disease. For example those with chronic kidney disease secrete more urea and creatine onto the skin's surface. This gives the skin the distinct odour of urine.

Shedding Skin
Your skin sheds approximately 30 to 40 thousand cells hourly. Herbalist Todd Caldecott speaks of how he feels dryer lint is the most toxic substance in a home. The toxins that float in the air everyday cling to our clothing. You would think that they are washed away in the washing machine, but not so according to Todd. They are fluffed off with the lint in the dryer.

I asked Todd if this is also true of shedding skin. Do those thousands of skin cells carry toxins from our body? He referred me to a study of people suffering with severe psoriasis, a condition in which skin cells replicate at stressed out rates forming an epidermis that is red, thick and plaque like. Those suffering with psoriasis shed more than the usual person. When these individuals spent time in areas with severe air pollution, their shedding increased.

To help your skin shed and increase its circulation to encourage a healthy glow, try dry skin brushing. Before a bath or shower, gently sweep the brush made with natural fibers over your skin. Be sure to always brush towards your heart.

Not only metabolic wastes smell. The interaction between sweat, bacteria and other flora on the surface of the body help to create your personal odour. Bacteria on the body live and die according to what its host eats and its state of health. An unhealthy diet or a lingering disease process determines the skin bacteria composition. When the bacteria mingle with sweat the body's scent reflects the diet or the illness.

However, I doubt that the Mayan's, the Cree or Samuel Thomas were interested in changing bacteria on the skin's surface when offering healing through sweating. Besides being a spiritual practice, sweating is about helping the body dispose of waste products.

Traditional therapies teach that when one organ of elimination struggles, the other organs of elimination help out. The sweat gland's affinity with the lungs and kidney takes some of the load off of both these organs.

Traditionally diaphoretics like yarrow, elderflower, and boneset are used to encourage sweating to remove deep-seated illness. Review the chapter 4 on circulation for more information on these herbs.

However, what happens when the toxic load in the body is too much to handle even with the skin's help? Traditional healers view most inflammatory skin conditions such as acne, eczema, and psoriasis as the result of the skin being overwhelmed by the body/mind's toxic load.

The following is a case history that illustrates the relationship between the skin, liver, kidneys, digestive tract and the mind.

Case History: Removal of toxins through the skin

When I first saw Lucy she had a number of health concerns. There was an ugly patch of burning, weeping eczema covering most of her lower right leg. It had been there for years. Her bowels were loose. Suffering with surges of adrenaline, she swung from fury to depression in any single day. Her mood swings made it difficult for her to shop and prepare food. She ate eggs and a few raw vegetables every day. Reading her eyes I saw low stomach acids and a constitutionally weak liver. Her tongue was fiery red.

I recommended Lucy make a poultice of powdered slippery elm bark and St. John's Wort infused oil and plaster it over the eczema every night. She kept the poultice in place with cheesecloth and a sock.

Lucy's initial tincture:	Her tea blend:
3 parts Hypericum perforatum	1 part Melissa
3 parts Silybum marianum	1 part Meadowsweet
2 parts Rumex crispus	1 part Chamomile
2 parts Articum lappa	1 cup three times a
1tsp twice a day	a day.

In this treatment I sought to relieve Lucy's depression and fury while supporting her digestion and liver.

Milk thistle is a hepatic and supports liver function

St John's Wort is also a hepatic and eases depression

Yellow dock is an alterative that resolves irregular, fluctuating bowels

Burdock supports both liver and kidneys, while nourishing and cooling the body

Melissa cools down the mind and digestion

Meadowsweet balances stomach acids while toning the bowel

Chamomile calms the mind and digestion and has a mild bitter activity

The poultice of slippery elm and St John's Wort oil cooled and calmed the inflammation while drawing excess fluid from the weeping tissue. St John's Wort infused oil is a traditional burn remedy.

I also advised Lucy to limit her eggs and add more variety to her diet.

Over a period of two months, the eczema on Lucy's leg cleared up, her bowels became regular, and her mood improved. Unfortunately her anger continues to rage and a new symptom appeared: a dry mouth. Lucy woke up parched several times in the night. She drank litres of water during the day.

I continued to encourage her to curb her temper and try to see the world from other points of view. I offered her cooling, nourishing herbs like marshmallow, plantain and chickweed and adaptogens like american ginseng. None of them relieved the thirst.

One day, complaining of an itch on her back, she lifted her shirt to show me. Thin red welts mark the area where she had been scratching, but what really interested me was a dark patch of skin over her kidneys. The discoloured skin was even

Conditions That Involve the Skin and Other Organs

Lupus - An autoimmune condition that can involve every organ in the body. On the face it presents with a red rash in the shape of a butterfly.

Celiac Disease - A stinging, itchy blistering rash can cover the whole body. It is also called gluten rash.

Amoxicillin Rash- Small reddish pink spots appear shortly after taking the antibiotic amoxicillin. This rash appears in 10% of children give the drug. It generally resolves quickly after discontinuing the antibiotic.

Rheumatoid arthritis - Vasculitis is an inflammation of blood vessels. Vasculitis can occur in a blood vessel. When associated with the capillary beds that nourish the skin there is sensitivity to cold, red patches or spots on the skin.

Itchy dry, scaly skin - This can be a symptom of advancing kidney disease, as the skin takes over the some of the kidneys workload in excreting wastes.

the shape of her kidneys.

Looking at the skin discolouration I thought of the plant goldenrod and offered her a tea made with its leaf and flowers. The symptom of thirst cleared up quickly, as did the itching. Over a period of six months, the patch of dark skin on her back faded. Goldenrod is a specific herb for poorly functioning kidneys due to inflammation.

All was well for some time. Lucy no longer needed the St John's Wort for her mood, her skin was clear and her bowels were regular. Her skin no longer itched and her mouth was not dry. Her temper continued to flare, but not with same fury. A year went by.

Then a crisis in Lucy's personal life threatened to takeall that she loved: her family and home. The crisis was demanding she stop the victim game that justified her use of anger. When the crisis deepened a rash appeared on Lucy's face. As it spread, it covered the entire lower half of her face, from her cheekbones to her chin. The skin became thick, as red as beets, and hot to the touch. It began to peel and shed.

Again we used St John's Wort oil and revived the previous formula. It did not help. I offered her some laying on of hands and drew some of the heat from her face. It was a temporary fix. Eventually I simplified the protocol and offered

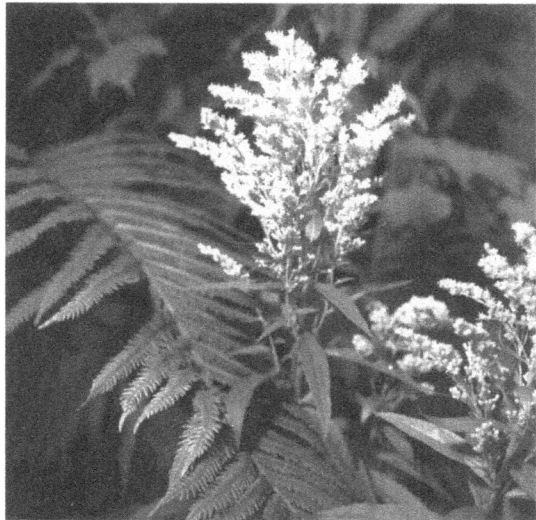

Golden Rod   Mark Arneson

her only burdock tincture and goldenrod tea. The herbs quieted down the inflammation, but did not resolve it.

The challenge was that every time Lucy lost her temper (which was several times a day) the red mask-like rash swelled and thickened. Then one day, desperate for relief, Lucy revealed the shame of her anger. The shame spewed from her mouth carrying the sound of a wild animal's desperate cry. The shrieking pain of shame came directly from Lucy's belly. Within ten minutes the mask faded.

A year has passed since Lucy expressed the visceral voice of shame. The mask has not returned. I have never seen Lucy so calm and agreeable. Overall her health is better than it has been for years. Although she occasionally complains of a lack of intensity in her life, she is discovering the health (both physical and mental) advantages to being peaceful with the world.

The Physiology of Regulation: The Nervous System and The Order of The Soul

My friend Ailo Gaup, a Sami Shaman from Norway, told me this story about drumming for a young man in a coma. The young man while in Greece on his honeymoon was in a car accident that killed his wife and the driver of the other vehicle. Doctors told the young man's mother that there was little hope her son would wake up. She sought out Ailo.

Ailo took his drum and visited the sleeping young man at the hospital. Ailo traveled on his drum to the place of the accident and found shattered pieces of the young man's soul still lingering about roadside. Ailo gathered up the young man's broken soul and traveled on his drum back to the hospital room. There, he carefully placed pieces of the young man's soul back in his body.

A couple of days after Ailo's visit, the young man woke up. Several weeks later, Ailo visited the now recovering young man. After the visit, the young man told his mother that he recalled some kind of unusual connection with Ailo but could not quite remember what it was.

In this chapter we will explore:

Fire: The Soul's Desire

Air: The Spirit Guards the Soul

Yin/Yang and the Nervous System

The Mint Family: Caring for the Nervous System

A Reductionist Approach to the Nervous System

Fire: The Soul's Desire

Hildegart von Bingen lived during the 10th century in the area of Europe we now call Germany. Hildegart was an abbess, musician and an accomplished herbalist. People journeyed long distances to be cured by her healings. Hildegart believed that the soul was responsible for the gestalt of life. Gestalt is defined as an organized whole that is perceived as more than the sum of its parts. Hildegart taught that the soul was the organizing principal in health.

Hildegart's understanding of the soul as the thread that stitches us whole is an idea I find most useful in my clinical practice of herbal medicine. The belief that the soul is the organizing principal behind a healthy life is particularly useful in understanding the nervous system.

Let's take a closer look at how Hildegart viewed the soul. She compared the soul to the sap of a tree.

Like the sun, the compassion of God's grace provides illumination for humankind; like rain or like dew comes the breath of the Holy Spirit; and in appropriately measured cycles, like those of the weather, comes the ripening of fruits (activities and products). The soul is for the body as the sap is for the tree, and the soul energies unfold as the tree unfolds its gestalt. Understanding corresponds to the greenness (viriditas) of the branches and leaves will (or desire) correspond to the flowers and blossoms, feeling is like the first fruit sprouting forth, and intellect like the fully ripening fruit. Sense perception is like the height and breadth of the tree. Thus, the soul provides the inner solidity and strength of the body. - Hildegart von Bingen.

Hildegart's mystical vision that the soul brings harmony to the many parts of life inspires within me tender reverence. To mouth the words, "The whole is greater than the sum of the parts," is not sufficient to bring the healing to the soul in a holistic practice. Healing the soul demands that both the healer and the person who seeks her help open their hearts to the deep truth of the interdependence of life. One can only do this by resting in the mystery of life and walk with faith in the journey called healing.

Hildegart described how the soul interacts with the body: *The human being has three pathways, on which life's activities take place: the soul, the body and the senses. The soul animates the body and brings the breath of life into the senses. The body attracts the soul to itself and opens the senses to the exterior world. The senses touch the soul and mediate the stimuli (of the sensory world) to the body" Wisse die Wege: Scivias, translation by Maura Bockeler. pg 131*

Hildegart experienced the soul as the force that brings life to body and then connects the body to the world. In today's language, we could substitute Hildegart's expression of the soul with the word desire. I would take this idea one step further and say the soul is the body/mind's desire it to breathe. Its

To Breathe
There is a Zen story that goes like this: A master and his student are in a small boat. The student tells the master his greatest desire is to become enlightened. The master grabs the student and plunges his head under the water. After a couple of minutes, the master pulls the student's head above the water. "What is your greatest desire now??," the master demands. Gasping for air, the student cries, "To breathe."

is our breathe that connects to all of life.

The breath connects all living beings. Plants inhale carbon dioxide and exhale oxygen while animals (including mushrooms) inhale oxygen and exhale carbon dioxide. In deep states of meditation the breath becomes a fine thread that weaves life together. It is the breath driven by the soul's desire that connects us with life and makes us whole within the whole. This beautiful story from the Hindu tradition glitters with the intimate relationship between the soul and breath.

Far away in the heavenly abode of the great god Indra, there is a wonderful net which has been hung by some cunning artificer in such a manner that it stretches out indefinitely in all directions. In accordance with the extravagant tastes of deities, the artificer has hung a single glittering jewel at the net's every node, and since the net itself is infinite in dimensions, the jewels are infinite in number. There hang the jewels, glittering like stars of the first magnitude, a wonderful sight to behold. If we now arbitrarily select one of the jewels for inspection and look closely at it, we will discover that in its polished surface that are reflected all the other jewels in the net, infinite in number, not only that, but each of the jewels reflected in this one jewel is also reflecting all the other jewels, so that the process of reflection is infinite. - The Avatamsaka Sutra

One could say that every living being in the universe represents one of the jewels in Indra's net. The threads that connect the jewels are the breath shared by every living being.

When people are emotionally overwhelmed, they instinctively hold their breaths. They stop breathing. I often wonder why this is, when breathing is one of the most wondrous activities of life. I wonder if when ceasing to breathe, we shut off the soul's desire for breath, allowing us to hide from the difficult emotion. When we stop our breath we are no longer glittering and reflecting all other life. Without the breath the soul's connection with existence is lost. When we release the breath, the overwhelming emotion is expressed and we return to being part of the whole.

Elena Avila, a psychiatric nurse and Curandera (a traditional form of healing specific to indigenous people of Central America and the southern United States) writes: *the soul is the part of us that includes all that we are: our talents, our hopes and dreams, our true voice, our nature, our identity. Because all souls are unique, each person's soul is his or her spiritual fingerprint. The soul is the seat of creativity. It does not just sit there unchanging, but is always in the process of evolving, wanting to finish one stage of development and go on to the next.* - Woman Who Glows in The Dark pg: 182.

So what does this have to with herbal medicine?

Let's face it: if the soul, the desire to breathe and the connection to life is unhealthy, disease takes root in the mind. Because the mind cannot be separated from the body, disease in the mind leaves traces in the body. It is essential that the soul be treated if health is to be restored. I strongly believe that there is not another physical system within the body that manifests soul sickness more than the nervous system and its relationship to mental health.

Consider these statistics:

1 in 5 Canadians will suffer with a mental illness in their lifetime.

70% of the time, mental illness begins in childhood or during teen years.

The World Health Organization predicts that by 2020 depression will be the second leading cause of disability in the world. Heart disease will be the first. There is a very strong link between heart disease and depression.

There has been a 114% increase in the prescription of anti-psychotics in children and teens from 2005 to 2009

Antidepressants are now more commonly prescribed to university students than birth control pills.

Mental illness (including the various forms of depression and anxiety, substance abuse, bipolar disorder, ADHD, etc.) are conditions that affect an individual's thoughts, feelings, and actions. Mental illness limits a person's ability to engage with their family, friends, coworkers and the world around them. Described with these broad strokes, mental illness sounds like the inability to connect with life, what Hildegart believed was the purpose of the soul.

Healing the Lost Soul

There was a time when psychoactive plants were used in rituals to reconnect the traumatized soul with life's purpose and meaning. Every traditional culture in the world uses psycho-active plants within the context of the sacred to heal the soul. American Indians in the South West United States heal shattered souls with peyote. First Nations living on the Canadian prairies prepare a combination of canary grass and other plants to mend the soul. In the Indes Mama Cocoa revives the soul while Cannabis is ritually smoked in Hindu Temples to enhance ones connection with the soul. Europeans used herbs like henbane to enter trace like states to heal tortured souls. During the burning times, these soul-healing rituals were extremely distasteful to the inquisitors. Many healers carrying this soul healing knowledge were burned at the stake.

These sacred soul healing plants are now illegal in civilized cultures. In the United States, plants like Cannabis are called enemies of the state. Bloated institutionalized religious sects continue to consider these plants the devil's tools. Since the very beginning human beings and their entangled relationship with plants, psycho-active plants have been used to reintegrate displaced souls into the matrix of human society. I have to

Bach Flower Essences
Doctor Edward Bach, M.D.(1886-1936), noticed that many
mental illness were intensified by fear. Because of this he
developed a number of flower essences to help ease fear and re-
root oneself in their soul.
Poplar flower essence helps overcome fears of the unknown.
This type of fear can manifest as paranoia and a sense of
sabotage. It can present as a vague other worldly sensation or a
full on sense of something coming that fills one with dread.
Mimulus flower essence is more specific to known phobias such
as heights, snakes, elevators, etc. Unlike Poplar where the fear is
nebulous, Mimulus fear has a focus and often the day is
organized around avoiding any contact with what will cause the
uncontrollable fear to rise.
Red Chestnut is the flower essence that eases obsessive worry
for another's wellbeing. It helps one detach from the chronic
worry and have faith in hopeful outcomes.

wonder: is the soul not helpful in a democratic society to
maintain order?

It is not surprising that more than 20% of those suffering
with mental illness (a number that I suspect is on the low side
because people do not like to disclose their use of illegal plants
to authorities) have co-occurring addictions associated with
these psychoactive plants or substances produced by plants.
Many addictions begin with self-medicating to limit the
paralyzing effects of anxiety or depression. Do humans carry
buried ancestral knowledge that turns to psychoactive plants to
heal the mind by renewing the soul's connection with life?
Demonizing these powerful healing plants, as our current
society does, seems to push those who seek their help even
further into the shadows of despair.

Having lost their psychoactive plants to legislation, traditional healers have become more reliant on songs, drums and rattles to alter states of consciousness and heal vandalized souls. But even these tools are viewed as suspicious.

There is one method of healing the soul that can never be shamed and outlawed: heartfelt listening. Heartfelt conversations can knit the lost soul back into life.

Heartfelt listening, not fixing or suggesting or diagnosing, is a powerful methodology for healing a broken or lost soul. Anyone with the intention of supporting the wholeness of another can do this type of healing. Hearing another's soul story is the most rewarding work I do in my practice.

It is important to remember that the soul knows what it needs. The healer, like the breath, leads the individual to the door to the room where the soul remains whole. It is up to the person to open door and enter.

The Nervous System: Mind/Body Medicine

The biomedical system of healing divides illnesses of the mind and diseases of the body into two distinct disciplines. You see a psychiatrist for depression and a neurologist for your headache.

Mental illness is viewed as a chemical imbalance while neurological illness is defined as a structural challenge within the body. For example migraine headaches are a neurological illness triggered by dilated blood vessels as are the tingling in a diabetics toes and fingers caused by damaged blood vessels limiting the flow of nutrients and oxygen to delicate nervous tissue.

An astute healer cannot help but notice that rarely is there a chemical imbalance (mental) that does not affect the physical body. The following are common symptoms of multiple sclerosis and anxiety.

Symptom	Multiple Sclerosis	Anxiety
Fatigue	Yes	Yes
Numb sensation on skin	Yes	Yes
Muscular weakness	Yes	Yes
Dizziness or Vertigo	Yes	Yes
Tingling sensations	Yes	Yes
Tremours/twitching	Yes	Yes
Clumsiness	Yes	Yes
Difficulty focusing	Yes	Yes
Depression	Yes	Yes
Difficulty forming words	Yes	Yes
Uncontrollable emotions	Yes	Yes
Constipation	Yes	Yes
Stabbing or burning pain	Yes	Yes

Although the drug regimes for MS are much more complex than drug regimes for anxiety, anti-anxiety and antidepressants drugs are prescribed for both conditions. Many suffering with MS find drugs that shift the balance of neurotransmitters in the mind/body reduce the pain and tremours associated with the disease. These mood-altering drugs do not cure either anxiety or MS.

Herbalists offer similar herbs to relieve the physical and mental challenges of both conditions. Plants do not distinguish between diseases of the mind and body. Traditional healers do not discriminate between diseases of the mind or body. Herbalists assess imbalances in both the mind and body with every person and offer plants to help regain harmony.

Plants Commonly Used to Relieve the Symptoms of Anxiety and MS

St John's Wort (*Hypericum perforatum*) is well known for its ability to alleviate moderate depression and anxiety. St John's Wort also alleviates muscular pain associated with a decrease in serotonin levels in the body, much in the same way the most favoured class of antidepressant of our time, SSRIs (Serotonin re-uptake inhibitors) do.. A traditional hepatic, St John's improves liver function. Weak liver function was once seen as the cause of depression. St John's is traditionally used to relieve inflammation within the nervous system, in particular the pain associated with burns. Studies have shown St John's increases cortisol levels in the blood. Cortisone, a drug that mimics the action of cortisol in the body, is one of the primary drugs used to combat inflammation in autoimmune conditions such as multiple sclerosis.

Fat and the Nervous System
In ancient medicine systems, the brain was believed to be made mostly of fat. Modern medicine now knows that essential fatty acids are critical for smooth development and proper functioning of the nervous system. Simply adding good fats to the diet can clear up both depression and foggy thinking and slow down the appearance of aging.

Wild Oat Seed (*Avena sativa*) is a gentle but powerful nerve tonic referred to as a trophorestorative in western herbal medicine. Trophorestorative herbs help restore organs after exhaustion has taken hold. For example, hawthorn is a trophorestorative for the heart, milk seed for the liver and nettle seed for the kidney. Oats seed replenishes a severely exhausted nervous system.

The shaped of the oat seed is reminiscent of the myelin sheaths. The Myelin sheath is essentially layers of fat that wrap around our neurons. These fatty coats are essential for smooth transmission of electrical impulses throughout the nervous system. It is the degradation of myelin sheaths that create the erratic and spasmodic symptoms of MS.

I think of oat seed as teasing out any tangles from within the nervous system. It is specifically used to clarify confused and unfocused thinking. Herbalists calm tremours and strengthen weak muscles with this little green seed. Wild oat seed is the demulcent for the nervous

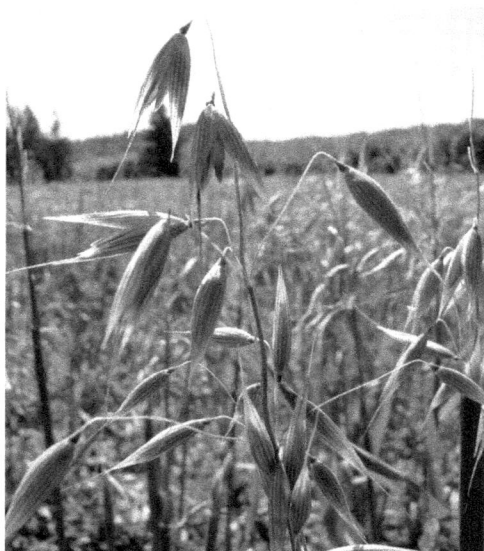

Oat Seed   Rosalee de la Forêt

system, soothing and cooling raw nerves. It is an essential herb in most conditions affecting the nervous system, whether physical or mental.

Gingko (*Gingko biloba***)** is often thought of as a circulatory herb. The leaves of the gingko tree increase cerebral circulation by dilating blood vessels and decreasing platelet levels in the blood. A decrease in platelet levels thins the blood and improves its flow. An increase of oxygenated and nutrient rich

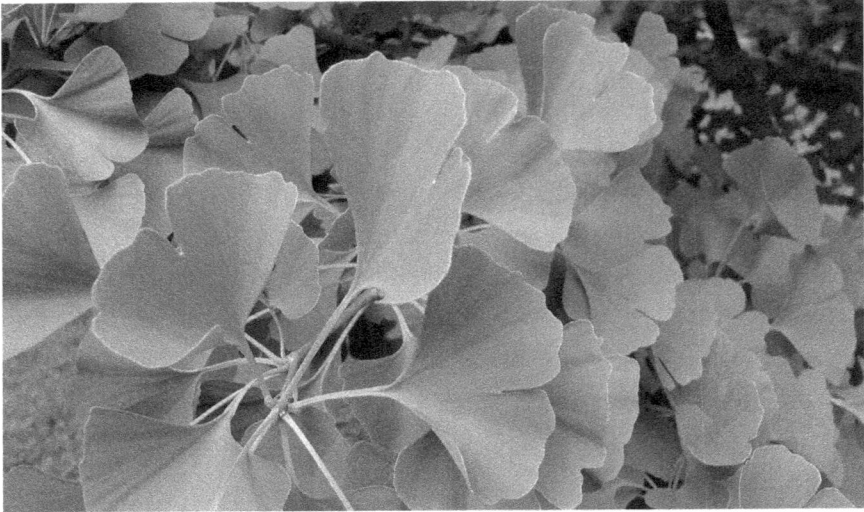

Gingko   Rosalee de la Forêt

blood to the brain improves an individual's ability to think clearly and enhances healing of inflammation within its delicate structure.

Gingko is a favoured herb for any condition associated with the brain including tinnitus, headache and vertigo, each a symptom of both anxiety and MS.

Air: The Spirit Guards the Soul

Hildegart envisioned the soul as a force that brings life to the body. Life is warm. Warmth is the fire element. Desire is the fuel for life's fire. The soul burns with desire to connect with life.

What happens when the soul's fire for connection to life is extinguished? Life loses its meaning. Dark loneliness fills the void where the soul's desired burned. Life goes on, but it feels empty. Traditional healers say those who suffer this way have lost their souls. They have lost their direction home. The fire that ignites the union with life dies out.

What extinguished life's fire? Fires that burn too hot suffocate themselves. When insatiable hunger erupts like a forest fire, and no discrimination is practiced, it is not long before the soul's fire vanishes and life cascades into meaninglessness. Many people suffer in this way. It is a syndrome called burn out.

Some of the symptoms of burn out are:

- Daily tasks are dull, mind numbing and meaningless
- Relentless exhaustion
- A cynical attitude as a cover for hopelessness
- No passion for life

Many of these symptoms are also seen in depression. Burn out is a situational depression. When someone is burnt out (most of

Adaptogens and Burn Out

When burn out threatens, choose adaptogenic herbs. We explored adaptogens in relation to the immune system in chapter five. Here let's look at the role of adaptogens in rebuilding the nervous system. Adaptogens act within the endocrine system. But do not let this fact blind you to their value to the nervous system. The nervous system and the endocrine system are entwined. Think of them like the symbiotic relationship between a trees roots and network of mycelium.

Many neurotransmitters are also classed as hormones. Neurotransmitters are the nervous system's messengers, while hormones relay messages to and from the endocrine system's organs.

For example the pituitary gland, found in the depth of your brain, is made uo of endocrine tissue that secretes hormones and bundles of nerve endings that release neurotransmitters.

. It is my experience in treating burn out that a formula combining adaptogens and nervines lead to the quickest recovery. Nervines generally act quickly by improving mental states and alertness within a week. Adaptogens deep inner work slowly shifts hormones, reestablishing circadian rhythms. The long term results promised by adaptogens require time and patience.

the depression I see in clinic) it is essential that a change of attitude towards life's purpose take place for health to return. Re-evaluating your life's purpose involves your spirit.

The spirit is aligned with the breath and the air element. The air element nourishes the thought process. Our thoughts are reflected in our breath. A person's thoughts reflect the health of their spirit.

Many people are confused about the difference between the soul and spirit. Basically the spirit is the envelope that protects that soul from harm. If the spirit is relatively healthy, the soul will be too. How do we keep our spirit in good health?....the spirit is the part of us that is the sum total of our nutritional habits, whether good or bad; it is the energy generated from our feelings, whether balanced or unbalanced; and the energy created by our thoughts. ---pg 172 Elena Avila in Woman Who Glows in the Dark

Thoughts are a manifestation of the spirit or air element in the body/mind. Our thoughts guard the fire burning in the soul. If the thoughts are dark, despairing and hopeless, the soul's fire will go out. If the thoughts are frenzied with endless possibilities, the soul's fire will be exhausted. If thoughts carefully feed the soul's fire and protect it with discernment, there will be health in the body, mind, emotions and spirit.

Herbal Medicine for Windy Minds

Let's take a quick detour and explore a similar idea found in TCM. In Chinese philosophy the body and the material world is the manifestation of yin. The immaterial, energetic realm of existence is the manifestation of yang. The symbol used to illustrate the relationship between yin and yang is the bamboo flute. The flute represents the yin element and the breath the energy of the yang element.

When playing a flute, if the breath is uneven the song is discordant. If the breath is too forceful the song is shrill. A weak breath creates a whisper of a song. If the breath is even and strong but not forceful, the flute's song inspires.

When thoughts blow here and there, without purpose or focus, I call this a windy spirit. A windy spirit needs grounding in the earth element, the body, or else actions are scattered like leaves on an autumn day. There are many herbs to still windy spirits.

I prefer herbal teas to rest windy spirits. The beauty of herbal teas is the few minutes you spend preparing it. I encourage clients to bring their awareness to their breath at the tip of their nostrils while the kettle boils and the tea steeps. I then suggest that they sit in a comfortable chair, breathe deeply, and just before taking the first sip, make a prayer, ask for the spirit to be calm and the mind a still pool. Deep breathing anchors the spirit in the body. Plants from the mint family brew tasty teas and are greater healers for driven spirits. My favourite mint for windy spirits is lemon balm (Melissa officinalis).

Lemon Balm (Melissa officinalis).Although most mints like to grow on the vertical axis, lemon balm tends to be lower growing and branches out more like a very small bush where I live in Alberta. My friend Dionne who gardened many years in Victoria, BC, a much milder climate, assures me it grow like other mints on the temperate west coast. In either case, lemon balm is a humble plant. Its scent has sweet lemon undertones. Lemon balm's delicate leaves

Emotions and the Breath

Sigh - Sadness or fatigue
Snort - Disgust
Flared nostrils - Rage
Gasp - Shock
Pant - Lust
Huff - Anger
Shallow - Anxiety

have scalloped edges. The season here in Alberta is not long enough for it to flower, but when lemon balm does flower the blossoms are quiet and soft.

Balm, as it is fondly called by Europeans, has thrived in herb gardens for a very long time. Charlemagne, considered the father of Europe in the 800s, ordered that balm be grown in every medicinal herb garden through his empire. This edict guaranteed his people a continuous supply of balm's soothing medicine.

Later, European herbalist John Gerard (late 1500s) suggested using balm to "comforteth the hart and driveth away all sadness."

Lemon balm's medicine is loved in the Middle East. 11th century Arab herbalist Avicenna wrote, "Balm causeth the mind and heart to become merry."

Today balm is favoured as a gentle but effective nerve tonic. When I hear the word hyper attached to any condition (hypertension, hyperthyroid, hyperacidity, hyperactive, hypersensitive, etc.) I think of lemon balm.

In traditional herbal medicine, hyper conditions are associated with

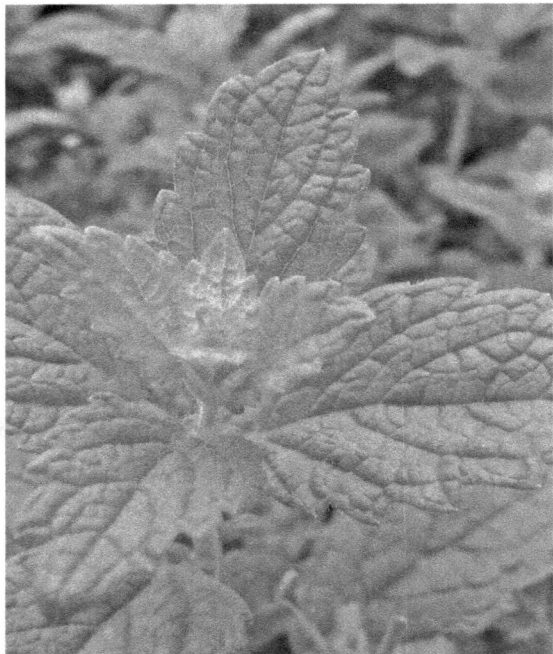

Lemon Balm   Rosalee de la Forêt

excess heat and tension in the body and mind. The seed of tension rides the gales of the windy mind until it takes root in the body where it grows into a hyper condition.

Lemon balm cools hot conditions, including hot guts and hot heads. Like many plants in the mint family, lemon balm calms upset stomachs and improves overall digestion while calming the mind.

Lemon balm is a great medicine for children. It has an anti-viral action and has a long history of being used as a compress to calm chickenpox and other herpes outbreaks. Offering an irritable, sick child a sweetened cup of lemon balm tea will quiet them down and ease them into sleep. Add a couple of cups of lemon balm tea to a bath to calm and soothe infants.

I recommend lemon balm tea during the last month of pregnancy. It settles heartburn and calms the mind in anticipation of labour. Many people like to use chamomile tea during this time, but I prefer the lightness lemon balm brings to the mind. It offers a feeling of hope to the heart and a sense of optimism that I find chamomile lacks.

For lemon balm's inherent optimism, it is also favored in formulas designed to ease depression. This is particularly the case when anxiety is depression's bed partner, as a result of the dreaded windy mind.

Lemon balm is perfect for those who have been living on coffee and adrenaline for months on end. It takes them off caffeine's cliff edge and gives them a foothold on calm ground.

The Bitter Taste and the Windy Spirits

Many bitter plants calm windy spirits. I think of these herbs as planting the spirit deep into the body. The bitter taste shocks the spirit back into the body much like a cold shower. It is after all the organs below the diaphragm that are primarily affected by the bitter taste. I think of the abdomen and pelvis which contain the liver, stomach, intestines, sexual organs, spleen and pancreas as the earthy/watery part of the body. Above the diaphragm, organs with an affinity with air (lungs) and fire (heart) are rarely treated with bitter plants.

Windy spirits do not rest. A windy spirit is like a kite that has broken its string. Bitter tasting herbs bind windy spirits to the body's earth element Windy spirits are addicted to adrenaline's fired that sends the sympathetic nervous system into a flury. Windy spirits cannot abide the calm offered by the parasympathetic system.

The vagus nerve, the manager of the parasympathetic system and stimulated by the bitter taste on the tongue, burrows into the body like a tap root. Sprouting from the brain stem penetrating the thorax to settle in the heart before moving on through the diaphragm the vagus nerve roots itself in the liver, stomach, pancreas and small intestine. (It is not surprising that many bitter herbs such as dandelion, yellow dock, oregon grape, and burdock all have significant tap roots.).

Cooling bitter herbs act like water on the adrenal gland's fire and offer the balm of discrimination to the soul's blazing desires. Understanding the primary needs of one's guts grounds windy spirits deep in the body.

Vervain (Verbena officinalis) is a bitter without a tap root and one of my favoured plants for a windy spirit. Vervain is a gangly plant. It has a tall thin

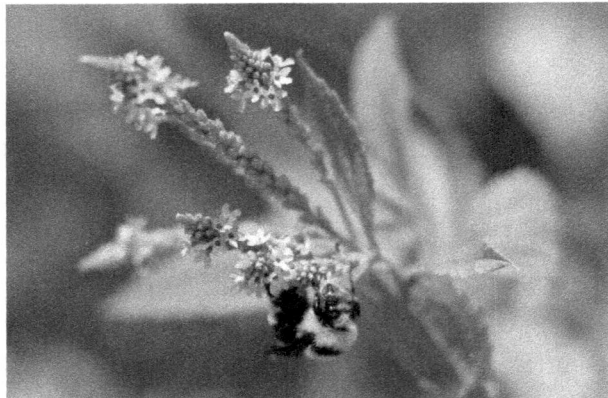

Vervain   Rosalee de la Forêt

stem, thin jagged leaves and lovely deep purple flowers. (Purple is the colour of idealism. Often windy spirits struggle with idealism and have a sense of how things should be. Their idealism constantly pushes them against how things are.) Vervain's fragile appearance is deceiving as it is a tremendously strong and flexible plant. Vervain's jagged leaves carry the bitter medicine. I think of vervain's leaves as medicine for jagged nerves.

Vervain is for people who spend their days busy making things "right". People who need vervain do not enjoy the morning light or refresh themselves with a pause during the afternoon. Vervain people bite off more than they can chew. They are people who live with a full plate. One of my friends who does very well on vervain says, "Every time I get a moments rest, I start dreaming up another great project." Vervain people are often insomniacs. They can't stop thinking.

The darkness of deep sleep heals the body. Sleep alight with dreams allows the spirit and the soul to digest the day. When one scurries about the day getting involved in too many conversations, conflicts, plots and plans, the spirit and soul become bloated. As over eating disturbs digestion, over consumption of activity disturbs sleep.

Vervain, with its bitter taste, helps the body to digest its food and the spirit to digest its day. Although not considered a hypnotic, vervain, is very important in formulas used to relieve insomnia.

Hops (Hummulus lupus) produces a bitter pollen that calms windy spirits.

Hops people are slightly different though than the idealistic vervain.

Every year the hops plant in my garden takes off in a new direction. One year it grows towards the house, another year it reaches out for the shed, the following year it tries to climb the fence. Every year I try to predict where it wants to go, and

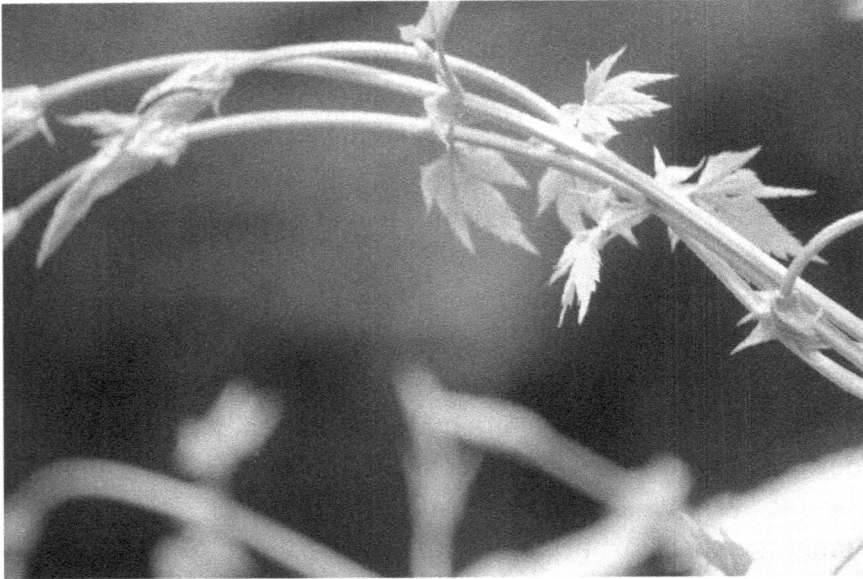

Hops   Mark Arneson

every year it changes its course. This year I found one of its roots, thickly coated in bark, leaping across the soil towards the back deck. Hops have a voracious appetite that cannot decide which direction to grow in.

Hops are a cholagogue. Cholagogues encourage the release of bile from the gall bladder. An increase of bile squirting into the small intestines improves digestion of fats and peristalsis. Cholagogues like hops are offered when digestion is sluggish.

TCM teaches that the gall bladder rules our ability to make decisions. The practitioner of TCM gives cholagogues like hops to treat the gall bladder when a person has a hard time making decisions.

Hops help those who lay awake at night worrying about what to do. Their soul is a tangle of knots. Their spirit, unable to take the direction their soul desires in order to connect with life, is left in limbo-- constantly changing directions, confused, and not knowing which way to go. By improving gall bladder function, the use of hops leads to better absorption of nutrients as well as the ability to make decisions. Hops calm the spirit (thoughts), allowing time for dreams and careful reflection upon awakening. The frantic worry that steals sleep settles as the spirit finds rest in the body.

Yin/Yang and the Nervous System

Nature thrives when contrary forces continually flow into one another: day into night, winter into summer, male and female, child and adult. In TCM the principal of two opposing forces flowing into on another is symbolized by the yin/ yang symbol. In chapter one, we explored the yin/yang symbol as a definition of health: the ability to continually adapt to the changing of the environment of the body, the mind, and nature. Let's take a closer look at the yin/yang symbol to come to a better understanding of the nervous system. Consider this passage:

At the extreme, yin and yang transform into each other, just as the moon, when full, begins to wane. This principal is depicted visually in ancient symbol of yin/yang. Here we see that when yang is at its fullest, the seed of yin is born (the black dot within the white area). Likewise, in the depth of the dark yin we find the seed of yang. Thus, the ancient Chinese, who understood the value of influencing things at their beginnings, point out that noon is the birth of the nighttime (as this the point when the light begins to fade), while the winter solstice "brings the victory of the light." - Archetypal Acupuncture: Healing with the Five Elements *by Gary Dolowich M.D.*

The yin/yang principal elegantly illustrates the nervous system's physiology. The parasympathetic system, known as "rest and digest", is a reflection of the yin force in nature. The sympathetic system, known as "fight or flight", is a reflection of the yang force in nature.

Yin and Yang and the Nervous System

The following illustrates the correspondence between yin/yang and the two divisions of the automatic nervous system:

Yang & The Sympathetic Nervous System	Yin & The Parasympathetic Nervous System
Active	Rest
Creative	Receptive
Fire and Air	Water and earth
Warm to Hot	Cool to Cold

Studying the nervous systems through the teachings of the yin/yang symbol nicely leads us back to the study of plant energetics. Most plants affecting the nervous system can be considered in terms of temperature.

Warming herbs stimulate the nervous system and relieve the cold and stagnancy associated with depression. Depression is an extreme state of yin. Warming herbs are yang in nature.

Cooling herbs(frequently bitters, although not always) calm the nervous system, easing tension and anxiety from the body/mind. Cooling herbs are yin in nature. Anxiety, associated with fear, is a state of yang. Using cooling herbs to calm anxiety or warming herbs to counter cold, stagnant conditions is called treating with opposites. Treating with opposites is in harmony with the teachings of the yin/yang symbol. Planting the seed of yin within the sphere of yang leads to a yin state. Seeding yin with yang, causes a yang.

Warming herbs used to bring a spark to the nervous system (Yang)	Cooling herbs used to dampen the nervous system's fire (Yin)
Damiana (*Turnera diffusa*)	Chamomile (*Matricaria recutita*)
Rosemary (*Rosmarius off.*)	Motherwort (*Leonurus cardiac*)
Peppermint (*Mentha piperita*)	Scullcap *(Scutellaria laterifolia)*
Basil *(Ocimum basilicum)*	Lemon balm (*Melissa off.*)
Valerian *(Valariana off.)*	Hops (*Humulus lupulus*)

Herbs that enliven the nervous system are often called stimulating nervines. Herbs that cool the down the nervous system are called relaxing nervines.

Notes on Cold Herbs

Traditional herbalists associated cold with illness and eventually death.

...I beseech you take notice of this, that seeing our bodies nourished by heat, and we live by heat, therefor no cold medicines are friendly to the body, but what good they do our bodies, they do by removing an unnatural heat or the body heated above its natural temperature.

The giving then of cold medicine to a man in his natural temper, the season of the year also being moderately hot, extinguishes natural heat in the body of man.

Yet have these a necessary use in them too, though not as frequent as hot medicine have; and that may be the reason why an all wise God hath furnished us with far more hot herbs and plants, than cold. - A Key to Galen's Method of Pysic

Galen's time and climate had very different needs than the time we live in. I know the climate I live in at 52.26N is very different from Greece. Our wired society is hot with multitasking and the instant gratification of button pushing. Therefore, more so than Galen's time, there is a place for cooling herbs in the apothecary.

The coolest herbs in the apothecary are the hypnotics. Hops, passion flower (*Passiflora incarnata*) and valerian have hypnotic actions. In clinic, I use these herbs to cool down an excessively tense body (hops if the digestive system is hot and tense, valerian when the muscles are taunt and painful) but only in low doses and in formulations with other herbs. I rarely find them effective sleep aids over the long term at higher doses.

Many people in our hectic society self-medicate with the cooling herb *Cannabis spp.* Although initially this plant is stimulating, over the long term is cooling to the body/mind. Pot smokers are famous for their lethargy and foggy brains. The expression "stoned" is used to describe the state of being after smoking cannabis, suggesting a cold state of being that lacks the intensity of feeling. Long term consistent use of cannabis weakens the libido (male sperm become stoned under the influence of cannabis). Cannabis impedes the ability to learn and grow and limits expectations for life on this wonderful planet.

In India, the original home of Cannabis, herbalists offer basil (*Ocimum spp.*) as the counter balance to over consumption of cannabis' intoxicating smoke. Basil is a warming, stimulating herb that creates enthusiasm in the mind. Basil is like sunlight burning through the fog left behind by cannabis.

The Mint Family: Caring for the Nervous System

Nature is elegant in her reuse of forms. Consider the cochlea's spiral, the curve of a wave and the snail's home. Branching systems are another of nature's favoured forms: brightly coloured coral, rivers with their tributaries and manipulating hands. Trees are nature's ultimate expression of branching systems with their central trunk, canopy and root system. Like the tree, the nervous system is a branching system.

The spinal cord has the canopy called a brain and a root system called the Cauda equine (Horse's tail). Where the nervous system differentiates from the tree is the branches off of the spinal cord. A better metaphor for nervous system might be a medicinal plant from the mint family. Plants in the mint family are characterized by a central stem, lateral branches and leaves, a flowering apex and a network of roots below. The mint family, with so many plants beneficial to the nervous system, mirrors the nervous system's brain, spinal cord, spinal nerves and caudal equine.

When the nervous system is fired up or burning with a low flame, other systems of the body are often out of balance. Thankfully we have dexterous plants from the mint family that temper minds, soothe tummies, settle grumbling gall bladders and bring peace to anxious hearts.

Motherwort (*Leonurus cardiaca*) is a handsome plant with a pronounced calming effect on both the mind and the heart. Motherwort is the favoured herb when anxiety and heart palpations occur simultaneously. Motherwort is useful in formulas designed to bring down blood pressure. A bitter plant, it also supports the release of bile from the liver.

Hyssop (*Hyssops officinalis*) is a member of the mint family that calms anxiety and dilates the bronchi. It is specific for anxiety with shortness of breath. I have found it useful for both anxiety resulting from shortness of breath and shortness of breath resulting in anxiety. I have also used it in congestive heart failure with anxiety to improve the depth of the breath.

Sage (*Salvia officinalis*) is another plant from the mint family that soothes the nervous system. Sage is an effective remedy for insomnia with bloating and abdominal discomfort. Salvia is a traditional liver tonic. Sage soothes irritated livers and quiets down grumbling gall bladders. It is useful to remember that if the liver is not happy the rest of the body or the mind is happy.

Scullcap (*Scutellaria lateriflora*) is an indispensable plant from the mint family when the mind needs calming and the spirits need lifting. Scullcap relaxes spasms

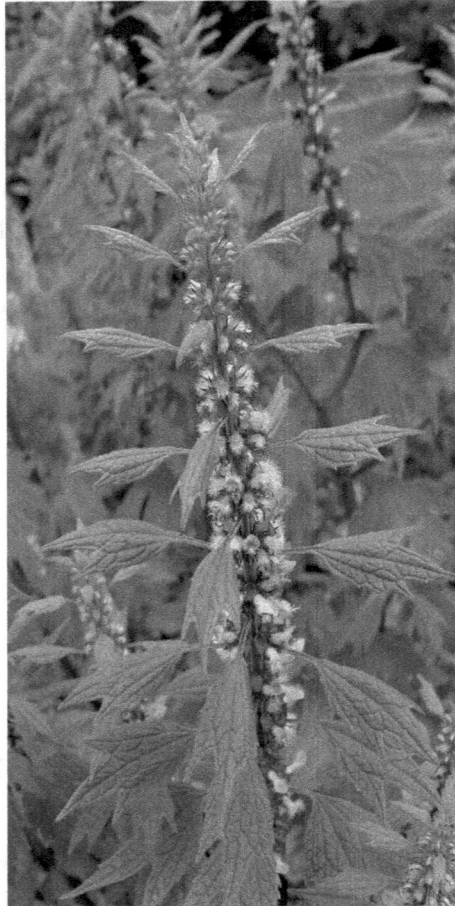

Motherwort   Rosalee de la Forêt

in the body resulting from chronic anxiety. I have seen it ease twitching and tremours when anxiety has been held in the body for several years.

Hedge Nettle (*Stachys palustris)* is a weed that planted itself in my garden. Like motherwort it calms an anxious heart but unlike motherwort does not interfere with thyroid function. Hedge nettle brings clarity, untangling a mind confused with disorganized thinking.

Peppermint (*Mentha piperita)* is the most famous medicinal plant from the mint family. There is a saying in India, "If one could name all the fish in the Indian Ocean, one could name all the medicinal uses of peppermint." Now I have never swum in the Indian Ocean, but I imagine there are a lot of fish in it.

Let's look at a few of peppermint's uses:

After over eating at the "all you can eat" Chinese buffet, peppermint tea is perfect. It quiets belching stomachs and signals the liver to release bile. The bile helps with digestion of fats from fried food. Bile also encourages peristalsis and moves sluggish digestion along, relieving bloating and gas.

Peppermint is the herb to offer when anxiety and a spasmodic bowel coexist, as in Irritable Bowel Syndrome (IBS).

Peppermint calms nausea, whether it's caused by morning sickness, motion sickness or migraine. When nausea lingers, try a strong cup of peppermint tea with a tablespoon of freshly grated ginger (*Zingiber officinale)*. A dab of honey makes this tea delicious.

Peppermint tea brings hope to a gloomy heart and inspiration to the lackluster mind.

When peppermint's volatile oils are distilled, an essential oil is made. Rubbing peppermint essential oil in the groove at the top of neck and the base of the skull replaces a headache's throb with a cool tingle.

Add a few drops of peppermint essential oil to an analgesic cream to melt tense and aching muscles. When first applied topically peppermint causes the blood vessels close to the skin to contract. This creates a cooling sensation. This is followed by the blood vessels dilating and a rush of blood into the area, creating a warming sensation. This effect is similar to applying heat and cold to pained joints. The quickly changing temperature and increased blood flow breaks up unresolved inflammation and promotes resolution.

Essential Oils and Carrier Oils

Essential oils are the most concentrated form of herbal medicine available.

Essential oils are made from a plant's volatile oils. Volatile oils are fiery. Essential oils have enough fire in them to burn the skin and when taken internally, mucous membranes.

For this reason, I never advise using essential oils internally and always recommend using a fixed oil as a carrier when applying essential oils to skin. The carrier oil dilutes the fire in the essential oil.

Properties of Fixed Oils

Peanut oil: Anti-inflammatory

Grape seed oil: Most quickly absorbed oil; good for oily skin types

Almond oil: Good for dry itchy, skin

Castor oil: Deeply cleansing

Olive oil: High in essential fatty acids; good for aging skin

Safflower oil: Specific to easing the pain of inflamed joints

Sunflower oil: Slow to absorb; keeps the medicine on the surface of the skin

A steam inhalation of peppermint combats sinusitis and eases its pain. Drinking strong peppermint tea and massaging peppermint essential oil over the sinus will resolve the infection.

A linament made with peppermint tea placed over the abdomen comforts menstrual cramps.

Peppermint tea needs to be avoided by breast-feeding Moms. But if a woman has lost a child and needs to dry up her breast milk, peppermint is one of the herbs that will assuage the grief of painful and dripping breasts. Parsley (*Petroselinum crispum*) and sage (*Salvia officinalis*) also have this action.

Combining peppermint with yarrow flowers (*Achillea millifolium*) and elder flowers (*Sambucus nigra*) is an effective cold and flu remedy.

A blend of green tea and peppermint, favoured in the Moroccan cafes, is a perfect morning wake up tea.

Be aware that peppermint is a hot, dry herb. This means that peppermint will bring heat to the body and dry up excess moisture, particularly in the digestive tract. If there is excess heat in the stomach peppermint causes heartburn.

A Reductionist Approach to the Nervous System

After spending 10 years traveling with my meditation teachers and living in meditation centres, I decided to go to herb school. I took my time considering each school. Some schools offered a spattering of classes with different herbal traditions from around the world. Others focused on traditions from India or China. In the end I decided on taking a science based program that is based on reductionist principals of medicine, whether pharmaceutical or herbal. The reason I chose this program was I had just spent ten years exploring the right brain, the intuitive function and the esoteric side of life. I felt I needed to study the scientific view of life to bring balance to my brain and life. I also thought that it was important to learn biomedical language. This is the language of healing in our time. At the time I made these decisions, I did not see yin and yang as being ideas that were easily translated into modern North American thinking about health and the body.

When I review my decision, I sit on the fence. In some ways, I wish my education in herbal medicine had more on the energetics of herbs and the body. At the same time, I believe that becoming familiar with a classic medical view (reductionist) of the body and health has enhanced my overall understanding of the body and herbal medicine as well as my ability to communicate with clients.

I find the study of neurochemistry and herbal medicine creates bridges between reductionistic principals of medicine and the holistic energetic principals traditional herbalist realizes on. With this in mind, please review the following information.

The Chemistry of the Nervous System

The neuron (there are 10 billion in the brain) is the basic functioning element of the nervous system. Neurons are single cells that initiate all activity in the body and receive all the information conveyed by the senses. Neurons are master communicators and the language they use are minuscule chemical packages called neurotransmitters. Neurotransmitters are responsible for every movement, thought, mood, heartbeat, word and secretion you make.

The following is a brief summary of neurotransmitters and how herbal medicine influences their ability to communicate.

Neurotransmitters and Herbs

Serotonin is a hormone called a neurotransmitter. It is also called 50-HTP. It is made from an amino acid tryptophan. Serotonin in turn is used to make the pituitary hormone melatonin (the sleep hormone).

Serotonin is found in the digestive tract, the CNS (brain) and platelets. It is made in the liver.

Its effect:
- Promotes cheerfulness and buffer for stress
- Plays a role in regulation of: peristalsis, circadian rhythms, body temperature and pH level

Signs of Imbalance
- Anxiety in typically low stress situations
- Impatience without explanation

- Fatigue with no obvious cause
- Inability to focus, poor memory, lack of mental clarity
- IBS type symptoms
- Chronic pain
- Sugar cravings
- Repetitive negative thoughts

Herbs that affect it

St John's wort, Skullcap, and passion flower.

Other interesting facts

Serotonin is found in many plants, mushrooms and insects. Because high doses of serotonin will cause diarrhea, it is believed that some plants coat their seeds in serotonin so they are quickly expelled from digestive tracts.

GABA Gamma Amino butyric Acid is an amino acid that is a neurotransmitter found only in the brain and is responsible for as many as 1/3 of all brain synapses.

Its effects

GABA is an inhibitory neurotransmitter. In other words, it is the off switch stopping neurons from over firing. It is often referred to as the "brake pedal"| neurotransmitter. GABA signals the muscle to stop once its activity has been completed. It is very important for rest.

Signs of Imbalance

- Feeling anxiety or panic for no reason
- Feelings of dread
- Feelings of "knots" in the stomach
- Feeling overwhelmed for no reason
- Feelings of guilt about decisions
- Restless mind
- Difficulty turning the mind off
- Disorganized attention
- Worry about things not previously thought of

- Feelings of inner tension and excitability

Herbs that affect it

Kava and valerian

Other interesting facts

GABA is made from a combination of B6 and glutamate. Glutamate is made from B6 and glutamine. Glutamine is made in the lungs, participates in protecting the lining of the bowel, and is inhibited by cortisol.

Norepinedrine is an amino acid that is considered a neurotransmitter when found in the brain and is considered a hormone when released from the adrenal medulla (more on this later). It is made with the amino acid tyrosine.

Its effects:

Norepinedrine arouses. This neurotransmitter is responsible for waking us from sleep. It gives us get up and go. It is active in the stress response. It increases heart rate, breathing rate and decreases digestive processes. It helps us think quickly and run fast.

Signs of Imbalance

- Racing thoughts
- Insomnia
- Chronically busy
- Intolerant to cold
- Abdominal weight gain
- Eating at night
- Hair loss

Herbs that effect it

Coffee, cola and ephdra.

Note: ephdra is a plant from TCM materia medica used to dilate the bronchi during asthma attacks. At one time it was used as a nutritional supplement to promote weight loss and increase energy The misuse of ephedra caused deaths and resulted laws that limit its use as a supplement.

Other interesting facts

Caffeine indirectly triggers norepinephrine release from the adrenal glands by inhibiting a calming neurotransmitter adenosine. Adenosine turns off a neurons firing activity. Caffeine fills adenosine receptors that turn off a neurons activity With extra neuron activity occurring, the pituitary thinks, "Oh something is up, I better get this body moving" and signals the secretion of norepinephrine.

Acetylcholine is a neurotransmitter found in both the CNS and the PNS. It is made from choline.

Its effects:

It has a paradoxical effect. It can relax a muscle such as the heart (a smooth muscle), or it can excite skeletal muscles causing contraction.

Signs of Imbalance
- Those suffering with Alzheimer's have a shortage acetylcholine
- Muscle weakness associated with chronic disease
- Parkinson's: acetylcholine is the counter balance to dopamine in the body.

Herbs that effect it

Lobelia

Other interesting facts.

The bacteria Botulinum blocks the movement of acetylcholine from neuron to on to muscle. This is why botox treatment (made from an injection of botulinum toxin) freezes the smile in place.

Dopamine is also an amino acid made from tyrosine. It is a neurotransmitter found in the brain and heart. Dopamine is closely related to norepinephrine.

Its effect:

Dopamine coordinates muscle movement (think of Parkinson disease which results in tremors and hesitancy of movement). It also plays a role in our emotional response.

Signs of Imbalance

- Depression
- Parkinson's Disease
- Fatigue
- Social Anxiety
- Heavy Menstrual cycles
- High or Low Blood Pressure
- Depressed libido
- Learning Disorders
- Need to use caffeine to get alert

Herbs that effect it.

Gingko and green tea

Other interesting facts.

Dopamine is the reward we receive when we are praised. Drinking beer and music also triggers it.

The Vessel: A Home for Transformation
Lady Slippers

In the beautiful book *Earth's Blanket* by ethnobotanist Nancy Turner writes about the relationship between the First Nations people who live in the southern Interior of British Columbia and grasses and small plants that inhabit the region. As the First Nations wandered across the land that sustained their lives, they referred to the low growing green plants as Earth's Blanket.

I wonder what they called the humans, particularly the greedy ones. You know the ones who reap so much and sow so little. Happiness appears to elude them.

Nancy Turner writes about the hooves of cattle trampling the delicate native grasses and wild flowers. Their massive collective weight hardens the soil. Fragile rootlets cannot penetrate in the calloused soil. The blanket's weave becomes thin like an old woman's skin.

My mind turns to violet, a shy flower seeking protection in the shade of other plants. Her heart shaped petals are purple or soft pink; pink the colour of the heart, purple the colour of inspiration. Both are so easily trampled.

I remember when the construction of the new subdivision began in the field behind my home. The field was dotted with Lady Slippers. "You can't stand in the way of progress", said the heir to the land. With my heart in my belly I dug up the Yellow Lady Slippers blooming yellow in the field. My friends were happy to receive them in their gardens.

Now where the erotic Yellow Lady Slippers hid in the tall grasses, bright petunias bloom. Every spring, the basements in the new subdivision flood. The homeowners stand on their lawns scowling and cursing the builder. They thought they would be happy. Walking past them, I become unhappy.

Previous years, in late spring, I walked in the same place, seeking Lady Slippers. Their raw feminine beauty enjoyed the sun while their roots sipped from the cool, damp earth. Finding them was not always

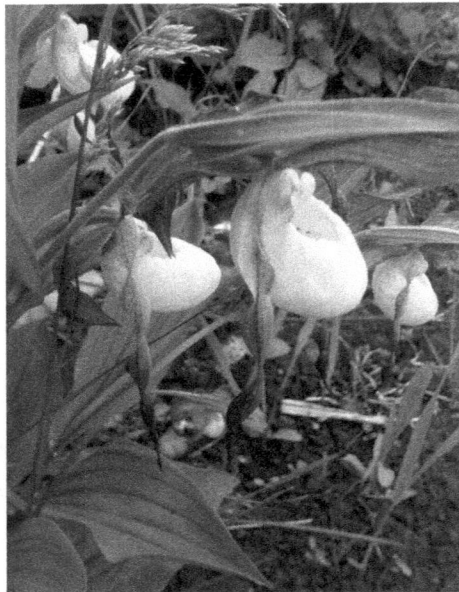

Lady Slippers Abrah Arneson

easy. They enjoyed their privacy. A moment with them always brought happiness. Knowing they grew so wild so close brought me comfort, like a soft blanket on cold winters night.

Happiness? Perhaps happiness is a quiet moment. It may not require loud noises, or bright colours. In my life, happiness often coincides with simplicity, like the lady's slippers irresistible braids.

In herbal medicine, Lady's Slipper's roots were used to calm female hysteria. I have been known to become hysterical; usually when something is terribly wrong and no one wants to listen.

A woman told me the story of her breast cancer. "I knew something was wrong," she said, "call it woman's intuition. But I found something else to keep my mind busy. Then it was too late. Now I have lost my breasts."

I told her about the Lady Slippers. Then we both knew what was wrong. The Lady Slippers have disappeared.

Perhaps I will take up knitting.

The Vessel

This central symbol is the vessel. From the very beginning down to the latest stages of development we find this archetypal symbol as essence of the feminine. This basic symbolic equation woman=body=vessel corresponds to what is perhaps mankind's - man's as well as woman's - most elementary experience of the Feminine.

The experience of the body as a vessel is universally human and not limited to woman. What we have designated as "metabolic symbolism" is an expression of this phenomenon of the body as vessel....Its entrance and exit zones are of special significance. Food and drink are put into this unknown vessel, while in all creative functions, from the

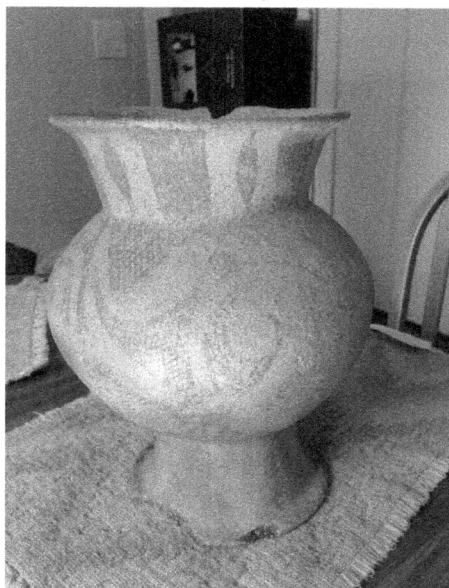

Loas Pot   Abrah Arneson

elimination of wastes and the emission of seed to the giving forth of breath and the word, something is "born" out of it. - The Great Mother: An Analysis of the Archetype by Eric Neumann

Standing in the chilled room, masked, gloved, and wearing white lab coat to protect me from the chemicals used to preserve the dead bodies surrounding me, the dissected body parts amazed and shocked me. The sciatic nerve was as thick as a strip of sinew, eyes glistened like pearls, ovaries were as soft as the flesh of a clam and the sooty blackness of a smoker's lung repulsed me. What astonished me, and I mean left me speechless, was the difficulty in finding a female body with an intact uterus. Approximately 600,000 hysterectomies are performed each year in the United States, the second most common surgery for woman of reproductive age. Caesareans take the number one spot.

The uterus is the vessel where life comes into being through the mysterious mingling of sperm and ovum. The uterus is the container where life is nurtured and from where it is birthed. The uterus is the centre of beginnings and endings of a woman's life. Conception, infertility, pregnancy, miscarriage, birth and blood loss, all events that take place within the uterus, profoundly influence a woman's life. They bring her great joy or devastating sorrow. One could say that the uterus is the vessel of a woman's creativity. Surely there must be more that can be done for a woman and her uterus than to cut into the soft flesh of her belly and rip out her container for life. Well guess what? There is!

In this chapter we will unearth the delicate steps of women's ancient endocrine system dance and come to appreciate the intimate relationship between sex hormones and the female body, mind, emotions and spirit.

Just as plants are more than "what they do", a woman is more than her hormones. Over the years, I have come to more fully understand the complex dance, the waxing and waning of a woman's hormones.

This journey began in the girl's change room at the age of 13 when our gym teacher, a woman who could do a hand stand and get the ball in the basket every time, tried to explain the "mystery" of a young lady's period. We giggled, and she shifted from foot to foot and I learned that tampons are less conspicuous than pads. Or in other words, your period is not something anyone else should know about. There is so much more to sex education.

To begin, the purpose of sex, contrary to popular belief, is not pleasure. It's all about reproduction. Perhaps sexual pleasure is a decoy that dupes humans into having offspring. The pursuit of pleasure has maintained the human population since the very beginning. The mind and heart seek pleasure. The body just wants to reproduce.

If the body's purpose is to reproduce, it has to live long enough to perform this function. This is where the intimate relationship between the nervous system and the endocrine system come in. The nervous system is about survival. It concerns itself with finding food for the body, while making sure the body does not become food. The endocrine system is about reproduction: make an egg, release an egg, and get said egg fertilized.

It is the role of the pituitary gland to choreograph the dance of the nervous and endocrine system.

Pituitary Gland: The Queen

The pituitary gland is a pea-sized queen who sits in the middle of the brain. She has two distinctive sides. One side, her posterior, contains 10,000 or so neurons that are concerned about hunger, thirst, rage, fear, etc. The posterior side of the pituitary ensures the gathering of life's basic survival needs.

One could say, the posterior gland is about keeping us alive long enough to reproduce. Her other side, the anterior, controls the body's metabolism, growth, development and homeostasis through the production and release of hormones. This side of the gland focuses on reproduction.

Like every queen, the pituitary relies on a messenger. Her messenger is the hypothalamus. He collects information about hormone levels in the body from the brain and the blood and relays the gathered data to the queen, who then decides which hormones to release.

Hormone secretion works on a negative feedback loop. When the hypothalamus senses a decline in a specific hormone, it messages the pituitary and she releases sequences of stimulating hormones. The stimulating hormones travel through the blood stream to their specific endocrine gland. After the stimulating hormone engages with the targeted gland, an action hormone is released. As the action hormone levels raise in the blood stream, the hypothalamus signals the pituitary to reduce the secretion of the stimulating hormone and the target gland slows the release of the action hormone.

Let's look at how the thyroid gland works. When thyroid hormones drop, the hypothalamus alerts the pituitary gland. The Queen secretes TSH (Thyroid Stimulating Hormone) that floats through the blood stream to the thyroid gland. When TSH interacts with the thyroid, it releases two hormones, T3 and T4. T3 affects all levels of the body's metabolism, while T4 is for spare parts and is sequestered away in the liver. T4 is later transformed into T3.

A Brief Outline of a Woman's Cycle

Day One: the first day of menstruation On this day, the hypothalamus notes the woman's sex hormones are low and forwards this information to the pituitary. The pituitary, interested in procreation, releases FSH, or follicle stimulating hormone--or as I like to call it, "Fresh Start Hormone". FSH causes follicles containing immature eggs to begin to develop on the ovary. Essentially, a follicle is a seedpod and the eggs are the seed.

From day one to ovulation: During this time, the follicles on the ovaries release estrogen. Estrogen has one purpose, and that is to make pregnancy possible. To do this, several bodily changes need to occur that estrogen takes care of:

- Building a welcoming uterus, rich in blood (nutrients and oxygen).
- Creating a gooey, thick cervical fluid that nourishes sperm and facilitate the swimmers' journey to the egg.
- Enhancing secretion of serotonin. Serotonin is a hormone that creates optimism. For most women, sex is more than just a physical experience. It is about possibilities, whether it is the possibility of a baby, a blossoming love affair, or an expression of deep hunger for pleasure. An open mind, heart and vagina is enhanced with the flow of serotonin between neurons. Depression, a shortage of serotonin, causes libido to go flat.
- Attracting men. Many studies have shown men find women with higher estrogen levels more beautiful than those in the second phase of their cycle when the estrogens levels taper off.

Many women are taught ovulation occurs on day 13th. This is not true. Ovulation occurs when the pituitary learns from the hypothalamus that there is a sufficient amount of estrogen in the blood stream to ensure a mature egg. She then releases LH, or luteinizing hormone. I call this hormone the "Getting Laid Hormone".

I have one client who says she always knows when LH is spiking in her blood stream and she is ovulating. At red lights, she develops the sudden urge to jump the guy in the truck next to her. Another woman told me that when she is ovulating she has to refrain from chasing men down the street. Luteinizing hormones, through sensitizing a woman to male pheromones, do everything they can to make sure she loses her head by falling temporarily and utterly in lust.

About a day after the LH"s release, the biggest and strongest egg bursts from the follicle and it floats into the abdomen to be swept up moments later by the fibrils of the fallopian tubes. Then, seeking sperm, it journeys to the uterus.

Ovulation to First Day of Bleeding: The egg leaves behind on the ovary a small hormone making corpus luteum (or in English "yellow body"). The corpus luteum secretes progesterone once the egg has been ushered down the fallopian tube.

Progesterone's job is to keep the ovum (a fertilized egg) growing in the uterus. I always think of progesterone as "pro-gestation." The second phase of a woman's cycle is a time of nesting. The second phase of the cycle is a wait and see period of time. Perhaps the pituitary has had her way and the woman is pregnant.

Progesterone is a more introverted hormone than estrogen. Progesterone is best friends with the neurotransmitters dopamine and GABA. Both these neurotransmitters create a pleasurable and calming effect on the body/mind. They both are used to bring on a deep, peaceful sleep. Where higher estrogen levels keep one up all night, progesterone promotes more REM time during sleep.

The second phase of a woman's cycle is her time for reflection and dreaming. It's her time for dreaming her baby into being, or perhaps dreaming herself into her next cycle of being. A woman's cycle is much like the waxing and waning moon: estrogen is the waxing moon, moving to the bright light in the night, whereas progesterone is the waning moon, with the night becoming darker and darker until there is no moon at all.

Two weeks pass and if the egg has not met up with sperm, the corpus luteum disintegrates, progesterone levels in the blood drop and the uterus begins to shed. If the egg is fertilized it begins to release a hormone called human chorionic gonadotropin (HCG). HCG prolongs the life of the corpus luteum sustaining the release of progesterone.

Because the pituitary gland is so intricately involved in the regulation of sex hormones for women, many begin a treatment to balance hormones with Vitex, an herb that specifically acts on the pituitary.

Chaste Berry *(Vitex agnus-castus)* If the pituitary is the Queen, Vitex (also called Chaste Berry), is the Queen of herbal medicine when it comes to hormonal balance. Vitex is a tiny seed that grows on a shrub from southern Europe. These days Chaste Berry shrubs also grow on the west coast of Canada.

Vitex is an essential plant in the herbalist's apothecary. It balances female sex hormones by enhancing the pituitary's secretion of LH.

Luteinizing hormone turns on the libido. Many women find taking vitex stimulates their desire. Vitex has the opposite effect on men. It decreases their libido. In the middle ages, monks sworn to celibacy took vitex to help them maintain their vows. This is how the tiny berry came by the name "Chaste Berry" or "Monk's Pepper".

Today, vitex is useful for boys entering puberty and suddenly diagnosed with ADD or ADHD. Boys entering puberty have ten times the amount of testosterone surging through their body than they did one year earlier. Testosterone coursing through a 14 year old's blood can cause aggressive behavior and an uncontrolled obsession with female body parts. Several times I have helped such young men refocus with vitex, calming the testosterone surges. Along with vitex I encourage martial arts training to discipline their minds. Without interfering with their overall sexual development, vitex makes life easier for boys in the throes of puberty.

In women, LH supports the corpus luteum. A healthy corpus luteum ensures sufficient progesterone in the blood stream. Progesterone is a counter-balance to the estrogens. As progesterone rises in the blood stream, estrogen declines.

I like to call estrogen the womb builder. When estrogen "over builds", women suffer with conditions like endometriosis, fibroids or heavy, heavy periods. By encouraging an increase in LH secretion, taking vitex promotes a larger, healthier corpus luteum. A strong corpus luteum results in an increase of progesterone in the blood stream, moderating the effects of estrogen. Vitex is very useful in slowing excessive bleeding caused by shedding layers of endometrium that were built by estrogen's enthusiasm for pregnancy.

Progesterone is also the "calm" hormone. Recall its preference for hanging out with dopamine and GABA. Vitex eases the storms of PMS as well as deepens sleeps and improves dreams.

Overall, I use Vitex for women in transition. Most hormonal imbalances occur during a life transition, such as from girl to adolescent, from birth control pills to the desire for pregnancy, from pregnancy to nursing, from nursing to weaning, from reproductive years to menopause, single to married, married to divorce and so on. All these transitions in a woman's life may bring on hormone imbalance, particularly when there is stress involved. At times of change in a woman's life I always think of Vitex.

Vitex is a safe herb, with few side effects. It is terrible tasting and can initially cause nausea. The one consideration to take into account when offering Vitex is that it generally takes 4 to 6 weeks before its effects become evident. This is why.Think of the endocrine system as a very old part of the body's physiology. While the reactive speedy nervous system travelling like lightening across synapses is all about survival, hormones flow. Hormones float through the blood, engaging cell receptors here and there, like tourists on a Caribbean cruise sailing from island to island. For this reason, changing the course of hormones with herbal medicine requires patience. This is true of both herbs affecting the sex hormones and the adrenal cortex.

What is a Hormone?

There are two types of hormones: water soluble hormones (similar to neurotransmitters) and fat soluble ones. Sex hormones are fat-soluble. Sex hormones are part protein and part fat.

Hormones interact with receptors on cell membranes much like keys turning locks to open doors. The fat part of the hormone is the key that fits into the cell receptor. Once the door is open, the hormone brings the cell under its influence. The cell follows the hormone's every whim. For example: fat cells grow when estrogens open their door. In the brain, estrogen asks neurons to be more receptive to serotonin. In the uterus, estrogen triggers arterial cells to grow and spread. (This process is called angiogenesis; we will look at this and the role of breast cancer a little further along.)

The protein part of the hormone is the fat's chauffeur. Wrapped in protein, the fatty hormone floats through the blood stream. Without the protein, the hormone would not be able to travel through the blood.

A diet low in fat or protein over an extended period of time leads to hormonal challenges. The body simply does not have the tools it needs to make hormones. This is why those suffering with malnutrition, whether through illness or anorexia, cease to have a period. This condition is called amenorrhoea.

A diet high in fat can also produce hormonal challenges. Remember, estrogens love fat and fat loves estrogens. Weight loss is recommended in conditions like polycystic ovary syndrome when multiple cysts develop on the ovary while they cease having periods. Women suffering with endometriosis should also look at their diet very carefully. On the other hand, adolescent girls need to be at least 100 pounds before they start menstruating. Just before a girl reaches the 100-pound mark would be a valuable time to begin explaining the changes her body is about to go through.

Another challenge to a woman's hormonal balance is exogenous hormones, synthetic estrogens found the environment she lives in and in the food she eats. Estrogens not produced by a woman's body are called exogenous estrogens. Exogenous estrogens enter a woman's body from cows fed estrogen in feedlots to fatten them up just before slaughter (remember estrogens build), air and water borne residues of pesticides and herbicides, and food stored in plastics. Remnants of synthetic hormones used in hormone replacement therapy and birth control pills also find their way into her drinking water.

Sufficient protein, good fats and cooking with organic, whole foods are essential for the health of a woman's reproductive cycle.

Estrogen and the Thyroid

Estrogens fill receptors on the thyroid gland that are meant for thyroid stimulating hormone, which is another hormone released from the pituitary.

Let's think about what is happening during the 1st half of a woman's cycle while estrogen is most active. Her body is preparing to get pregnant. Estrogen is building a womb. It is also increasing the size of fat cells in case the woman needs resources to support two lives. To do both of these activities, estrogen needs to slow down the woman's metabolism. The thyroid gland is in charge of the body's metabolism. To accomplish the slowdown, estrogen fills receptors on the thyroid meant to receive thyroid-stimulating hormone (TSH). Estrogen blocks the work of TSH. This temporarily slows the production of T3 and T4. After ovulation when progesterone levels start to rise in her body, estrogens detach from the thyroid and metabolism speeds up. The woman now needs a quicker metabolism, because her body may be supporting two lives.

The Liver

The liver's role in hormonal balance is substantial. I frequently refer to the liver as the body's factory. Like many factories, the liver receives raw materials to make new products. A prudent factory owner gathers as much raw materials from recycled material as possible. Doing business this way is sustainable. If the liver were a business, it would be a sustainable one. The liver receives previously used hormones and dismantles them. It then recycles some hormone parts, stores others, disposes of the left overs, and makes new ones. The liver essentially sorts everything that comes into your body or is made by your body. This includes food, drugs, alcohol, enzymes, amino acids, etc. The liver is a busy place.

Now if the liver is hyper busy with pesticides, alcohol, pharmaceutical drugs, fatty fried junk food, etc., the hormones that need to be processed are put on the back burner. This is why most hormonal formulas include some liver herbs.

Vervain (*Verbena officinalis* - European or *Verbena hastata* - North American) likes tall, nervous, thin women. Or perhaps if she is not tall and thin, she relies heavily on her head and has a finely tuned nervous system. Vervain helps the organizers of the world. It loves the women who create lists and keep things moving tickity boom. Just as a little vervain makes the liver's job of sorting out the necessities for life by unclogging its channels, vervain helps women ease up on their endless lists and enjoy a little spontaneity.

Vervain also contains plant medicine called phytoestrogens. What are phytoestrogens?

Phytoestrogens come in many forms. Sometimes they are isoflavones, as in red clover, sometimes lignans, as in soy, or sometimes they have a steroidal component as in licorice's saponins.

Essentially phytoestrogens are similar in structure to the estrogens the human body makes. Just like the estrogens found in plastic or meat from feedlots, phytoestrogens are called exogenous estrogens, as they come from outside the body. Estrogens that the body makes are called endogenous estrogens.

The difference between the estrogens the body makes and the estrogens that plants make are that phytoestrogens are smaller. Just like endogenous estrogens, phytoestrogens fit the lock and key mechanism on the surface of the cell. However, because of phytoestrogen's smaller size, they do not have the power to turn the key, open the door and change the cell's activity. With fewer estrogens attached to cell membranes, more endogenous estrogens are floating around in the blood. The hypothalamus reading the blood makes note of the excess estrogen floating around and signals the pituitary to do something about it. The liver also becomes busy disassembling the extra estrogen floating around. Succinctly put, phytoestrogens keeps the body's own estrogen (endogenous estrogens) in circulation, supporting their removal.

Vervain's phytoestrogens help reduce the effects of estrogens on the cells, and supports the liver in clearing it from the body.

Just as a note: vervain, like many bitters, is a traditional anti-depressant. Recall that excess estrogen interferes with the activity of the thyroid gland producing the symptoms of hypothyroidism.

The Adrenal Glands

Adrenal tonics (adaptogenic herbs) are the darlings of alternative health practitioners these days. But what are the adrenal glands and what do they have to do with female hormonal balance?

Adrenaline - A Review

Adrenaline is the fight or flight hormone released from the interior portion of the adrenal glands called the medulla. Adrenaline is blaring red lights and survival at all costs. Under the influence of adrenaline, long term planning, digesting food or ideas or pausing for a moment to clear up thinking is not possible. Adrenaline leaves two options: duke it out or run.

Historically, adrenaline surges into the body/mind were short term, as in BEAR=RUN. When running from bears, one is not particularly concerned with having children. Long-term adrenaline hits have a profound effect on a woman's hormonal balance. Today many live life as if it is a long fight or flight. Besides painful periods complete with severe mood swings, these women often/typically present with headaches, weak digestive tracts and insomnia. Adrenaline fries a woman like too many hair dyes. The key to helping woman soaked in adrenaline is to help them relax and let go of the fight. Try flower essences, nervines and cardio exercise.

Cortisol

The cortisol secreted from the adrenal cortex is a long-term stress hormone. Unlike adrenaline which burns calories, cortisol is into long term planning. One could say cortisol fills the pantry. Cortisol makes belly fat.

So why are these little caps so important in female hormonal balance? Let's take a look at progesterone.

In the evolutionary process, it is speculated that progesterone is the oldest hormone on the planet. A conservative estimate for progesterone's age is 500 million years. Some believe progesterone first came into being with vascular plants. Progesterone is recycled to make other hormones including estrogens and cortisol. When stress is unrelenting, free progesterone floating around in the blood stream is used up to make cortisol. This results in less progesterone in the blood stream to moderate the effects of estrogen. Estrogen without progesterone's restraint builds the uterus' endometrium and results in conditions like endometrioses, fibroids, heavy periods, difficulty losing weight and a sluggish thyroid. Many female cancers also love estrogen. Estrogen helps cancer build networks of blood vessels to feed its ravenous habit.

Case History: Estrogen Excess with Progesterone Deficiency

Louise was 51 years old and in menopause. Menopause was being gentle with Louise. She was experiencing a few hot flashes, unpredictable periods, and some moodiness. Over all, Louise considered herself lucky. Then her son had a car accident. He was in the ICU for months. She was at his bedside day and night. The day after he moved out of the ICU, Louise woke three times in the night with soaking wet sheets. During the day, she began carrying extra shirts to change into after debilitating hot flashes. She felt like she was losing her mind. She was happy, sad, and angry all at the same time.

The adrenals relied on her progesterone stores to make the cortisol she needed while she sat at her son's bedside. Now that the stress had eased, her body sought balance, manifesting in imbalance.

Wild Yam (Dioscorea villosa)

The steroidal saponins in wild yam do not act as "hormonal precursors" inside the body, despite what can be read in some marketing literature. The human body lacks the enzyme to convert these compounds into sex hormones. However, steroidal saponins may influence hormones in other ways.   Herbal Constituents: Foundations of Phytochemistry,   - Lisa Ganora

Mexican Yam root was originally used to synthesize the first birth control pill as well as many other synthetic hormonal drugs such as prednisone and cortisone. Today the pharmaceutical industry prefers the soybean to make hormone replacement drugs. Many herbalists consider wild yam both an adaptogen and a hormonal regulator.

Herbalists use wild yam root to ease the symptoms of menopause, principally insomnia and hot flashes. Wild Yam root contains a constituent called diogenin which is a steroidal saponin.

No one knows exactly how diogenin and the other constituents contained in wild yam's root effects a woman's hormonal balance during menopause, but it does. Some say wild yam potentiates progesterone. Others think it may be due to wild yam's cleansing effect on the liver. The one thing I know is that it works. It helps menopausal women sleep, balances their moods, and moderates night sweats.

I tend to offer wild yam alongside an adaptogen because stress has such a profound impact on how a woman's body/mind is handling menopause. I also pair it with vitex, which you will remember is the herb for female transitions. A formula may look like this:

20 Wild Yam (*Dioscorea villosa*) Liver support, possible progesterone support

30 Rhodiola (*Rhodiola roscea*) Adaptogen (adrenal tonic)

20 Chaste Berry (*Vitex agnus-castus*)Hormonal balancer via the pituitary

30 Scullcap (*Scutellaria lateriflora*) Nervine for physical and mental tension

The Uterus - The Vessel

Let's begin by debunking a myth about the uterus. Many people believe that once a woman has had her children the uterus is no longer of value. This is not true. The uterus secretes a blood thinning hormone well into a woman's 70s.

The uterus (Latin for womb) is a sensitive environment. Some believe a woman's uterus is intimately and energetically bound to her heart. Wounds to the uterus are wounds to her heart. Unfortunate life events such as miscarriages, abortions, infertility, the loss of a child, or sexual abuse or misconduct leave deep wounds on a woman's heart and her uterus. These events are often shrouded in taboo and some believe speaking of them is to invite further misfortune.

In my family there is a belief that to announce a pregnancy before the beginning of the second trimester is to tempt a miscarriage. Wrapped in the cocoon of this belief, miscarriages become secret life passages to be hidden away. Why do women not talk about miscarriages? Perhaps a miscarriage reflects on the woman's inherent value; women do after all give their partners children. Perhaps the profound sadness that can occur with a miscarriage is too painful for most people to witness. Whatever the reason miscarriages are hidden, it is essential for a clinical herbalist to have a heart to heart and womb to womb talk with every woman she sees who is experiencing hormonal challenges. Often once the grief concerning the uterus' loss is expressed, there is a profound shift in hormonal balance.

Motherwort (*Leonurus cardiaca*) It's minus 26 degrees this morning. Over my morning coffee, I flip through seed catalogues, dreaming of spring and consider growing exotic herbs this summer, like something from China perhaps. An image of Chinese herb gardens surrounded by old stone walls and women wearing wide, flat hats drift through my mind. In the distance, I hear a lute. I turn the page of the catalogue to find motherwort seeds for sale. It does not require much imagination on my part to dream up motherwort. Motherwort commands one corner of my garden. This spring, I know she will try to take over again.

If I could only have fifteen plants, motherwort would be one of them. Motherwort is one of my teaching herbs. I use it to demonstrate the Doctrine of Signatures. The Doctrine of Signatures is found in every traditional form of herbal medicine. Traditions that are faith-based believe that God left a mark on every medicinal herb to guide humans to its use. Others believe that the Doctrine is a device used by budding herbalists to remember the uses of herbs. The Doctrine of Signatures is not for literalists.

In the garden, motherwort grows tall and stately. Like other plants from the mint family, motherwort's stem has four flat sides. Motherwort is strong and sturdy yet flexible. From the stem, soft leaves reach out. They are dark grayish green and shaped like hands with fingers spread. After nibbling on a leaf, a bitter taste lingers on the tongue. Motherwort's small, nondescript pink flowers are sweet. Bees hover about them, satisfying their thirst for nectar. Motherwort is not a beauty. She is a handsome plant.

This description of the plants informs quite clearly its medicinal uses. Motherwort above all is medicine for the anxious heart. It is specific for soothing the overwrought heart of caregivers. When anxiety grabs hold of the heart, a flurry of activity is created as superwoman tries to take care of too much. Or sometimes anxiety stops one from acting at all, and stuck in worry, the caregiver lays awake at night fretting.

A simplistic but effective definition of anxiety is the loss of one's centre. Recall motherwort's tall, sturdy, but flexible stem. The stately stem rising up through the centre of many hand shaped leaves is a metaphor for a steady centre, the heart, and caring hands. Motherwort calms hearts. It brings a pause to the day and peaceful sleep in the night. Motherwort helps one re-centre. Under the influence of motherwort all one's actions stem from the heart.

Motherwort is added to formulas designed to relieve high blood pressure associated with anxiety. Motherwort tincture also settles heart palpations caused by anxiety attacks, and/or menopause.

While motherwort soothes a worried heart, it is also indispensable in easing uterine cramps. Many doctors and healers who work with women's gynaecological challenges such as endometriosis, fibroids and infertility, intuitively feel that illnesses associated with uterus and ovaries reflect back to a time when the heart was broken.

This is a holistic point of view, or mind/body medicine. Motherwort is a perfect example of mind/body medicine. It eases the emotional turmoil of the mind, quiets a struggling heart and soothes a uterus in physical pain.

It is my experience that many women, fearing surgery, leave uterine concerns too long. Few women welcome the idea of having their uterus scraped or removed. Uncertain about all their available options, women hope something changes, gets better or just goes away. As most uterine conditions involve heavy bleeding, women will bleed and bleed and bleed before deciding on a course of treatment. Postponing research and decisions about their fibroids or endometriosis, women succumb to the depression of anemia and are left with no energy to make an informed decision. I think the learned secrecy that cloaks issues surrounding the womb come into play here.

In my practice I have rescued more than one uterus from a hysterectomy. In one case, a twenty-six year old woman with severe cramps was told after birth control pills failed to reduce

Abortion

The wound of abortion is cloaked in a profound darkness for many women. The moral ambiguity of terminating a pregnancy leaves a smear of shame on many women's hearts and wombs. Although Canada is one of few countries in the world where a woman can decide to terminate a pregnancy in a safe, professional environment, there are complications that she should know before making this difficult decision.

Abortion is a procedure called Aspiration D&C or dilation & curettage. During an abortion the cervix is dilated, the contents of the womb are sucked out, and then an instrument called a curet is used to scrape the endometrium. This is a common medical procedure used not only for abortions but also to remove any remaining placenta after a miscarriage or conditions of uterine overgrowth such as endometriosis, fibroids and uterine cancer. If a D&C is performed without extreme care, the layer of the endometrium (called the basilis layer) can be removed. This is the underlying layer of the endometrium that is responsible for the growth of the uterine walls with each cycle. When the basilis layer is removed the endometrium will no longer thicken and will be too thin to support a fertilized ovum. This condition is called Asherman's Syndrome. Ninety percent of all cases of Asherman's Syndrome are due to a D&C. No matter how common a surgical procedure is, there are always risks. I strongly recommend seeking several opinions before accepting surgery as the only way to care for your uterus.

the pain with her bleeding, that her only option was a hysterectomy. She arrived in my office hysterical. She had always dreamed of having five children! After two months of herbs and getting off the prescribed birth control pill the pain resolved. She now has a beautiful but challenging three year old daughter.

Sometimes overcoming uterine challenges with herbal medicine and nutritional changes requires patience, determination and perseverance to undo years of estrogen's enthusiastic overgrowth but it is possible.

Raspberry leaf *(Rubus Sp.)* is probably the most pleasant hormonal herb in the apothecary. It is a lovely tea.

Herbalists say Raspberry leaf tones the uterus. Toning involves astringency. Raspberry's astringent action is due to its high tannin content.

I generally like to combine raspberry leaf with nettles in a tea and use it for all conditions affecting the uterus. Raspberry and nettles are high in calcium, iron, folic acid, potassium, phosphorus and magnesium, as well as Vitamin A and C, just to name a few. I consider this beautiful green tea nature's prenatal vitamin and excellent for replenishing mineral stores after prolonged bleeding. Adding some rosehips will make the minerals even more bioavailable.

When a woman is struggling with fibroids or endometriosis, drinking several cups of raspberry leaf and nettle tea a day will heal the womb. I recommend drinking raspberry and nettle leaf tea throughout pregnancy. Many of the Moms I work with report fewer if any cravings when taking this pregnancy tea and have all had very good births. Raspberry leaf has never created a challenge.

Why is there so much controversy around when to drink raspberry leaf tea during pregnancy? Perhaps it is the alkaloid fragarine found in rich concentration in raspberry's leaf. This alkaloid, along with the plant's tannins, relaxes and tones the pelvis and uterine muscles. It makes the uterus stretchy without losing elasticity. Plants containing alkaloids are generally contra-indicated in pregnancy as most can affect the developing fetus' nervous system. Famous alkaloids are nicotine and caffeine. (Note that alkaloids usually end in "ine"). But this is not the case for fragarine. Personally, I think as most doctors and orthodox health care professionals know next to nothing about herbs, they decide to play it safe and caution against them. This is certainly the case with raspberry leaf and pregnancy.

Just another testimonial about Raspberry Leaf from herbalist/midwife Willa Shaffer:

"It prevents morning sickness, strengthens the uterus, prevents miscarriages "in most cases", makes delivery more rapid and prevents tearing of the cervix."

Raspberry leaf is not just for women. It is used in China to promote fertility in men. Chinese herbalists use it to stop leaking fluids. I suspect that its action on the prostate is toning,

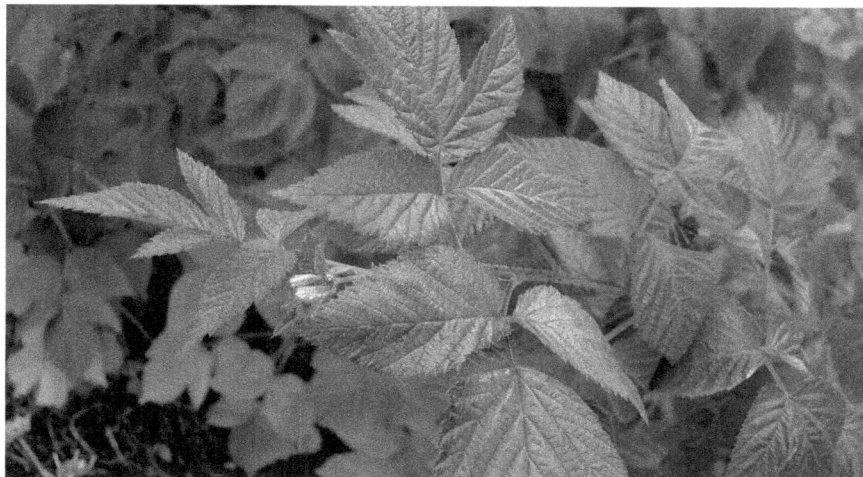

Raspberry Leaf   Rosalee de la Forêt

just like it is on the uterus. Raspberry leaf protects the prostate from becoming boggy. I think "boggy" is a perfect signature for raspberry leaf. It protects tissues from becoming boggy. A leaking uterus is one of the initial signs of a pending miscarriage.

The Ovaries

The Taoists, an ancient wisdom tradition from China, believe that a woman's life force flows from her ovaries.

When a female child is born, her ovaries are formed and within them contain all the possible lives she may birth during her life. This means the ovum from which you received half of your DNA grew inside your Grandmother's body. Like life moments cocooned within memories, ovaries carry knowledge of other times and other places from when your Grandmother carried your mother within her uterus.

In biology, there is a study called Epigenetics that considers inherited traits that are not necessarily defined by one's DNA.

Some who study epigenetics suggest that when an illness comes on at a young age (for instance lung cancer at age 42 with no history of smoking, second hand smoke or being exposed to carcinogenic substances over an extended period of time) it may be beneficial to consider what was going on in the grandmother's life during the time of her pregnancy with Mom. There is speculation that unknown toxins or severe stresses in her life may dramatically influence the long term life force or DNA sequencing of not only her children's lives, but also the lives of her grandchildren.

The First Nation's people believe that one needs to consider the effects of one's actions on seven generations into the future. This belief is currently used to express concern over the long-term effects on the environment. Considering the profound effect a grandmother's life has on her grandchildren's health, it is not such a stretch to see deeper implications of one's activities on future generations.

During the cadaver anatomy class we were fortunate to see ovaries. They were like clams; delicate and complex in their smallness. Vulnerable. One condition herbalists frequently treat is ovarian cysts. Cysts can interfere with ovulation and result in fertility challenges. Sometimes the woman has not had a problem becoming pregnant, but the cysts are a source of extreme pain. In either case, there is a herb that will dissolve ovarian cysts: red root (*Ceanothus americanus*). I first learned about using this herb for ovarian cysts from American herbalist Meryl Ann Kastin Flacchoni. In clinic I have used it several times successfully in conjunction with *Vitex agnus castus* to regulate periods and remove cysts from ovaries.

Black Cohosh (*Cimicifuga racemosa*) is a famous menopausal herb and is a best-selling herb. It is reputed to stop hot flashes and calm irritation in menopausal women. Irritability and moodiness are the plant's keynote indications.

In 1876, Lydia Pinkham, a herbalist homesteader in Massachusetts, introduced Lydia Pinkham's Vegetable Compound. This herbal formula was marketed as a remedy for "female weakness". Taking this foul tasting formula, many women were relieved from the burden of dramatic hormonal swings. The remedy contained several herbs but black cohosh was the principal ingredient. Critics of Lydia Pinkham suggested that the high alcohol content in the herbal compound was the real reason for its popularity. In the 1800's, few women drank openly. The critics felt the formula relieved a woman's "thirst" for alcohol.

Today, clinical studies conducted in Germany have shown black cohosh regulates female hormones via the pituitary gland. Being the Queen of hormones, if the pituitary gland is not happy, no one is. Herbalists offer black cohosh not only to menopausal women, but also to women of every age who succumb to the darkness of hormonal swings.

Black Cohosh is an elegant perennial with wine coloured, feathered leaves. It graces Central Albertan gardens under the name of Bug Bane. This particular common name refers to the unpleasant odour the long spike of fairy-like white flowers produces. Bugs don't like the smell. This is also reflected in Black Cohosh's Latin name, *Cimicifuga* . *Cimi* in Latin means bug, and *fugare* means to take flight. The name also reflects the needs of women who do well on it. When a woman tells me that she just can get a moments peace and says, "-- they say, "Don't bug me!", I think, "Black Cohash."

Black Cohosh is not native to Central Alberta. Its natural home is the moist woodlands of Eastern Canada and the US. It needs a lot of water in prairie gardens to bloom. Black Cohosh has entered Western Herbal Medicine via the First Nations of the east. The word Cohosh comes from the Algonquin word for labour. Along with Blue Cohosh (*Caulophyllum thalictroides*), black cohosh was used to induce and shorten labour. For this reason, pregnant women should not use black cohosh

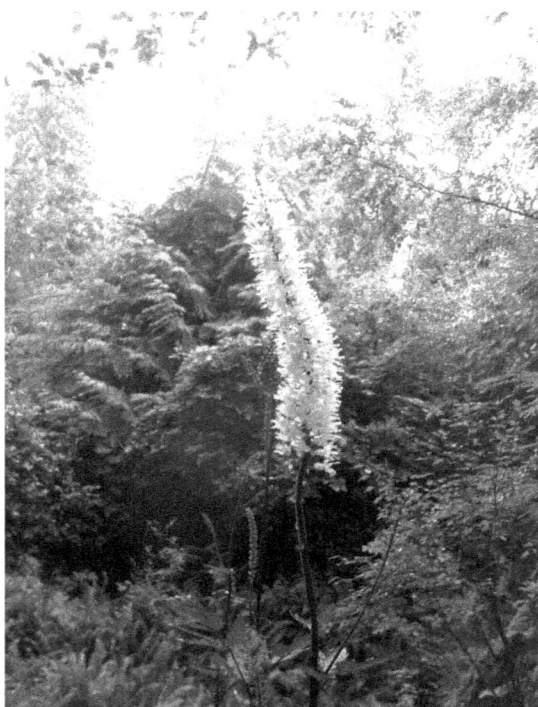

Black Cohosh   Abrah Arneson

during early pregnancy. It will bring on a miscarriage.

Besides bringing on labour and calming hormonal swings, black cohosh is a valuable remedy for relieving dull aching pain anywhere in the body. This is particularly true for pain associated with rheumatoid and osteoarthritis, neuralgia and fibromyalgia.

Black Cohosh relieves pain in three ways. First, it is an alterative with an anti-inflammatory effect. It supports the body in cleaning up the debris caused by inflammation. Secondly, it is calming to the nervous system, reducing the spasms that cause of the pain. For this reason black cohosh is also frequently added to formulas for bronchitis and other spasmodic coughs. Finally, black cohosh alters perception of pain in the brain. It calms the mind. A calm mind does not feel pain as intensely as an anxious mind.

Black Cohosh's root contains the medicine. I caution against going out in the backyard and digging up some root. Although some herbalists swear by a fresh root tincture of Black Cohosh, I advise against this for herbal dabblers. Black Cohosh belongs to the *Ranunculaceae* family, commonly called the Buttercup family. The plants in this family have very strong medicine and most are too toxic to be of medicinal value. To help the medicine settle, the root is dried before use. In the drying process, the root loses its toxic quality, making it good medicine. A prolonged use of over 6 months of large doses of Black Cohosh is still not advised. Large doses of this plant can cause nausea and headache. In any case, like most plants with strong medicine, Black Cohosh has a very repugnant flavour. The taste will limit the amount of Black Cohosh any one person can take at any given time.

Because of the medicinal strength of Black Cohosh, small amounts of it are generally used in a formula to augment the effects of other herbs. For example, a teenage girl with menstrual cramps may be given Black Cohosh with Cramp Bark (*Viburnum opulus*). A menopausal woman will find her anxiety decreases with Black Cohosh and Motherwort (*Leonurus cardiaca*). A man with rheumatoid arthritis may find Black Cohosh combined with Angelica (*Angelica archangelica*) relieves the inflammation and pain.

Black Cohosh is a complex and versatile herb. It is a plant of beauty and strength that helps the young, the middle aged, and the elderly. It is an essential plant in any herbalist's apothecary.

Breasts

Let's consider breasts. By the way, your breasts are for your pleasure, not his. They are right just the way they are! Hmmm, and this leads us to pleasure. Did you know the clitoris has over 8,000 nerve endings? That's twice as many as the penis! But we are getting off topic.

Nothing strikes fear in women like the words "Breast Cancer". Women whisper fears about breast cancer amongst themselves, terrified of having to cope with the scars it leaves on chests, the loss of hair, and perhaps the death. They also sell hot dogs and soft drinks in front of grocery stores and run car washes in bikinis on sunny hot days to raise money for breast cancer research. Is there a disconnect between fundraising for breast cancer research and preventative self-care? I feel a serious rant coming on about self-care and education as the key to prevention of breast cancer, as opposed to no self-care and little education when billions of dollars are raised to cure it through the sale of soft drinks, hot dogs and bikini's. Is not prevention the best cure?

Let's have a little education. Early detection is considered the most effective protection against breast cancer. But when is early detection too early?

Mayo Clinic supports screening beginning at age 40 because screening mammograms can detect breast abnormalities early in women in their 40s. Findings from a large study in Sweden of women in their 40s who underwent screening mammograms showed a decrease in breast cancer deaths by 29 percent.

But mammogram screening isn't perfect. Another study concluded that despite more women being diagnosed with early breast cancer due to mammogram screening, the number of women diagnosed with advanced breast cancer hasn't decreased. The study suggested that some women with early breast cancer were diagnosed with cancer that may never have affected their health.

Unfortunately doctors can't distinguish dangerous breast cancers from those that are non-life-threatening, so annual mammograms remain the best option for detecting cancer early and reducing the risk of death from breast cancer.   Mayo Clinic

There is something very unscientific about treating a cancer that may or may not grow to kill a woman. The side effects of cancer treatment are horrific and deadly. After cancer treatment a woman wears the scars of a mastectomy, suffers heart disease due to chemotherapy, and has brittle vertebrae due to radiation unnecessarily. When radiation is part of treatment, the majority of cancers return within 20 years. So much for the young woman growing old. Herbalist Chancel Cabrera who specializes in helping those with cancer using herbal medicine speaks of a curious finding in the States. In some states it is mandatory that an autopsy be done when there is an unexpected death, including car accidents. During these autopsies the coroners were finding scar tissue in breast tissue that suggested the resolution of cancer. Further research found that few of the women showing resolved breast cancer had ever been diagnosed.

Now that being said, women under 40 are at the highest risk of an aggressive, life-threatening cancer. This age group of women requires intensive education about prevention and signs of breast cancer. Women diagnosed in the 50's diagnosed with breast cancer and treated are likely to live into their 80's (many eventually die of breast cancer). It is this population that early diagnostic techniques are encouraged.

This population of women who are going through menopause are still offered hormone replacement therapy (HTR) for menopausal symptoms (which are not really symptoms, as symptoms are associated with disease and not natural changes due to aging). The longer a woman is on HRT the higher her risk of breast cancer (and uterine cancer if she still has her uterus, as well as ovarian cancer). A study involving one million women suggested that there will likely be 19 extra breast cancers diagnosed for every 1,000 women taking a combination of estrogen and progesterone over a period of 10 years. After a woman comes off HRT, the risk of developing cancer returns to "normal" after a five-year period.

Overall, I find the advice women are given about caring for their bodies and the prevention of breast cancer confusing and emotionally charged. Even though research now suggests that self-breast examinations are ineffective in discovering breast cancer, I think they are empowering for women. Particularly when a woman knows what kind of lump to look for.

Different types of lumps found on breasts
Fibrocystic Breast Disease

Despite its name, this is not a disease. These lumps are fluid filled cysts that appear with monthly hormonal cycles. Frequently (but not always) women who develop cysts also experience breast tenderness. During a breast exam, cysts squirm under fingers as gentle pressure is applied. Cysts are round, feel like a bubble and vary in size. There may only be one cyst but more frequently several are found.

Fibroadenomas

Fibroadenomas occur in women of every age. Unlike cysts, a fibroadenoma is not tender and they are singular. They first feel round during a self-breast exam but frequently change shape as a woman ages. Once a fibroadenoma forms, it does not come and go. Fibroadenomas, like cysts, move under fingers. A fibroadenoma rarely become cancerous.

Cancer

Just as a cyst and fibroadenomas have specific characteristics, so do lumps formed by cancer. Cancerous lumps are not round or smooth. They have irregular shapes and do not move under fingers. These lumps feel fixed to the breast. A cancerous lump does not change with hormonal cycles. They are not tender, but the breast, the back or chest may ache.

Red Clover (Trifolium pretense) If you use your imagination, red clover resembles a lymph node. Lymph nodes are circular maze-like structures that filter and vet the fluid of the body. Within the maze's nooks and crannies lie white blood cells waiting for nasty pathogens. Lymph nodes do their best work when fluid is flowing freely in the body. When the fluid becomes backed up, cysts develop.

Breasts are high in lymph nodes, which is why they are susceptible to cysts. When a node discovers a pathogen, it swells as the white blood cells they house multiply in preparation for the immune system's battle. When lymph nodes swell, whether due to fluid back up or as an immune response, red clover is the herb to choose (along with a little echinacea.) Red clover clears lymph nodes and has a particular affinity for the nodes of the neck, chest and breast.

In the meadow, the sphere-shaped red clover clings to moisture. Dew burrows deep into clover's cluster of flowers, making the flower a thirst-quenching treat on a hot day. Most flowers and leaves are picked for medicine once the morning dew has evaporated under the summer sun. I prefer to pick red clover after a couple of hot dry summer days. Then I lay the clover out on a thin metal mesh, careful that the flowers do not touch and leave them for a couple days. It is important to carefully feel the flowers before storing. If there is any moisture left in the flowers, they will turn mouldy in storage.

Unscrupulous herb gathers will use heat to dry red clover flowers. If heat is used the flowers will turn brown and lose their pink/purple colour. For good medicine, it is essential that the flowers retain as much as of their original colour as possible.

Red clover is an alterative herb. Alteratives were once called blood cleansers. Cleaning blood is now considered ridiculous in the medical world, for if the blood is dirty, one would be dead. We now know it is not the blood that stores toxins. Toxins are stored in interstitial fluid. This is the fluid which cells float in. Interstitial fluid is the body's ocean. Alteratives clean this fluid. Because interstitial fluid is cleansed via the lymphatic system, many alteratives have the ability to remove lymphatic stagnation.

If a toxin is really nasty, the body will build a wall around it. These swellings are also called cysts. Cysts form within interstitial fluid and again call for use of alteratives to limit their growth and gently allow the body to re-absorb and eliminate their contents.

Red Clover is an alterative with an affinity for the lymph nodes in the breast. Because of this, red clover has been a traditional breast cancer remedy for centuries. Cancer spreads through the body in two ways: via the blood and/or lymph. When cancer moves through the lymph, as it most frequently does in breast cancer, the herb of choice is the humble red clover. It has the ability to clean the lymphatic system. A tea of red clover flowers taken several times daily is an important remedy for breast cancers. Please be aware that it is not a matter of simply drinking the tea for a couple of weeks, but for months and months.

Red Clover is high in genistein, a flavonoid with significant anti-oxidant properties. It protects cells from mutation and improves the integrity of connective tissue. This is important in the treatment of cancer. Cancer eats through connective tissue and through a process called angiogenesis builds weak blood vessels to feed itself. It spreads when the weak vessels break or the connective tissue gives away.

Genistein also have the properties of phytoestrogens.. This is significant in the treatment of breast cancer. Most breast cancers live on the estrogen the body makes. The cancer puts out feelers, calling the estrogen hormone to turn the lock and key mechanism on the cell walls of the tumor. Estrogen gives cancer cells the energy to replicate.

Red Clover's estrogen also attracts to the cancer's feelers and

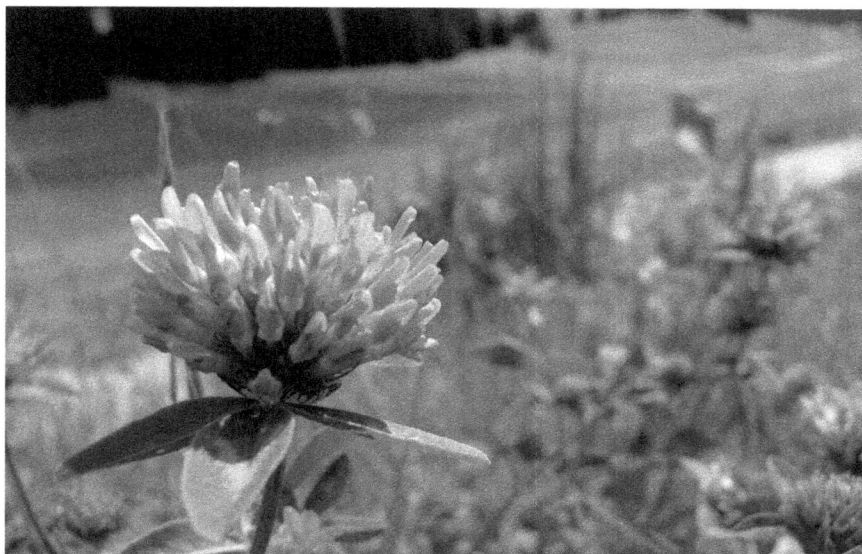

Red Clover   Rosalee de la Forêt

fits into the lock and key mechanism. However, it is not big enough to turn the lock. Genistein blocks the larger estrogen that the body makes from entering the lock. Hence the cancer does not eat and it does not have the energy to replicate.

Finally, Red Clover is very alkaline in nature. Cancer, along with most inflammatory diseases including eczema and psoriasis, prefer an acidic environment. Taking a tea of red clover with nettles and alfalfa will create an alkaline environment in the body.

Libido

Demeter herself no longer bathed. Her robes were mud drenched, her hair hung in dreadlocks. Even though the pain in her heart was staggering, she would not surrender. After many askings, pleadings, and episodes, all leading to nothing, she finally slumped down at the side of a well in a village where she was unknown. As she leaned her aching body against the cool stone of the well, along came a woman, or rather a sort of woman. And this woman danced up to Demeter wiggling her hips in a way suggesting sexual intercourse, and shaking her breast in her little dance. And when Demeter saw her, she could not help but smile just a little.

The dancing female was very magical indeed, for she had no head whatsoever, and her nipples were her eyes and her vulva was her mouth. It was through this lovely mouth that she began to regale Demeter with some nice juicy jokes. Demeter began to smile, and then chuckle, and then gave a full belly laugh. And together the women laughed, the little belly Goddess Baubo and the powerful Mother Earth Goddess, Demeter.

And it was just this laughing that drew Demeter out of her depression and gave her the energy to continue her search for her daughter...The world, the land, and the bellies of women thrived again.   Women Who Run with The Wolves Clarissa Pinkola Estes

Libido is such a challenge for so many women. A woman's libido is really all in her head! Perhaps that is why in Alice in Wonderland, the Queen of Hearts cuts off heads!

Let's peer into the complex tangle that is the female libido,starting with the brain. Are you surprised to learn that there is a difference between a man's brain and a woman's in relation to sex?

In men, the sexual experience is interpreted in the hypothalamic nucleus, which is the primitive part of the brain. An average man's hypothalamic nucleus is two and halftimes larger than a woman's.

A woman's brain is much more involved in sex. Like the male brain, areas driven by hormones (the primitive brain) are involved, but so is the cerebral cortex. The cerebral cortex is the "thinking brain." This is the part of the brain that surveys its surroundings, assessing possibilities and noting trouble or opportunities. The cerebral cortex has difficulty relaxing. To enjoy sex, a woman's cerebral cortex needs to turn off. Men can enjoy sex and still have their cerebral cortex up and running. The implication here is that a woman needs to surrender to the man. Or in other words, trust him to survey the surroundings while she lets go.

If a woman does not feel safe, has had a sexual trauma in life, or simply does not feel loving, the cerebral cortex turns on during sex, as opposed to turning off. Instead of surrendering to the pleasure of the moment she is thinking.

All this takes place in a woman's brain because of one little neurotransmitter called dopamine. It may be possible that all the woman needs is a little more dopamine to make her more amorous. Many women find good dark chocolate to be an aphrodisiac. Interestingly enough, chocolate encourages the release of dopamine.

My favourite herb for releasing dopamine is kava (*Piper mysticism*). Is the perfect herb to quiet down the over thinking cerebral cortex and promote loving feelings. If Kava sounds dangerous, passion flower (*Passiflora incarnata*) will help relax the cerebral cortex and let the dopamine flow.

I always assess a woman's adrenal glands when she is troubled by low libido. The primitive brain (limbic brain where the hypothalamus lives) has a very close relationship to the adrenal glands. Both are completely wrapped in the fight or flight response of stress. When a woman is flying from one task to another, forgetting to take time for herself and constantly taking care of every one but herself, the result is adrenal fatigue. The adrenal glands use up the sex hormone progesterone in making stress hormones. Low progesterone equals low dopamine levels and results in no libido. This is why holidays make for great sex; no kids, no parents, no cooking, cleaning, or emails, etc. and etc.

And for The Men: Prostate Health

Every November, we have a new addition to my household and it is prickly and thick! My husband grows a moustache. I don't like moustaches. They are messy and itchy. Yet, I applaud every man who is wearing a moustache through the month of November.

I love Movember. All the curious bursts of facial hair on bankers, teachers, plumbers, store clerks and my husband bring the touchy subject of prostate health to greater awareness with both humour and sensitivity.

The downside of the Movember is the focus seems to be on the moustache, with little information on the prostate itself. So here are some facts about the prostate beyond moustaches.

Exactly what is the prostate?

The prostate is a walnut size gland that sits below the male bladder and wraps around the urethra. It secretes the white fluid that sperm travel in during ejaculation. The prostrate thrives on testosterone. Without this male hormone, it shrivels up. Estrogens have a similar effect.

Benign Prostate Enlargement or Benign Prostatic Hyperplasia (BPH)

BPH occurs in 50-60% per cent of men between the ages of 40 and 49. BPH is the gradual enlargement of the prostate. For some men BPH is completely asymptomatic. In others it causes a number of challenges.

The first symptoms of BPH are:
- Hesitancy: Difficulty getting the stream started.
- Urgency: A strong need to urinate. This includes frequent trips to the bathroom at night.
- A thinner stream: Winning peeing contests becomes more challenging.

As the prostate continues to enlarge, complete emptying of the bladder becomes increasingly difficult. This can result in back pain, chronic bladder infections and in the worst cases, kidney damage.

Most believe BPH is caused by the accumulation of testosterone. Some suggest the best way for a man to avoid BPH is to have sex at least 3 times a week. Herbal medicine has lots to offer BPH. These include nettle root (*Urtica dioica*), horsetail (*Equisetum arvense*) and corn silk (*Zea mays*).

Prostatitis

Prostatitis is inflammation or an infection of the prostate. This can result from the spread of infection from another part of the body like an abscessed tooth, Sitting too long on hard surfaces, not letting go of stress and drinking too much beer can also cause it. Hard surfaces include bicycle seats.

The symptoms of prostatitis are similar to BPH, with the addition of pain on sitting and/or a dull ache in the area of the prostate.

Prostatitis can lead to bladder and kidney infections.

Malignant Prostatic Enlargement

This is commonly referred to as prostate cancer. Current estimates are that one in nine men will be diagnosed with this disease. One in three of these men will die from it. Although commonly a disease of the older man, it was often left untreated because of the advanced age of the man; it is occurring more frequently in younger men.

Many of prostate cancer's symptoms are similar to BPH. A visit to the doctor's office involves similar tests. These include a digital exam in search for unusual lumps and a blood test for PSA.

PSA means Prostate-Specific Antigen. Elevated levels of PSA are found in both cancer and BPH. It has recently been discovered that there are two different PSAs. One PSA is bound to a protein while the other is not. A low ratio of unbound PSA to bound PSA suggests BPH. A high ration suggests cancer.

Caring for the Prostate

- Regular sex (other than when suffering with prostatitis. Abstinence is best until the infection clears up).
- Eat fruits and veggies. The tomato with its high lycopene is the prostate's best friend.
- Quit smoking and drink moderately.
- Exercise. Sports with a competitive edge are best for the prostate as competition engages testosterone.
- Drink green tea and eat garlic.

- Wear boxers.
- Learn to do Kegel exercises during TV commercials.
- Substitute pumpkin seeds for peanuts and snack on oysters. Both foods are high in zinc.
- Take a water bottle to work.
- Pick up James Green's *The Male Herbal* for loads of ideas on herbal care for men.
- Saw palmetto berries (*Serenoa repens*) are commonly taken for prostate health. These berries are one of the worse tasting herbal medicine used in practice. I strongly recommend capsules.

Dreaming: Preparing to Create Plant Medicine

"Are you sure
That we are awake?
It seems to me
That yet we sleep, we dream" – William Shakespeare, A
Midsummer's Night Dream

There is increasing reason to suppose that this "primitive" world-view may also be the most accurate and sophisticated scientific hypothesis as well. The so-called "Gaia Hypothesis" proposes that the earth itself appears to behave like an immense living organism that regulates its planet wide metabolic activities with large-scale ecological mechanisms that parallel and mimic (and may be the original paradigm for) the homeostatic, self regulating metabolic activities and systems of individual animals and plants. Thus hypothesis may be seen as a revival of the ancient matriarchal agrarian theology of the earth as the living body of the Great Mother, which in turn grew out of the hunter-gatherer "animistic" theology of shamanism.

Contemporary physics and cosmology tells us that every atom of the physical universe was apparently first born in the undifferentiated heart of the "Big Bang" that now appears to be the most likely origin of the universe. As Carl Sagan puts it, we are all "star stuff." The fact that some of those undifferentiated and supposedly "inanimate" atoms formed organic molecules and evolved over the millennia into all the living things on the plants suggests strongly to me that the most useful way to view those atoms may be that were alive (or at the very least carried the potentiality of aliveness) all along. ...

For the practicing shaman in a nontechnological culture, such suggestions are only stating the obvious. No one can get a verbal answer from a stone or a star with our limited waking ears. But in the timeless world of the dream, healing trance, and the collective myth the "subtle" spirit energies that are the life of rocks and water and wind and stars can be touched and communicated with. Viewed as an expression of basic human consciousness, "animism" begins to echo with Carl Jung's formula of the archetypes of the collective unconscious." - The Wisdom of Your Dreams, Jeremy Taylor Page 199.

Our Green Friends: Learning From the Teachers

Traditional societies believe dreams contain initiatory experiences for those who seek to heal using plant medicine and are essential for a healer's credibility. For this reason, I decided before we get into the nuts and bolts of medicine making that we journey into realm of dreams.

In contemporary culture, dreams are scoffed at or at the very least considered weird. But then again healing weeds are sprayed with cancer-forming chemicals. Is it possible that in a world where we are taught that forests and wild places are to be feared and one should only walk in straight lines on the sidewalk that a healer can rely on her dreams more than research from the sterile laboratory? Many times in my life, I have felt the sensible thing to do was ask for a dream.

Thyme - The Little Warrior

After the second TIA (Transient Ischemic Accident) and a long night in the hospital emergency, as dawn chased away the darkness of night, I lay in my bed thinking of all the people I know who have been paralyzed by stroke. A TIA can be a precursor to a stroke. Frightened, I asked for a dream to guide me during this difficult time.

When sleep finally came, I had a simple dream. In a garden grew a thyme plant.

Upon waking I questioned the dream's logic. Thyme? Using thyme to treat or prevent strokes made no sense to my herbalist's brain. The dream confused me. I had used thyme in my practice for its powerful antibacterial effect on respiratory and urinary tract infections. I dismissed the dream and spent the rest of the day moping about in a fog, a thin veil masking the terror of the long-term consequences of stroke.

The next day, a friend who is skilled in the language of dreams interpreted the thyme plant's meaning as suggesting slowing down and practicing patience. I am not known for my patience, particularly with medical tests and doctor appointments. We pondered the possibility of the old saying, "Time heals all wounds". The healing cliché did not settle the anxiety I felt about the TIA, and I was sure the dream carried another meaning.

The next morning I spread a blanket out under the poplar tree that graces my herb garden and let the dabbled light guide me into dreaming with the garden. This is a favourite summer pastime of mine. I don't fall asleep when dreaming with the garden; it's more like I merge with its many shades and shapes of green. Dreaming the garden is like acknowledging I am part of the community of plants that have settled there over the years. I dream the softness of their leaves, the buzzing of the insects and prickly nature of their thorns.

Eventually I took a walk around the garden, greeting each plant: my skinny friend vervain, my gentle friend motherwort, and my shy friend violet. Some of the plants have been in the garden since my first year of living in the house (when we moved in, there was only a patch of dirt where the previous owner parked motorcycles). Like old friends, we have had boundary disputes. Raspberry and valerian will not settle in one area of the garden. Borage has annoyed me with her love of spiders and I have lamented skullcap's disappearance during drought and rejoiced at her return with rain.

Near the house, I found my thyme plant and recalled the dream. I sat close to him, took a small sprig, crushed the leaves and held them under my nose. The fear I had been holding at bay flooded my body. Just when I thought it would overwhelm me, it passed and I was left with a quiet strength I had not felt since the TIA. I nibbled on a leaf. The burning, piercing sensation of thyme's powerful volatile oils brought clarity to my mind, waking me up from the fog I had been shrouded in since TIA had temporarily stolen my sight.

Thyme's effect on my mind/body amazed me. I turned the small sprig of thyme over in my fingers and found a thin red stem from which delicate clusters of leaves emerged. Red stems, particularly thin ones, are signatures for fine blood vessels like the ones that feed the brain. A plant's signature suggests its medicinal uses.

The other curious signature was the singular root emerging from the stem. The root reminded me of the close relationship between the nervous system and the circulatory system. The root connects the plant with the intelligence and nutrients of the earth. The nervous system provides the pathways for the exchange of information between the body and the brain: a process that gets totally messed up when one suffers a stroke.

Sitting next to the thyme plant, I felt I was getting closer to understanding the healing dream. I decided to research the history of thyme in medicine a little further. Here is what I found:

The word thyme is derived from the Greek for thumos, or spirit. Curiously, in pre-western medicine, strokes were considered an illness of spirit.

In the folk medicine of England, thyme was used to restore and strengthen the mind.

Finally, in the days of the Crusades a lady embroidered a sprig of thyme with a bumblebee hovering over it on a scarf to give to her knight for protection. Thyme is a plant of protection.

The TIA had certainly left me feeling very vulnerable, without protection.

With this new knowledge, I returned to sit next to the thyme plant and named it "The Little Warrior". My encounter with the thyme plant in my garden and dream told me everything was

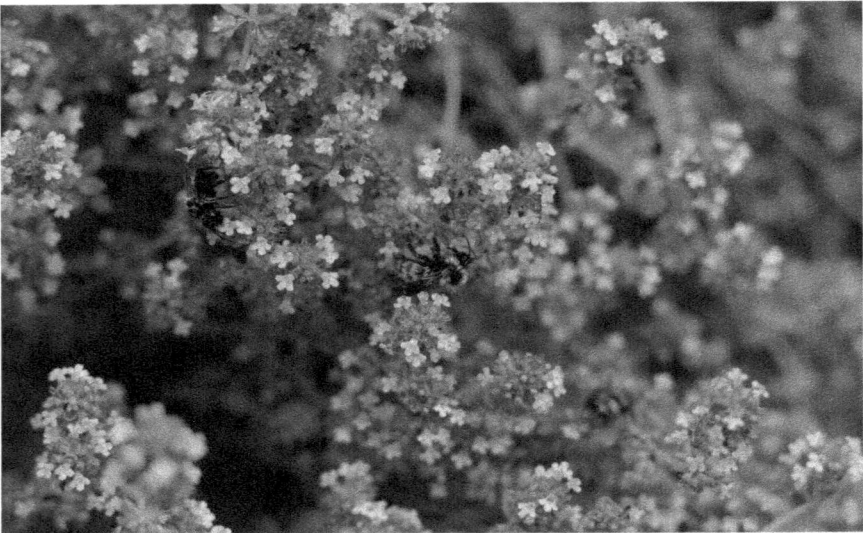

Thyme   Rosalee de la Forêt

going to be all right. For the next six months I wore a sprig of thyme everywhere I went.

How to evoke the dream?

To access plant dreams, begin by walking where there are no sidewalks and preferably in bare feet. I have found the First Nations saying, *"May you walk on uneven ground,"* quite appropriate for studying plant medicine. It is on uneven ground where one finds dreams.

The word dream here is used loosely. One may have a night dream or a day-dream, or perhaps there is a sudden knowing while drawing or watering a plant. We all have different ways of coming to an understanding of plant medicine that transcends books and lectures. Find yours and trust it.

Here are a few ways to encourage dreams of the green teachers.

A Pledge:

Make a pledge to the plant world. I find this particularly important if you are planning to make a living with plants. The pledge will define your relationship with the plants. The pledge should contain all that you will give back to the plant world in exchange for the knowledge and support the plants will offer you.

As a student in herbal medicine, I made a pledge to the plants in a nearby forest (as representative of all plants around the world) that I would protect them from exploitation. To fulfill my pledge I speak, write, and use whatever medium possible to help people come to a personal understanding of the profound relationship between plants and humans. My intention is to foster greater understanding and respect for the natural world. I believe that by doing this, there will be less exploitation of nature. I work daily at supporting this pledge in one way or another.

Tania says that you need to feel the plant when you begin to work with it. "Talk to it, asking permission to work with it. The plant may have other plans. Let the life force of the plant go through you, touch the tree, embrace it, feel its energy through your body. You may feel warmth or tingling. Each tee has its own separate life. The plant or tree gives a certain kind of strength, which we need. A knowledgeable person can tell which tree or plant relates to a person or to an organ, and ask that to help.

"Then that the tree after it has given you strength, ask forgiveness for coming onto its territory. Maybe leave a cloth, a coin, or food. I can go into one forest with complete comfort. Another may treat me like an enemy, scratching and bumping. Always speak to the area, go with an open mind." All this indicates that it is not just the pharmaceutical properties of plants that make them effective. Petya Topoev, a musical-instrument make in Khakassia, told me that he know a person who listened to plants that to him how to find someone who was lost. He also knew of a woman who learned how to find her lost cow by listening to a stone. This is similar to the way shamans get information from the forty one pebbles and they way they can listen carefully and get information about the weather. – Singing Story, Healing Drum: Shamans and Storytellers of Turkic Siberia by Kira Van Deusen.

When making a pledge, look deeply into your heart. Ask for a dream from your heart. Perhaps this question will help: How does your heart wish connect you with the plant world, people and society?

Breathe with the plant or plants

Breathe with a single plant or a forest. As you exchange carbon dioxide and oxygen with plants, become conscious of it. Offer your "out" breath to the plants. Accept your "in" breath as a gift from the plants. Let yourself relax into the flow of exchangeand enjoy the connection with our green friends.

Breathe a gentle breath of exchange until there is no separation between you and the plant that nourishes you.

Draw the plant

Creating a literal drawing of a plant is a lovely way to spend a morning. Let your eye untangle a maze of leaves and sketch the subtle curve of a leaf as it parts from a stem. Carefully record the numbers of petals on a flower. Drawing plants is satisfying and helps you see the plant with greater clarity.

If you are not comfortable with realistic interpretations of plants through drawing, try an abstract representation of the plant. Breathe with the plant for a while, let your eyes go blurry and then when you are ready, without thinking, draw the plant. You will be surprised!

Write about the plant

As Susan Weed does so well in her book called *Healing Wise* (the first herbal I purchased) imagine the plant's voice and write in it. Write about what it enjoys, what it does not enjoy, and what it is good at.

You may also want to write your way into the plant's dream (or your dream depending on which side of the looking glass you are on). This is the technique I often use to access the plant's dream. Sit quietly listening for the whispers from the plant world and follow the twisting well-worn path to the place where the plant and human meet in spirit. Then dream the plant's story into being.

Photograph the plant

Before you photograph a plant, spend a moment taking in its beauty. Engage the plant while you photograph it. Ask it to pose and smile, or show you a side you have never noticed. Return again and again to photograph the plant. If you have different types of lenses, photograph it from micro to macro. Don't forget to photograph it from different angles.

Talk to the plant

Talk to the plant and take time to listen. Most plants will happily take the time to have a conversation with you if you walk on uneven ground long enough.

Give the plant gifts

Plants love gifts. Offer your healing plants water, or perhaps tobacco, or a ribbon or a shiny marble, or even a whisper of air from your hand. Tug a strand of hair from your head and gift the plant a piece of yourself. Sing the plant a song and do a dance or recite a poem proclaiming its beauty. Give the plant your heart and you will not be sorry.

I am not sure if the following story is myth or truth; I would like to ask His Holiness the Dalai Lama one day if this story is true, but in many ways it does not matter.

The Jewel Garden

Every spring, the Dalai Lama left the Grand Potala and all his serene and serious rituals to spend six months at the summer palace, where his only duty was to keep the plants of the Jewel Garden happy. The farmers of Tibet depended upon these plants to keep their lands flourishing.

So every day, the king went out to sing and dance for the plants, to stroll amongst them showering them with loving praise, to pray for them and tenderly admonish them not to be stingy in their yields of fruit and flower.

Sooner or later, every Tibetan farmer made his pilgrimage to the Jeweled Garden there to receive a handful of seeds which, when sprouted and full-grown, would become the spiritual kings and queens of the farmlands. One could look at a Tibetan field so blessed by the Dalai Lama and see that plants grew taller according to their proximity to the holy ones. Fields of barley, rice, buckwheat, maize, potatoes, turnips, onions and radishes resembled undulating mounds at harvest time, peaking wherever

*a seed from the Jeweled Garden had sprouted and flourished. -
Tales of a Dalai Lama by Pierre Delattre*

Become sensual with plants

Enjoy plants with your senses: smell them, taste them, and
caress them. Notice how the scent of your plants changes in the
moonlight or after a thunderstorm. Study the change of colour
rain brings to their leaves and petals. Nibble their leaves after a
few days of hot dry weather. Taste them again after a couple of
wet days. Let yourself become totally sensually immerse in
your plants.

Dream the plants

Ask plants for a dream. If you are have a challenge dreaming,
perhaps make yourself a dream pillow.

Dream Pillows

Bears are astute herbalists with an uncanny ability to find
medicinal plants and use them for their well-being. Bears are
also gifted dreamers. Sleeping through long winters on a bed of
leaves, bears dream of seasons yet to come. I wonder if the bear
chooses leaves from plants known to enhance dreaming to
slumber on through the cold and dark time of year? For this
reason, to dream of a bear is auspicious for someone studying
herbal medicine.

Every fall, as I harvest the last of the roots the garden has to
offer, I become a bit of a grumpy bear. My mind turns to a long
winter's dream of spring. As I prepare for winter, I make myself a
dream pillow for long dark nights. The gentle scents of dream
pillows, embroidered with stars and moons, have long been used to
deepen sleep and guide the sleeper and herbalist in her dreams.

From Europe a Prophesy

William Blake

Five windows light the cavern'd Man: thro' one he breathes the air;

Thro' one, hears music of the spheres; thro' one, the eternal vine

Flourishes, that he may receive the grapes; thro' one can look.

And see small portions of the eternal world that ever growth;

Thro' one, himself pass out what time he please, but he will not;

For stolen joys are sweet, & bread eaten in secret pleasant.

So sang a Fairy mocking as he sat on a streak'd Tulip,

Thinking none saw him: when he ceas'd I started from the trees!

And caught him in my hat as boys knock down a butterfly

How know you this said I small Sir? Where did you learn this song

Seeing himself in my possession thus he answered me:

My master, I am yours. Command me, for I must obey.

Then tell me, what is the material world, and is it dead?

He laughing answer'd: I will write a book on leaves of flowers,

If you will feed me on love-thoughts, & give me now and then

A cup of sparkling poetic fancies; so what I am tipsie,

I'll sing to you to this soft lute; and shew you all alive

The world, where every particle of dust breathes forth its joy.

I took him home in my warm bosom: as we went along

Wild flowers I gatherd: & he shew'd me each eternal flower:

He laugh'd aloud to see them whimper because they were pluck'd

They hover'd round me like a cloud of insense: when I came

Into my palour and sat down, and took my pen to write:

My Fairy sat upon the table, and dictated EUROPE.

And what herbs does one use in a dream pillow?

Although there are many dreaming herbs, my favourite is mugwort (*Artemsia vulgaris*). A common meadow plant, mugwort is one of the seven sacred herbs of the druids. She belongs to a family of plants named after the Greek goddess of wild places, Artemsia. I frequently give Mugwort to women who have lost touch with their wild place within.

In dream pillows mugwort helps the sleeper find her way with dreams. It enhances dream recall and brings the gift of lucid dreaming to those who seek this skill. For some, mugwort offers prophetic dreams. Some say mugwort guides women during their moon time into a deeper understanding of the cyclical nature of life. Others use mugwort to enhance daydreams and ritual journeys. Wherever you are at in your dream world, mugwort will help you understand and learn from the gifts of the night.

Lavender (*Lavendula angustifolia*) is a favoured plant for dream pillows. Some people are afraid of their dreams. Dreams for them come from dark places. These dreams are difficult to understand and their messages are feared. Lavender in a dream pillow helps us let go of the anxiety associated with these dreams. The lovely calming scent of lavender eases the stress of the day from our thoughts and allows us to approach our dreams with a sense of well-being. Lavender helps you to wake refreshed.

The final herb most frequently added to dream pillows is Hops (*Humulus lupus*). Hops are used in herbal medicine to bring on sleep. It is a very bitter herb and a difficult tea to drink. In a dream pillow, the scent of hops will bring the peace of sleep to you and help you find sleep again if you wake in the middle of the night.

For those who consider Plant Dreaming flaky

Some of my friends who enjoy plant medicine cringe when ask to talk with a plant. These are my friends who have strong analytical minds. They always blow me away with their ability to recite complex laws of chemistry or explain the ATP cycle's interaction with arsenic and apple seeds without referring to notes. I always think their remarkable analytical abilities beautifully compliment my more intuitive personality.

So I ask my more analytical friends who squirm at the thought of having to become spiritually intimate with a plant to consider the following idea: the most significant healing plant medicine offers is firm understanding of the interdependence of all life. Or as some call it: the web of life. Here is a short meditation on the interdependence of life.

What is a Seed?

A life is a wish. The wish is a seed.

Imagine in your hand you hold a seed-- perhaps a sunflower seed or a rose hip. Maybe the seed grew inside a sweet tangerine or an apple. In any case, in your hand you hold a seed, even if it is only a wish.

Image you can see a cloud in the seed. Clouds carry rain across the sky. It is the rain that softens the soil and nourishes the plant so it can birth the seed. Some see the wind in the seed. The wind pushed the cloud across the sky to release the rain above the plant that produced the seed. If there were no wind, there would be no clouds, no rain and no seed.

Some see a ray of sunlight in the seed. The sun warmed the earth where the seed slept, awakening it to spring, just as we awaken in morning's light with a wish.

Some see their breath in the seed in your hand. The plant that birthed the seed used sunlight to make chlorophyll, the life-blood of the plant. In making the chlorophyll the plant exhales oxygen into the air. We inhale this oxygen and our blood carries it to every cell of our body, bringing life.

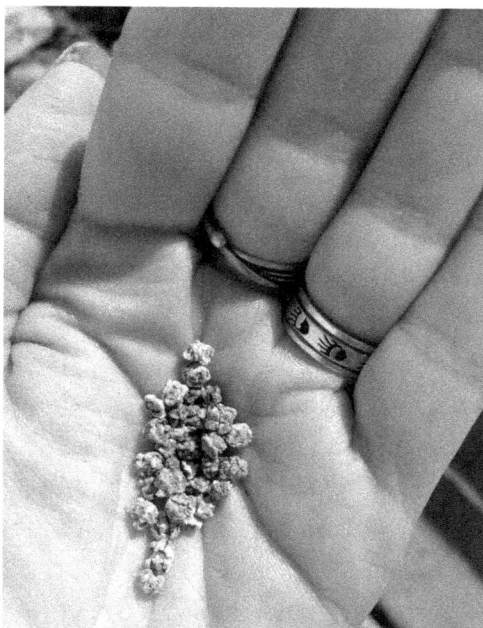

The seed contains your breath. Each exhalation you make offers carbon dioxide to the plant. It combines carbon dioxide with sunlight to make a beautiful green, refreshing your eye. The green chlorophyll is the life-blood of the plant.

Some say they see mountains and the ocean floor in a seed. The prairie was once an ocean and the mountains were once tectonic plates buried deep in the earth. The roots from the plant that birth the seed in your hand sought the minerals left behind by oceans and stirred by shifting tectonic plates: calcium, magnesium, selenium, iron, copper, zinc. With these minerals, the plant build strong cell walls, like the bricks of clay used to build your home. When you prepare a tea or salad or soup with plants, the minerals drawn from the ancient ocean floor become your bones, hands, legs, toes and skull.

Look at the seed in your hand and see a flower. It may have been an inconspicuous flower; tiny, green and yellow, not the rambunctious blooms of a peony or the seductive petals of a rose. No matter its size, the flower knows how to catch the eye of a butterfly or a hummingbird, or a bumblebee that seeks pollen for the honey that sweetens your tea. Perhaps the flower's lover is the pesky housefly of late August. The seed knows the intimate meeting of flower and animal on its journey to your hand.

Maybe the flower exchanged caresses with the wind, and it is the wind's soft touch you find in your hand.

If in the seed in your hand is a strawberry, you can see a crow. Crows love juicy, plump, sweet berries. Spying the shiny red jewel of a berry (inside the seed is the colour red, standing out in a sea of green, making it easier for crow to find), the crow swoops down and gobbles up the luscious berry before the gardener can come out her back door waving a tea towel, shooing the sly black winged one away.

Then, sitting on a branch in a quiet poplar grove, the crow poops. In the poop are strawberry seeds. Approximately 200 seeds safely pass through the crow's gullet, stomach and intestine (yes the seed you hold in your hand contains the journey through the crow's gizzard. Hidden in their little pile of fertilizer crow poop, the seeds pass a winter.

Let's look again deeply into the seed in your hand. In this seed are your ancestors. My ancestors came from cities and grew roses and pansies. Sometime before cities grew up around this seed called Earth, our ancestors gathered seeds very carefully every fall and over wintered them in a safe dry place. Our ancestors understood that their life and the lives of their children depended on the seeds they collected. The plants relied on our ancestors to keep their seeds safe. Every spring gardens bloomed with the future. There was a mutual respect for life. Generations of human families and plant families nourished each other in the most intimate matter, creating each other's bodies, each other's histories, lineages and tomorrows. Your ancestors are found in the seed in your hand.

Now consider this: because of its journey through time and its dance with water, air, fire (sunlight) and earth, the seed knows how to grow. No one has to tell it. It just knows what to do. It knows that in the warm damp spring it is time to wake up and begin its tentative reach into the earth with its first fragile root. It seeks sunlight with its tender sprout. It is not frightened by the darkness beneath the surface of the earth. It knows it cannot make its wish bloom if it only preferred the light. The seed understands the value of both. No matter how you place the seed in the soil, it knows the direction to put down its roots, and the way to reach for the light of sun.

The seed knows how to grow in the community. It makes friends with bacteria and worms, offering them food and drink. With others, it sets up boundaries with scents and tastes that are not particularly friendly. The seed knows to grow into a flower that blooms under the moon to call the moth that pollinates in the darkness. The flower may bloom in the early morning, trapping dew for a sip of moisture during the hot dry afternoon. The seed knows to create a plant that leans out of the shade and into the sun, or to stay hidden within the dappled shadows of the aspen tree. It knows what to become, because it always is its future.

The seed knows how to grow, because it contains all the knowledge of the past, and the whole of the future. It contains this eternal present moment. What will your seed, your wish, your life become? Do you know?

There is an expression, "It is easy to count the number of seeds in an apple, but only God can count the apples in a seed."

Now one final consideration: if you took away the sunlight, would the seed still be a seed? If you took away the wind, would the seed still be a seed? If you took away the earthworm or crow, would the seed still be a seed? Or if there had never been an ocean or mountains, would the seed still be a seed? If there were no humans, would the seed still be a seed? Would the seed still be a seed if there has been no flower, chlorophyll, or tentative first root? The seed is all of this and much more.

For now, be confident that the seed knows how to grow, just as wishes know how to grow.

This is the nature of plants. Plants are the sun, rain, the earth's minerals, wind, insects and the fur of a dog that transports the plant's seed. The plants are the humans who care for them. The plants are the bones of the dead and the lightening flash on a summer evenings.

Our bodies are the green of plants, and their roots, leaves, flowers and seeds. Our bodies are the animals that feed on plants. Our bodies are the sun, rain, and minerals from the earth, wind, insects and fur of the dog that carries the seeds within the burr. Our bodies and the plant world are interdependent.

It is for this reason, which now calls for a leap of faith, that humans, when still and listening, can hear a plant speak and understand their language. Plants are in every cell of our being. Plants are rooted in our DNA.

Doctrine of Signatures (Doc of Sigs)

The Doctrine of Signatures is a well-worn pathway to understanding the language of plants. There are many thoughts on the origin of Doc of Sigs. I enjoy Matthew Wood's definition from his book Herbal Wisdom:

Each plant is a personification of a pattern, of vitality brought together into a configuration. As such, there are certain patterns in the plant – the way it grows, where it grows, and what it is like to our senses – which reveal its medicinal properties. Each is signatum or sign which shows what the medicine is for and how it is to be used.

Nature is economical. It finds patterns that work and sticks with them. This is particularly true of the shapes nature makes.

Nature finds great value in the circles, squares, and triangles, and the variations on them such as spirals, rectangles and ovals. Each of these shapes intuitively speaks to the human mind. For example: squares suggested stability, while circles suggest wholeness.

Nature is fond of re-using colour. Although there are many shades and hues of each colour, everyone is familiar with the primary colours of red, blue and yellow, and the secondary colours, green, purple and orange. Each of these colours, like the shapes, intuitively suggests meaning to the human being. For example: yellow suggests sunshine and joy while green is the colour of the forest and intuitively suggests protection.

When studying a plant's doctrine, begin uncovering the basic patterns and shapes of the plant. You will find co-corresponding shapes and colour within the human body.

For example: blueberries resemble eyes while thin red stems are reminiscent of blood vessels.

Colour is important in understanding a plant's medicine: red often represents blood or blood vessels and yellow symbolizes the bile from the liver or the jaundice of liver disease.

Next, consider the environment the plant prefers to grow in. Plants that thrive in wet areas often help the body resolve fluid imbalances. Plants sprouting from sandy/rocky soil, such as parsley, are often used to break up stones. Frequently in the wild I see plants growing together that combine well in formulas, such as uva ursi (*Arctostaphylos uva ursi*) and yarrow (*Achellia millifolium*) for bladder infections.

Consider this reflection on yarrow's doctrine of signature.

To be a medicine man you have to have to experience everything, live life to the fullest. If you don't experience the human side of everything, how can you teach or heal? To be a good medicine man, you've got to be humble. You got to be lower than a worm and higher than an eagle. – Archie Fire Lame Deer –Gift of Power.

Yarrow grows tall in meadows. Its white umbrella of tightly knit flowers hovers above the swaying grasses. In the mountains, yarrow grows stout amongst the wild sage and pearly everlasting. Down in the badlands it rises boldly from dry cracked earth, its grey white flowers contrasting *Monarda's* flaming petals. In all these places, yarrow's odour is pungent like that of a wild animal.

In my garden, yarrow grows long. The umbrella of flowers is lacy, not the tightly compact economy of her wild sisters. The stems lack strength and lean over into the walkway. The garden yarrow has no scent. It is in the yarrow's scent that one finds the medicine.

Native people say harsh growing conditions make medicine. This belief has now been confirmed by science. The medicine the plant yields to relieve the sickness in humans, is the medicine the plant makes for itself. In the dry badlands I find the strongest yarrow. These plants have the harshest growing conditions where the sun is brutally hot and water is scarce. Yarrow's pungent bitterness fills my body with warmth and

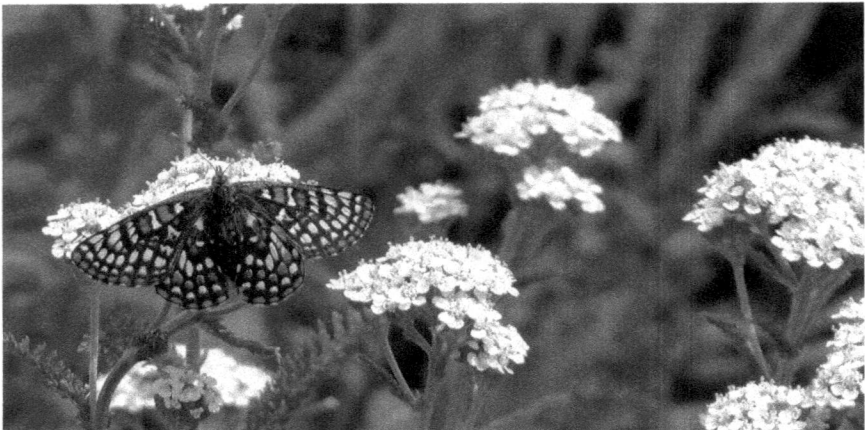

Yarrow   Rosalee de la Forêt

carries with it the timelessness of the badlands. I feel strong. I am disappointed by the yarrow in my garden. It is useless but for its beauty.

Matthew Wood, an American herbalist, says yarrow is the herb for the wounded healer. Yarrow's history of healing wounds goes back to ancient Greece where it was carried into battle to staunch the bleeding of war. It is considered a warrior's herb. When I read Matthew's musings on yarrow, I was puzzled by the inherent contradiction between the healer and the warrior. So I sought yarrow's story from the plant itself.

Clearly, yarrow prefers wild places. The healer cannot be too domestic or polite. The healer must be ready to discuss unpleasant sides of life openly without embarrassment or judgment. The healer must be able to speak with kindness and confidence of things that need to be spoken of and that have been left unsaid. This makes the healer a little unpredictable and beyond societal norms. Perhaps a better word to describe a healer would be wild.

A healer must wake to her own life. If she has some wisdom she will accept the guidance of others but she knows that it is not the same as waking to her life. She accepts her life with its dreams and disappointments, joys and sorrows, losses and blessings, scars and beauty. The healer's medicine comes from her challenges. If she is raised in a garden she will have no scent.

Medicinally, one of yarrow's properties is to bring blood to the periphery of the body. It is in this way yarrow nourishes the whole body. In many ways this is the healer's role: to nourish the whole, to bring wholesomeness.

In these four ways: its ability to close up wounds, its fearlessness in the wild, its ability to make the strongest medicine in harsh conditions, and its ability to nourish the whole, make yarrow the healer's herb.

One more thing about yarrow: yarrow's flowers reach directly for the sun. Yarrow's flowers do not form a hierarchy like a spike or grow off to one side like roses do. They spread themselves open so each petal receives an equal amount of light. This is a humble way to grow. As she moves through life a healer is humbled by the light she finds in so many. She knows a person who appears ordinary on the outside is extraordinary on the inside. She is deeply moved by the light that shines through on the most difficult days at the most challenging times.

A healer cannot be a rose. She would get lost in her own beauty. She cannot be a timid violet or a towering valerian. St John's Wort is too soft and mellow. It is yarrow with her sturdy stem, understated flowers and pungent scent of the wild that is the healer's plant.

The study of a plant's signature requires a playful, imaginative mind. After discovering a plant's signature, write it down and then do some research in the plant's known medicinal properties. Do they fit?

Making Medicine Pragmatics

...if we could actually 'see' a molecule, we might be surprised by how exotically and curiously beautiful it is. We might see colourful, blooming, interlaced patterns of perpetually moving energy which nevertheless retain a stable spatial relationship with each other. I like to say that rather than thinking of molecules as tiny objects, we might better conceptualize them as being patterns of energy in relationship. This way of visualising phytochemicals introduces the intriguing possibility of perceiving them as fluid expressions of a plant's energy or spirit.
- Lisa Ganora in Herbal Constituents Foundations of Phytochemistry

Everything, decided Francie after that first lecture, was vibrant with life and there was no death in chemistry. She was puzzled as to why learned people didn't adopt chemistry as a religion.
— Betty Smith, A Tree Grows in Brooklyn

Overview

I love the idea of chemistry. I think of chemistry as the continued response of every molecule in every cell in every being to every other molecule, cell and being. The idea of the dynamic transformation of life via molecules beyond my

355

limited perception thrills my imagination, stimulating the sense of the mystery of what it means to breathe, eat and love. Chemistry to me is the continued dance of matter in and out of being. Do not be fooled that chemistry is concerned only with individual molecules with impossible names and complex classifications. It the study of the vast interactions of fire, water, air, earth and space, with space being the container in which all this transformation takes place.

To understand chemistry it is essential to keep in mind that chemical transformation occurs in response to the environment. For example, an egg is fried in a pan when the stove is hot enough. It is not possible to fry an egg in isolation without the heat and pan. Chemistry does not happen in isolation. It is about the interaction of the universe.

In Phytochemistry, a plant adapts and responds to its environment through complex chemical changes that protect it from diseases and predators, nourish it, and bring it lovers for sex. It makes use of earth (obviously we are talking of beings who have visible roots), wind, heat and water to create a life. It arises in space.

A plant, not being able to run away or engage in negotiation, only has one way to respond meaningfully to its environment. It changes its chemistry.

Plants are continually creating medicine for themselves. Most of the medicine a plant makes is also medicine for humans.

Although in this chapter we will look at individual phytochemicals in medicine making, please do not be fooled that the individual phytochemicals are the medicine. It is the transformative power of the chemical interactions between the phytochemicals and the human chemicals that create medicine.

Secondary Compound made by plants to avoid being eaten by grazers.	Human Pharmacological effect
Alkaloids (Lobelia, oregon grape root, california poppy)	Antibacterial, stimulants, sedatives, vaso-constrictors and dilators, diuretics, expectorants, anti-diarrheal
Cyanogenic glycosides (Wild cherry bark)	Cough suppressants, calms digestion, slows metabolism.
Saponins (Wild yam, licorice, rhodiola)	Expectorant, diuretics, hormone balancing
Cardiac glycosides (Lily of the Valley)	Regulates heart activity
Tannins (Raspberry and blackberry leaf)	Astringent for wound healing and diarrhoea
Simple phenolics (Sage, thyme, rosemary)	Antihelmethics, anti-microbial

Amazing Phytochemical Facts

Plants growing in a pasture will have a different chemical make-up than the same plants growing in an open meadow where few animals feed. The plants in the pasture shift their chemistry to create unappealing tastes for the grazers.

Plants communicate with each other using scented molecules called volatile oils. When an predator or infecting fungus attacks, the plant releases a volatile oil to let the other plants in the area know not only what it attacking it but also what chemical change it needs to make in order to survive the invasion.

The birch's beautiful white bark, like a Canadian on a Mexican beach in February, has to protect itself from the harsh rays of the sun. Like the pale Canadians, the birch tree slathers itself in a self-created sunscreen called betulin, a wax mingled with plant steroids. Currently, lab techs are applying betulin to rats to measure its effect against skin cancer. This research will eventually lead to humans.

Chaga mushrooms which look like a black offensive growth, loves to perch on birch trees. Chaga is one of the most powerful immune-modulators in the apothecary and is a favoured remedy for breast and lung cancers. Chaga looks like a tumour on a birch tree. But the interesting thing is that it is partially the butelin content in the chaga that gives it neoplastic activity. Chaga derives it butalin from the birch tree it lives on.

Birch also protects its lovely fresh spring leaves from the sun's radiation. Young leaves are high in anti-oxidants such as quercetin, a darling of supplement industry. In high doses, quercetin reduces inflammation and eases allergies. A tea of the birch leaves in the early spring might be a solution to itchy eyes caused by poplar fluff.

Synergy

A rose combines approximately 400 chemicals to create its seductive perfume. There is not a single chemical with the allure of rose's scent. The sought after scent of rose is a synergistic blend of 400 plant chemicals that cannot be reproduced in a lab.

Physics defines synergy as "the whole is greater than the sum of its parts".

Synergy in plant medicine is a beautiful thing. It is the complex weaving between the phytochemicals in a single plant, the harmony of several herbs in a formal focused on a single outcome, and the interactions between the human body and plants. Synergy may also take place between a group of phytochemicals and a pathogen.

Synergy within a plant

St John's Wort's medicine is an example of a synergetic effect encompassing a wide range of phytochemicals to produce a beneficial effect on human beings.

Research into St John's Wort suggested that "hypercin" was the active chemical behind this weed's anti-depressive powers. A standardized version of St. John's Wort was created with elevated levels of hypercin. Clinical studies were organized to face the standardized (and patentable) version of the plant medicine off against a traditional preparation using the whole plant as found in the meadow. The studies were halted mid-way through. The results were stunning and humbling. The standardized version performed poorly while the traditional preparation relieved depression.

Now it is known that the flavonoids in the St. John's Wort facilitate the absorption of hypercin in the gut. The standardized product had a high hypercin level but low absorption rates along with compromised levels of flavonoids. Today it is also known now that St. John's Wort contains trace amounts of melatonin and at least four other chemicals that contribute to its anti-depressant effect.

Traditionally St John's is used as an anti-viral and heptoprotective herb. In cases of depression, both these actions may have a beneficial effect. Chronic, low-grade viral infections can present as depression. Some psychologists feel depression is repressed anger or rage. In TCM, the liver is associated with these emotions. Improving liver function is a traditional method of treating depression.

In wholistic medicine, synergy is important as it helps us consider the whole plant and the whole person. Perhaps St

John's Wort is trying to tell us that depression does not just happen in the head.

Synergy amongst plants and humans

The interaction between plant salicylates and the human body demonstrates synergy between plants and humans.

Salicylates are found in many plants as a glycoside called salicin. Salicin has little effect on the human body.

Willow bark, meadowsweet, poplar and birch all contain salicin. Salicin is a combination of a salicyl alcohol and a glucose molecule. Salicin passes through the stomach and most of the small intestine where it is converted into alcohol called salicyl by the flora of the distal ileum and the colon. As an alcohol it is absorbed into the blood steam. The pH of the blood stream transforms the alcohol into an acid. Thus salicin becomes the medicinal salicylic acid. At this point, it achieves a number of effects on the human body.

Some of its effects on the body are: anti-inflammatory actions due to its antagonistic properties towards prostaglandins and bradykinnins, and anti-pyretic actions directly associated with its effect on the hypothalamus. Its action on the liver increases the amount and concentration of the bile. Its anti-septic actions occur as it passes through the hepatocytes and urinary tract. It has an analgesic effect on the CNS.

Because it does not become an acid until it directly interacts with the blood stream, tincture of willow, poplar, or birch have never caused stomach ulcers.

Synergy amongst plants within a formula

I recall as a student I was asked to study the following formula and try to explain its actions. This is the formula:

Oak bark (Quercus alba)
Comfrey leaves (Symphytum officinale)
Marshmallow root (*Althea officinalis*)
Mullein leaf   (Verbascum thapsus)

Black walnut husk (*Juglans nigra*)
Gravel Root   (Eupatorium purpureum)
Wormwood   (Artemesia absinthium)
Lobelia   (Lobelia inflata)
Scullcap   (Scutellaria lateriflora)
Pluerisy root   (Asclepias_tuberosa)

The formula made no sense at the time. There are herbs used to relax, heal lungs, clear up soft tissue injury, work against parasites, and break up stones. The formula is a hodge-podge of actions and with no apparent focused intent. Baffled, I surrendered and was introduced to the famous Bones, Flesh and Cartilage formula created by Doctor John R. Christopher., an American herbalist.

The story behind this formula goes like this:

A teenage girl came to see Doctor Christopher because she was suicidal. She was suicidal because her face was covered with thick, red, pitting, oozing, and peeling skin. She would not leave her house because she felt so horribly ugly. She believed her only hope after trying everything else was suicide.

Doctor John R Christopher was born in 1909 in Utah, USA. Although Doctor Christopher never received a doctorate, his kinds and gentle manner as well as his knowledge of plant medicine lead many of his patients and students to call him doctor.

Doctor Christopher developed between 50 and 60 formulas still used by herbalist today.

Studying Doctor Christopher's formulas will help the budding herbalist learn about combining diverse herbs in order to treat a specific condition.

Skin issues are not always so simple, and particularly with teenage girls. Not knowing what to do, Doctor Christopher raised his eyes to heaven and prayed. The above formula appeared in his mind's eye. He mixed it up for the girl. Soon after applying it, her skin began to clear up. Within months she had radiant skin and the miraculous BFC formula came into being.

Looking at this formula now after practicing herbal medicine I can see some sense in it. Mullein, pleurisy root, comfrey and marshmallow have healing properties for connective tissue. Skin is essentially connective tissue. Gravel root softens hardness in the body, something needed to soften the thickened skin and hard pustules. Oak bark is a powerful astringent, binding the excoriated skin. Wormwood kills everything; with all of the tears in the skin, oozing and pussing, some kind of pathogen must have been involved. As for lobelia-- well, Doctor Christopher put lobelia in everything. But black walnut husks and skullcap? Who knows?

One thing I do know is this formula works for any injury to connective tissue. Whether it is broken bones, slipped discs, misaligned ribs, torn ligaments, tendonitis bruises, etc., it is amazing how effective it is when everything else has been tried. The incredible results of this formula can only be attributed to some mysterious synergy between all the herbs in the formula.

Synergy amongst plants and pathogens

MSRA (*Methicillin-resistant Staphylococcus aureus*) is a stubborn anti-biotic resistant bacterium. Goldenseal and barberry, two herbs known for their anti-bacterial actions are quite effective against it. The alkaloid berberine, is common to both and known for its anti-bacterial activity. Yet when berberine was used in a petri dish against MSRA bacterium, its action was mediocre. This led to the discovery of other phytochemicals within these plants called pheophorbide and 5'-MHC-D.

Berberine enters the bacteria on a mission to kill it. The crafty MSRA bacteria senses berberine's ill intent and spits it out. The pheophorbide and 5'-MHC-D set up a road block at the sites where berberine is forced to exit the bacteria. This maintains deadly levels of berberine in the bacteria, killing it and resolving the stubborn infection.

Practical points for Making Medicine
There are few important questions to ask when making medicine:

What is the purpose of the medicine?

What form will the medicine take? For example: an infused oil vs. a tincture?

Who is taking the medicine? Compliance needs to considered when making medicine.

What phytochemicals need to be extracted from the plant need to create the specific action?

It is upon asking the last question that we begin the rich and complex study of chemistry in medicine making. Different plants have different chemical make-ups. The chemicals in plants are called constituents. Each constituent has specific actions on the body. It is important to know how to extract specific constituents to make medicine, or how to leave certain constituents behind.

For example: Calendula is a plant with many uses in the apothecary. How a herbalist uses calendula is determined by the constituents that are extracted from the plant.

Calendula has saponins used to balance hormones.

The resin found on Calendula's flowers and leaves have anti-microbial properties.

The orange of Calendula's flowers is created by a mix of carotenes that are anti-oxidant.

The volatile oils that give Calendula its scent are bitter and microbial.

The polysaccharides (sugars) Calendula uses for food are immune stimulants.

The flavonoids that protect the delicate tissues of Calendula from sun damage are anti-oxidant in the human body.

Each of Calendula's phytochemicals has different soluble properties.

Ultimately, medicine making is all about solubility. Solubility is essentially the concept of "like attracts like". A very general rule of thumb is that if a phytochemical likes water, it does not like fat or oil. If a phytochemical likes oil, then its likes alcohol and does not like water.

Again let's look at Calendula:

Saponins are for the most part fat soluble, but may also be water-soluble.

Resins are fat-soluble.

The carotenes are fat-soluble.

The volatile oils are fat-soluble.

Its polysaccharides are water-soluble. (Sugar dissolves in water.)

Its flavonoids may be water or fat-soluble.

Heat and cold are also variables in this mix. Think of peppermint tea. Delicious, right? This flavour is largely attributed to its volatile oils. Being fat soluble, volatile oils do not like water. However, the heating process during infusion agitates the oils causing them to move out of the plant material and into the water.

Here is a quick look at a few common plant constituents used in herbal medicine and their solubility.

Volatile Oils

How plants use volatile oils.

These plant constituents are part of the plant's mating ritual. A plant mingles a variety of volatile oils to create a scent that attracts their one and only insect. Loving the plant, the insect travels from blossom to blossom, moving pollen from stamen to ovary.

The volatile oils also keep microbes that the plant does not like away or more aggressively kills off any unwanted pests that may have arrived on the plant's doorstep.

Volatile Oils in Medicine Making

This is a large complex family of chemicals. Volatile oils are classes as either phenolic compounds or terpenes. However, for our purpose, all volatile oils are oil soluble and dislike water. They can be pulled into medicine using a medium to high percentage of alcohol. Many can be extracted with a hot infusion and taken as a tea. When infusing plants with volatile oils, alwaya keep the lid on otherwise the volatile oils will escape into the air.

For example, if you want the medicine from garlic's volatile oils to be present in your food, do not sauté it. When sautéed, garlic's stinky medicine evaporates into the air. If garlic is added just before the meal is served, then the volatile oils do not have a chance to escape the food and you and your guest get to digest garlic's medicine, as opposed to just smelling it in the room.

There are many types of volatile oils and many classes of these plant constituents. For our purpose we will lump them all together and call them volatile oils.

Saponins

How plants use saponins

Plants make saponins for medicine. They protect the plant from invasion of fungi and insects. They are generally unpleasant in the mouth. Animals avoid munching on plants high in saponins.

Saponins in Medicine Making

Saponins are classed as either triterpenoid saponins or steroidal saponins. In medicine making each class has a different solvency so it is important to differentiate them.

Triterpenoid saponins belong to the same family as volatile oils (the terpenes), but are quite different in nature. Like volatile oils, triterpenoid saponins alone are attracted to fat and dislike water. However, they often travel around in plants on a sugar molecule (glycoside). Sugar likes water. Therefore, when a plant is dried, the triterpenoids that are attached to a glycoside are water-soluble. We can therefore access this plant medicine with water preparations or a low percentage alcohol tincture.

Plants containing triterpenoid saponins: licorice, eleuthrococcus, ashwagandha, astragulus.

Steroidal saponins, like triterpenoid saponins, enjoy a bath with fat and dislike water. However, they too travel around with plants on sugar molecules and therefore can be extracted with a low percentage alcohol, a water infusion or decoction.

Plants with steroidal saponins: wild yam, fenugreek seeds, american and korean ginseng, devil's club.

In my personal experience of making medicine with plants containing both types of saponins, a tincture with 45%-60% alcohol is best for extraction.

Note all the plants that contain saponins are classed as adaptogens.

Resins

Resins are like a very thick volatile oil and strongly dislike water. To pull resins from plant material, either an oil is needed or an 80% – 90% alcohol tincture. Resins are typically strongly anti-microbial and willing to take on fungal, viral and bacterial infections.

Poplar balsam buds are a perfect example of resinous medicine. The resin provides a protective layer over the young buds insulating them from cold. In the heat of the sun, they soften, giving off their distinct sweet musky aroma, strongly associated

What is a menstruum?
A menstruum is the solvent herbalists use to extract the medicine from plants. Menstruums are usually a combination of substances, in paticilar the alcohol and water of tinctures. But honey, vinegar and glycerine may also be part of a menstruum.

with the first day outside in a t-shirt after a long winter, the sun kissing everything alive. Poplar resin also protects the young delicate bud from water damage that may occur during spring's thaw/freeze cycles.

Infusing the buds in oil creates a warming topical remedy useful in soothing aching joints and relieving inflammation.

Macerating the buds in 90% alcohol creates a strongly anti-bacteria tincture, particularly useful for lung infections. Recall that the trees are by many considered the lungs of the planet.

Carotenes

Carotenes are orange, as in carrots. There are over 600 identified carotenes in plants. It is estimated that 50 of them are common in our diet. Plants use carotenes to protect themselves from the radiation of the sun. Plants use flavonoids in a similar way.

Carotenes differ from flavonoids in that they like oil and dislike water. Carotenes specifically protect fat from oxidation. This includes human cell membranes. The endocrine system organs such as the testes, adrenal glands and ovaries store carotenes and many herbalists use plants high in carotenes to balance hormones. Recall that hormones, although made from protein, travel through the blood stream on fat. Perhaps this is part of the relationship between the carotenes, endocrine system and hormone balance.

Carotenes are also good for eyes.

To access the carotenes in medicine, it is necessary to either use oil as a solvent or a medium to high percentage of alcohol.

Polysaccharide

Polysaccharides are a big group of plant constituents that is similar in size to the volatile oils. Polysaccharides are a group of different types of sugars. Plants make sugar, also called carbohydrates, to live on. Animals (including humans) eventually also turn all sources of nutrients into sugar to be used for energy. In making medicine, polysaccharides are extracted from plants using all water.

Let's look at the different types of polysaccharides.

Immune-modulating polysaccharides

These sugars are either a very complex sugar molecule or a sugar attached to a protein. In either case they stimulate the immune system. How they act on the body in not well understood. Calendula contains polysaccharides engaged with a protein. Consider the other plants with similar polysaccharides, and it easy to see the immune modulating similarities: echinacea, arnica, wild indigo, plantain, shiitake mushrooms.

Mucilage

Mucilage is all sugar. Mucilage loves to thicken up and get slippery in water. Mucilage is found in plants called demulcents. They include: marshmallow, comfrey, slippery elm, plantain.

A cold infusion is the recommended method to extract mucilage from a plant. To prepare a cold infusion combine one cup of cold water with between 1 tsp to 1 tablespoon of herb, cover and put in fridge overnight. In the morning, you will find a thick, gooey substance that will heal an irritated digestive, respiratory, urinary, and reproductive tract.

Personally, I recommend cold infusions of mucilage herbs. Mucilagenous plants can also be tinctured in a lower percentage of alcohol (15-35% or whatever the number actually is), but personally, I recommend cold infusions. Low alcohol tinctures of plants with a high mucilage content are just too thick."

Flavonoids

Like carotenes, plants make flavonoids to protect themselves from the sun's radiation. Unlike carotenes, flavonoids come in a rainbow of colours and in some cases, like the volatile oil, the specific colour of the flavonoid is used to attract the perfect insect for pollination.

Like carotenes, flavonoids generally prefer oil to water when it comes to solubility. But unlike carotenes, flavonoids are usually attached to a sugar (glycoside) making them water-soluble. Because of flavonoids affinity for sugar, it makes it difficult to discern the appropriate water to alcohol ratio in a tincture.

For example, the flavonoid rutin is a fat-soluble flavonoid that requires a high percentage alcohol for extraction into medicine. When rutin attaches itself to a glycoside, it becomes quercetin, which is water-soluble. One trick a herbalist can use when wanting to encourage extraction of fat-soluble constituents is to add a little honey to the menstrum. The honey provides the gylcosides needed to create water soluble flavonoids.

In formulation of medicine, adding a plant high in flavonoids will improve absorption of other medicinal constituents, such as saponins and volatile oils.

Alkaloids

This is a very important group of plant constituents to be aware of when making medicine. Some alkaloids can be quite harmful to the human nervous system and liver. Plant alkaloids are a diverse group of chemicals and many have very little in common with each other. However, for the most part, alkaloids dislike water and require a medium high or high percentage of alcohol to be extracted into medicine.

A skilled medicine maker can control the amount the amount of harmful alkaloids in medicine by using a water based preparation or a low alcohol tincture undermining the plant's toxic effects.

The common garden plant Borage is a perfect example. There is an old saying:"Borage for courage". This could be used as a definition of an adaptogen. Borage with its calming effects and willingness to grow almost anywhere would seem to be a perfect herb for the apothecary. However, Borage contains pyrrolizidine alkaloids that are toxic to the human liver. So what to do? A tea or low percentage alcohol tincture will not contain the pyrrolizidine alkaloids. These alkaloids are soluble at around 70% alcohol.

There are many commonly used alkaloids, in particular nicotine and caffeine. The medical profession makes wide use of morphine and codeine. The illicit drug industry enjoys profits from cocaine. Notice two themes developing here. Names of alkaloids end in "ine" and alkaloids generally affect the nervous system.

Berberine from goldenseal and Oregon grape is an alkaloid frequently used in the apothecary. Berberine is from the isoquinoline alkaloid group and does not affect the nervous system. Berberine is strongly anti-microbial. To access the alkaloid berberine, a tincture needs at least 60% alcohol. Other plants with isoquinoline alkaloids are barberry, bloodroot, and celandine, all anti-microbial with effects on the liver and bowel.

Another commonly used alkaloid rich plant is lobelia.

Lobelia was the darling of Dr. Christopher, the 19th century American herbalist. Recall the BFC or "Bones/Flesh/ Cartilage" formula.

Lobelia is complex mix of at least 14 alkaloids, some of which are relaxing and some some of which are stimulating to the central nervous system. Herbalists primarily think of lobelia as a relaxant and make particular use of it in formulas designed to relax the bronchi as in asthma and chronic irritated coughs.

Lobelia in large doses is poisonous. However, in large doses (and even in not so large doses), it is an emetic. Lobelia forces people to vomit. There is little fear of giving too much lobelia and it causing lasting harm.

Because lobelia's alkaloids relax smooth muscle tissue, it is useful as a carrier herb in a formula. Personally I add it to a formula when a stressed out client complains of tight neck and shoulder muscles. The chronic state of tension in the muscle (apart from the mind) causes sleeplessness. A little lobelia eases the muscular tension.

Tannins

When thinking of tannins, think about binding. Tannins bind proteins. The tannins in a raspberry leaf spit poultice binds cuts on the knee. A

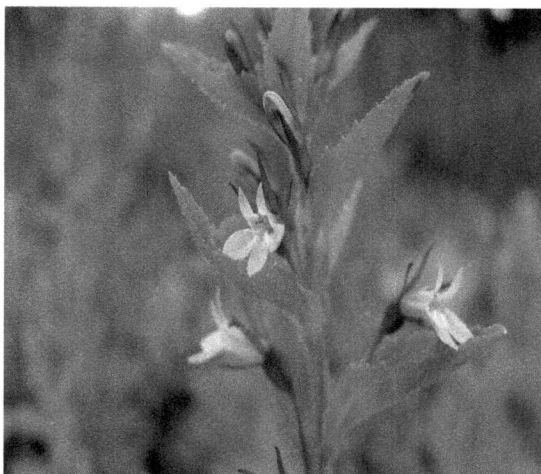

Lobeila   Rosalee de la Forêt

tear in the skin is ripe with loose proteins flowing from blood and torn tissue. Chewing a leaf of raspberry mixes it together with the enzymes in your salvia, breaking down the plant's cell wall and releasing its tannins. When the chewed up leaf is placed over the cut, the tannins knit together the loose proteins by forming a scab and speeding healing along.

Historically plant tannins were painted on animal skins to tan them and create leather. This is another example of how tannins have been used to bind proteins.

Two classes of tannins

Hydrolysable tannins are composed of an alcohol and a sugar. This creates a unique molecule that is both water and alcohol soluble. I use plants with hydrolysable tannins in teas to ease loose stools.

Tannins in tinctures are a bit tricky, as their binding property will become active. Tannins bind or precipitate out alkaloids in a tincture. Tannins neutralize alkaloids. This can be both useful and not so useful for the herbalist. If the alkaloids are not helpful to the formula, tannins will lift them out. If both the tannins and alkaloids are needed in the formula, a good shake before pouring will separate the tannins and alkaloid increase their bioavailability. If there is an accidental poisoning with alkaloids, plants with tannins can be used to counter or nullify their toxicity.

Tannins also precipitate out sugars. Tannins travel throughout living plants bound to sugars. In a formula, the tannins will seek sugars because that is there natural tendency. Shaking the tincture before taking it will make both the sugars and tannins bio-available.

The following traditional formula is used to settle inflamed bowels. The formula makes use of alkaloids, tannins and sugars. This is an important example to demonstrate how multiple and seemingly conflicting plant constituents can work together in a formula to support healing.

Goldenseal (*Hystrastic Canadensis*)   Alkaloids

Bayberry   (*Mycaria cerifera)*Tannins

Fenugreek   (Trigonella foenum-graecum) Mucilage

Turkey Rhubarb (*Rhuem palmata)* Mucilage and anthroquinones

Camellia sinensis (green and black tea) is high in tannins. I recall one English herbalist commenting that many of the digestive issues facing the English population may be due to their addiction to black tea. Although milk (loose proteins) binds many of the tannins in the tea, he wondered if the extreme amount of tea the English consumed was not turning their guts to leather causing malabsorption and its assorted challenges. In any case, tannins desensitize guts.

Tannins are anti-bacterial and anti-inflammatory. They clean up loose proteins and remnants of both white blood cells and the invading bug after a battle between the immune system and a pathogen.

Hydrolysable tannins are found in: raspberry leaf, strawberry leaf, grapes, wild geranium and blackberry leaf.

The second class of tannins is called condensed tannins. These tannins are quite large molecules that enjoy becoming bigger molecules. Condensed tannins are not soluble in water. Condensed tannins are soluble in alcohol.

Condensed tannins are called oligomeric proanthocyanidines (OPCs). (I truly wish for simplicity sake plant molecules only had one name.) These tannins are frequently classes as anti-oxidants and used to support the cardiovascular system. They have similar anti-inflammatory and anti-microbial properties as hydrolysable tannins. Hawthorn, green tea and gingko are all high in OPCs.

Cranberry is also high in OPC. The OPCs in cranberry bind bacteria in the urinary tract, facilitating the infecting organisms' ejection from the body.

Ratios and Percentages with Tinctures

This is a guideline for different amounts of alcohol to use in your tinctures.

Ratio	%	Portions	Original alcohol	Amounts
1:4	25%	100 grams herb 400 ml menstruum	40%	250 ml HO 150 ml H_2O
1:4	60%	100 grams herb 400 ml menstruum	95%	250 ml HO 150 ml H_2O
1:4	70%	100 grams herb 400 ml menstruum	95%	320 ml HO 80 ml H_2O
1:5	45%	100 grams herb 500 ml menstruum	95%	237 ml HO 263 ml H_2O
1:5	25%	100 grams herb 500 ml menstruum	40%	310 ml HO 190 ml H_2O
1:4	35%	100 grams herb 400 ml menstruum	40%	350 ml HO 50 ml H_2O
1:3	75%	100 grams herb 300 ml menstruum	95%	237 ml HO 63 ml H_2O
1:4	40%	100 grams herb 400 ml menstruum	40%	400 ml HO

Note: HO = alcohol and H_2O = water

Summary

There are many other types of phytochemicals. Most have value to both plants and humans. This is just a brief introduction to a few of the larger classes of phytochemicals used by the herbalist in order to elicit specific physiological responses. This is, however, enough to get you started in medicine making.

I encourage you to continue your study of phytochemistry, as it will broaden your appreciation of the incredible elegance of nature and the dynamic interdependence of life.

Thoughts on Standardization of Herbal Medicine

Standardizing herbal products does not necessarily guarantee potency because the medicinal activity is often not due to a single chemical but to a mixture of constituents (many still unidentified), and often to the additive, synergistic (or antagonistic) activity of several components inherently difficult to control all factors that affect a plants chemical composition. - The Clinical Guide to Herbs - Mark Blumenthal

In a culture that believes survival of the fittest is the law of evolution, it is difficult to come to the realization that all beings, plants, animals, humans, and the earth live in dependent and indeed mutually supportive relationships. In a world that uses expressions like "dog eat dog" (although I have never seen a dog eat another), it is difficult for humans to experience the interconnection of life and surrender to the Earth's wisdom. It is almost impossible for humans to believe everything is just fine and doesn't need to be fixed, improved or changed.

I am challenged by belief systems that seek continued improvement and change. When we have only vague glimmerings of the immense interplay between all living beings, perhaps manipulating plants to create patented medicines for profit is not in the best interest for life on the planet.

There are many applications of the word "standardization" in herbal medicine. Some believe that by using standardized names such as the Latin binomial to record the plants used in medicine creates standardized medicine. As you already know, plants have many names! Using one agreed upon name is useful and practical form of standardization.

Others suggest standardization is a set of practices used religiously to prepared plant medicine. These practices include methods of growing, harvesting, drying, solvents and length of maceration, etc.

Typically though, the word "standardized" is most often used to describe a type of plant medicine that carries with it a specific amount of plant compounds (or a singular phytochemical) from batch to batch. These compounds are referred to markers that are measured each time the medicine is made. The marker does not necessarily have any specific medicinal property; it is simply a plant constituent that is easy to measure.

The other form of standardization is an increase in a specific plant constituent that has physiological effects. The process of extraction for this type of pseudo-plant medicine is beyond maceration in a water/alcohol bath or any other traditional solvent. Often isolated plant constituents are added to the medicine. Some herbalists feel this type of standardized medicine can no longer be consider herbal medicine as the focus on isolated chemicals negatively affects the synergy of a complex group of chemicals. In any case, plant medicine made in this manner is patentable. There may be deeper underlying ethical concerns about undermining the universality of plant medicine when the goals of medicine making are patents and therefore, profits.

Creating a Formula

Focus of the Formula

The most important question a herbalist needs to ask when creating individualized formulas for her clients is: what is the focus of the formula? Most people who seek support from a herbalist have multiple health concerns. Often these health concerns overlap andare recognizable layers of unresolved illnesses and/or injuries that have occurred over a lifetime. Deciding where to begin treatment and the focus of the initial formula can be difficult.

I often begin with the client's primary concerns, even when I feel that underlying issues are the true challenge. It is my experience that if a client does not see resolution of their initial complaint, he will not return to work on the underlying challenges. Each herbalist must find her way with this clinical challenge and work on a client-to-client basis. One of the keys to gaining the client's confidence while making headway with treatment is to focus your initial formula on the client's primary concern while using plants with layers of actions.

Case Study

A young man who is a hockey player comes in to the clinic. He suffers with insomnia. He wakes several times a night. He also suffers with lower back pain. The pain is worse in the winter during hockey season; however quitting hockey is not an option. He notices the pain is worse at night and has a hard time getting comfortable. When examined, his lower back shows no signs of redness and heat, and it is cool to the touch. The tension in the muscles was palpable. He has taken over the counter anti-inflammatories for three years two to three times daily. He smokes cigarettes and indulges in binge drinking once or twice a month. He strives to quit smoking, yet has not been successful up to this point. Previously his diet was primarily fast foods, carbs and processed meat. With a recent new love interest, his diet has improved and includes morning smoothies, salads and soups. He notices he is feeling better with the changes in diet. He has come to the clinic because he wants better sleep.

I, the herbalist, know that as long this young man plays hockey (he is a heavy hitting defense man) he will have lower back pain. I also know that it is probably the pain that is waking him. I have concerns for both his liver and lungs due to the toxic load his body carries. I wonder if there is a relationship between the health of his liver and his ability to sleep. I make a mental note to support his liver as we move deeper into the treatment. To begin I decide on an anti-inflammatory formula to ease the back pain. In conversation with the client, I review how his sleep should improve as the pain resolves.

I prepare a tincture of the following plants:

Curcuma longa   Moderates cortisol levels and encourages resolution of inflammation; also a hepatic   protectant.

Populus balsamifera   High in salicylates. Will limit the amount of over-the-counter anti-inflammatories while dulling the pain.

Polygonatum multiflorum   Demulcent for joints and ligaments. Soothes, moistens and heals inflamed joints.

Valeriana officinalis.   Anti-spasmodic; relaxes tension in the muscles and in the mind.

Lobelia inflata   Diffusive; encourages circulation through the lower back.

Effectors vs Tonics (of Physiological Enhancements)

Another way to think through creating a formula is to consider whether the mind/body needs stimulation or relaxation.

Stimulation includes increasing processes of elimination, enhancing circulation and mental processes, waking up the immune system, etc. Herbs that are stimulants can be referred to as effectors. In other words, they affect a specific physiological response from the body. Some effectors are: turkey rhubarb on the bowel, elecampane on the respiratory tract, peppermint on the upper digestive tract, coffee on the nervous system.

Plants that create relaxation calm overactive physiological process due to a pathogen or because the body has been overcompensating due to a prolonged period of stress or illness. This is achieved by using herbs with "anti" as the suffix of their actions, such as anti-microbial or anti-spasmodic. These herbs are also effectors.

Generally, effectors are used for a short time and are discontinued once their effect is achieved.

Tonics (Physiological enhancements) on the other hand replenish the body/mind's resources. They are plants you offer your clients over an extended period of time. These herbs retrain the body/mind while offering deep cleansing and nourishment. Tonic herbs include: nettle, eluethrococcus, oat seed, and dandelion root.

To consider whether a system needs enhancement or quieting down ask the following questions:

Is elimination weak or overactive?

Is circulation overactive and weak?

Is the nervous system underactive or over-stimulated?

Remember though, often the body compensates for a weak system through overstimulation, as in autoimmune diseases. Inflammation can look like over activity when in fact the immune system has stalled. In this situation, herbalists use the immune stimulating and moderating effector plant echinacea to bring the inflammation to resolution.

The Landscape of the Body

Another essential consideration when choosing plants for your formulas is the balance of the element in the body's landscape. Ask the following questions:

Is the body too hot or too cold?

Is it dry or wet?

Assessing the landscape of the body is most easily done through your senses. Does the skin feel hot and dry, warm and moist, cold and dry, or cold and moist? Is the tongue bright red or a lavender colour? Is it dry with cracks or wet with a thick coat? Is the cough productive? Does the chest have a wheeze? Are the stools dry or are they moist?

Dry conditions require demulcents and nutritive herbs.

Wet conditions are helped with astringents.

Cold conditions require circulatory stimulants while hot conditions can be helped with diaphoretics.

Compliance

The best formula in the world cannot resolve illness if the herbs are not taken by the client. Different herbalists have different views on compliance. Personally, I consider it my responsibility to make the medicine easy for the client to take. After I have done everything in my power to facilitate the client's ability to take the medicine, it becomes their responsibility.

When creating medicine consider who the client is. What are her preferences and lifestyle?

A child who prefers bland food requires a mild tasting medicine while someone who frequently uses herbal teas and tinctures can take the most bitter medicine in the apothecary.

Someone on a number of medications may prefer a tea to capsules. More pills may overwhelming him.

When a client is a recovering alcoholic, does not use alcohol due to spiritual beliefs or is just uncomfortable with alcohol in general, the herbalist needs to think outside the tincture bottle.

If the client is in a hurry in the morning and can barely eat breakfast (or does not eat breakfast), tinctures are quicker to take then making a tea.

Many herbs taste wonderful. Many herbs taste horrible. When making a medicine that is not particularly good to taste, warn your client. Make it sound really bad. Give her the space and the right to complain about the taste of her medicine to you (not her friends, this is bad for business!). This helps with compliance. Be sure to also offer several strategies to get the medicine down! Do not ask your clients to sip on a tea of unpleasant tasting herbs.

Start simply. Your clients, like you, are busy. If you begin with too many changes and herbs to take, compliance will fall off. Know what your client can do and offer your medicine accordingly.

Your personal beliefs systems will influence his ability to take plant medicine. For example, sometimes client referrals come only to please a loved one. This can have a profound effect on her ability to take the medicine. This is important information to gather during the consultation so these challenges can be talked about before they burden the healing process.

The Art of the Formula

This system of formulation is borrowed heavily from Traditional Chinese Medicine. It is a template. As with most of herbal medicine, particularly when creating individualized formulas and working holistically, the template must be adaptable to the diverse needs of client, the herbalist and the plants present in the apothecary.

Let's begin with a five herb formula. Personally, I try to stick to between three and five herbs in a formula. (Although it seems like often in student clinic I am continuously recommending six herb formulas!) Different herbalists are comfortable with a varying number of herbs in their formulas. I find when I use more than five herbs, the formula loses its focus. I know exceptional herbalists who regularly use ten herbs in a formula.

The Queen Herb

This is the herb that focuses the formula. The queen makes a statement about the effect the formula will have on the body.

For example: Vitex in the case of adolescent PMS
Meadowsweet in the case of heartburn
Turmeric in the case of chronic inflammation

Note: The Queen is not necessarily the herb with the highest quantity in the formula.

The Ministers

This may be one or two herbs that support the effect of the Queen.

For example:

Vitex is well supported by either vervain or black cohosh. Both plants aid hormone balance and cleansing in the body.

Meadowsweet is supported by licorice and chamomile. These plants both have a cooling effects on the body and improve liver function.

Turmeric is supported by willow and meadowsweet. Willow and meadowsweet contain salicin which offers anti-inflammatory activity.

The Secretaries

This herb helps the plants in the formula work together.
For example:

When creating a formula for adolescent PMS, skullcap eases the tension of teenage angst.

When cooling digestive heat as in heartburn, hops calms the liver and encourages the release of bile and coordinates peristaltic contractions. Hops also quiets down the nervous system when anxiety is disrupting digestion.

During chronic inflammation, echinacea supports the lymphatic system in its role of clearing up the dead cell bits caused by the inflammatory process.

The Messengers

The messenger herb supports the distribution of the medicine throughout the body. Dr. Christopher's favourite carriers were:

Lobelia for relaxing tissue and improving the body's ability to absorb the medicine

Cayenne for increasing circulation to assist the movement of the medicine through the body

Quieter circulatory stimulants such as ginger, rosemary and American prickly ash are also useful messengers.

Plants high in flavonoids are great messengers in a formula. Flavonoids improve the bioavailability of the other plants in the formula. Plants from the rose family are useful here: rosehips and hawthorn berries are my favourites as I grow rosehips and have a hawthorn in my garden. Most circulatory stimulants are also high in flavonoids.

Ratio of Herbs in a Formula

Many North American herbalists determine the amount of each plant in a formula by measuring in parts. A part can be a teaspoon, cup, gram, or kilogram. A formula using this system looks like this:

A tea for heartburn

2 parts meadowsweet   Queen, balances stomach acids

1 part marshmallow leaf   Minister, cools heat in the stomach

3 parts chamomile   Messenger, relaxes the digestion, allow digestive flow

½ part hops   Secretary, enhances bile secretion, improving peristalsis

I was not trained in this method and find it cumbersome. For this simple reason I prefer to take everything to either a 100 millilitres (ml) or a 100 gram (gr) total.

When using the metric system the above formula looks like this:

Meadowsweet	25 grams
Marshmallow leaf	15 grams
Chamomile	50 grams
Hops	10 grams

----

100 grams

Note: grams are for dried plants, while milliletres (mls) are for plants extracted into liquids, such as tinctures.

When working out the amount of each plant in a formula, use these questions as a guideline:

Do any of the plants have a toxic effect in higher dose?

Do any of the plants create unpleasant side effects at higher dose?

How much of the plant do I need to achieve the desired mind/body effect?

What is the sensitivity of the client? Their age? Health? Weight? Constitution?

Are any of the plant actions overlapping? (This will influence the ratio of the plants in the formula.)

Compliance? (Will a higher dose of one of the herbs limit the client's ability to take it?)

Dosing

The science and art of dosing is called Posology. The longer I practice herbal medicine the less standardized my dosing practicing becomes. Each seems like I am continually lowering my doses. There are however a number of considerations to make when dosing herbal medicine.

Chronic vs Acute

We already learned in the chapter on the immune system that when a client suffers with a chronic illness, the general practice is a relatively low dose over an extended period of time.

During an acute illness, herbalists tend to dose quite high over a short period of time.

Age

The following is a general formula for arriving at an appropriate dose of of herbal medicine for children. It is called Young's Formula.

Young's Formula:

Age + 12 / age = dose

Examples: 4yrs + 12 = 16/4 = 4. Therefore, the dose is 1/4 that of an adults

3yrs + 12 = 15/3 = 5. Therefore, the dose is 1/5 that of the adult dose.

I do not always use a child's age for this formula. Some kids are big for their age while others are small. Use common sense here and round the child's age up or down according to their size.

Frail individuals, either seniors or those plagued with long-term illness, need to be initially offered a lower dose.

Finally, as to clients who tell you they are sensitive to herbal medicine: believe them and dose low. Or if you suspect someone is sensitive to herbal medicine, believe yourself and dose low.

You can also increase a dose if the desired results are not being achieved.

Toxic Plants

Know your toxic plants. These herbs have strong physiological effect with low doses. A reliable book for determining which plants require very cautious dosing is *Bartram's Encyclopedia of Herbal Medicine* by Thomas Bartram.

A few toxic herbs in my apothecary are:

Poke root (Phytolacca decandra)

Lobelia (Lobelia inflata)

Mistletoe   (*Viscum album*)

Cedar   (Thuja spp.)

Pasque flower (Pulsatilla vulgaris)

Appendix 1

Type of Preparations

Wherever the art of medicine is loved, there also is love of humanity. - Hippocrates

There are many methods of preparing herbal medicine. Herbal medicine encompasses everything from soups to teas made with milk to high percentage alcohol tinctures. I strongly recommend you try all sorts of methods, solvents and forms of medicine making. Keep good notes and taste all the medicine you make. In this way, you will become very close friends with the plants you use to help others. Making your own plant medicine will give you a special kind of confidence that only comes when your hands are scented with aromas of healing plants.

Tincture

Definition: A water/alcohol extraction of plant medicine

Advantages:

The percentage of alcohol in the tincture will determine the plant constituents extracted. This allows the herbalist control over the chemistry of the tincture and can leave harmful constituents behind in the plant material.

Tinctures do not require large areas for storage.

For the most part, the medicine in tinctures does not degrade with time.

Many people are familiar with tinctures and they are for the most part not difficult to take.

Disadvantages:

Alcohol is not a friendly substance to many people.

Alcohol is expensive and it is very difficult to find alcohol made in a manner that is conscious of the well-being of the planet and all its inhabitants.

It can mask the flavor of plants.(This maybe a benefit, but remember taste is part of a plants medicine.)

Glycerites

Definition: A water/glyercine extraction of plant medicine

Advantages:

Friendlier substance than alcohol. (Be sure to purchase food grade vegetable glycerine.)

Tastes good.

Has emollient and demulcent properties.

It's cheaper than alcohol

Will extract some fat-soluble constituents from plant material.

Disadvantages:

Does not have the same power as a solvent as alcohol does. (Try decocting your plant material before maceration, this seems to help.)

Does not have the same preservative qualities as alcohol, so its shelf life will be much shorter.

Teas (Infusions and decoctions)

Definition: A water extraction of plant medicine.

Infusions are prepared by steeping plant material in cold or hot water. Infusions are primarily used for leaves and flowers.

Decoctions are typically simmered longer and are used to extract the medicine from roots, bark and seeds.

Advantages:

The client is actively involved in preparing her medicine.

The ritual of preparing it can be a moment of rest in the day when she sits and sips her tea.

Tastes pleasant if blended well, and can be immediately nourishing and refreshing.

Disadvantages:

Water will not extract fat-soluble constituents.

Some clients just will not make tea or do not enjoy tea.

Can be difficult to take consistently when travelling.

Capsules

Definition: Powdered plant medicine encapsulated in gelatin capsules.

Advantages:

Clients are familiar with capsules.

Disadvantages:

Lose the medicine in the taste of the plants(particular important with the pungent and bitter herbs. (Review chapter two for details on this.)

Labour intensive to make.

Powdered plants lose their potency.

Oxymel

Definition: A honey/vinegar extraction of plant medicine.

Advantages:

Inexpensive preparations.

Both honey and vinegar have medicinal qualities.

Excellent for extracting alkaloids.

Disadvantages.

Does not extract many fat soluble constituents.

Does not have the same preservative qualities as alcohol, particularly with fresh plant medicines.

Essential Oils

Definition: Industrial extractions of volatile oils from plant material

Advantages:

Concentrated medicine, only a small amount in needed.
Many are entrancing and inspiring to the nostrils and mind.
Strongly anti-microbial.
Many people find the scent of essential oils alluring.

Disadvantages:

Burn the skin when used without a carrier.
Can burn the esophagus, stomach and cause liver damage when taken internally.
Extremely large amounts of plant material are required for making essential oils.
Not a medicine making process available to most herbalists.

Salves

Definition: A topical remedy made from an infused oil and beeswax

Advantages:

Allows medicine to slowly penetrate the skin while protecting the surface from further abrasions.
Easy to make, inexpensive and portable

Disadvantages:

Can leave skin feeling greasy.
Cannot mix water-soluble substances with a salve.

Creams

Definition: Combined oil soluble and water-soluble constituents in topical remedy.

Advantages:

Medicine is quickly absorbed through the skin.

Can combine many different types of plant medicine in one jar.

Disadvantages:

Does not leave a protective barrier on the skin

Can go mouldy over time.

Appendix 2

Harvesting and Drying Medicinal Plants

Harvesting and Drying

Imagine, we are out in the mountains. There is a gorge to our left with quick, cold running water. To our right is a mountain. The ground is dry, reddish grey, and covered in bearberry-- thick green leaves about the size of your baby fingernail with red mealy berries. Intermixed with the bearberry are scrubby juniper bushes with prickly needles and pungent purple berries.

Now, as we know something about herbal medicine, standing here on this ledge we think of urinary tract infections (UTIs). Both herbs are famous for relieving UTIs. And knowing that the antibiotics that are frequently used to treat UTI's are ineffective, we decide to collect some of each plant to help our friends and families with this very common ailment. So here's what we do before we get started....

- -Never gather an endangered or threatened species (and in this example we know that neither bearberry or juniper are).
- -Identify the plant before harvesting it; be absolutely sure that you know what you're harvesting!

- -Ask the plant for permission. If permission is given, offer thanks and acknowledge the connection between all of life. You may decide to offer a gift to the plants.
- -Leave mature and seed producing plants. These are called the Grandparent plants. Seeds run downhill, so if harvesting on a slope, work your way up.
- -Harvest no more than 10% the plants and gather only in abundant plant stands.
- -If wild crafting on public or private land, ask permission.
- -Stay away from downwind pollution, roadsides, high tension electrical wires, public parks, and areas where there have been heavy fertilization and/or pesticide/herbicide use
- -Use gardening techniques such as root division, thinning, and top pinching.
- -If harvesting the leaves, don't pull out the roots.
- -If digging roots, be sure to scatter the seeds of the plant and replace the dirt you have removed.
- -In wild places, plants which complement each other's medicinal activities choose to live in close proximity. Perhaps this is a key to understanding synergy. The bearberry and juniper are an interesting example of this. They both are effective at providing relief for UTIs but from very different angles. Bearberry contains a chemical call arbutin which creates an alkaline urine. Bacteria that prefer an acidic environment suddenly find the urinary tract inhospitable and leave. Juniper on the other hand will not change the pH balance of the urine, but its powerful volatile oils have anti-microbial effects. Juniper is so powerful that one never uses it for more than a 2 week period. Herbalists therefore may

choose to combine these two plants along with others to relieve the infections.

These are guidelines for harvesting herbs.

Harvesting

General Rules of Thumb:

- -Harvest aerial parts in the morning on a sunny day soon after the dew has dried.
- -Harvest leaves and stems just before the plant flowers.
- -Harvest flowers on the morning they open.
- -Harvest roots in the fall when the above ground plant has died back. Or harvest in the spring before growth begins.
- *Harvest your plants when you have time to garble (prepare them for drying). Do not under estimate the amount of time garbling takes!

Drying

Herbs are generally dried in a dark place which is cool and not too moist. Moisture stalls the drying process and the plants will be susceptible to molding. Light and heat degrade the medicinal properties of plants. Some people like to have a gentle breeze which facilitates the drying process. Garden sheds, attics, and closets can be used. Herbs should dry rather quickly; usually no more than a week.

The herbs are ready for storage when they are dry to touch but not brittle. Leave the herbs as whole as possible. Do not break them into bits. Store them in glass jars in a cupboard away from a direct light source. Whole herbs do not lose their medicine as quickly as bits and pieces of herbs.

Different methods

Bundles (For plants with stems which are easy to bundle)

Make a bundle of five to seven stems. You want each stem to be exposed to air. Use a twist tie for binding the herbs. Make it tight, because sometimes when drying the stem contracts and the bundles tumble.

You may choose to place the bundle in a paper bag. (Lunch bags work well, as do paper bags from the liquor store, and being a medicine maker you will have plenty of them). The paper helps absorb the moisture, keeps the herb in the dark and protects it from dust, spiders and what not. Use another twist tie around the bag and hang. Check the herbs in a week.

This is the optimum method.

If you don't have bags and you have time to garble and process them, the bags can be added later or possibly not at all if you have a good drying room.

Paper bags placed over the drying plants is also a useful method for collecting seeds. As the plant dries, the seeds fall into the bag.

Some plants are very long and it is difficult to fit them in a bag. If this is the case, do not cover with a bag.

Laying out flat method.

This method I use for flowers, pieces of root, bark, and single leaves such as comfrey. In a loosely woven basket or a tightly woven wire rack place the flowers or the single leaves until they are dry. I used to spread cheesecloth over the racks, but the plants get caught up the cloth and it becomes a nuisance to untangle the cloth from the herbs.

With really wet plants like comfrey, I place them on a flat basket and leave out in the shade for the day. This quickens the drying process. Do not forget to bring them in before bed, as the dew in the morning will spoil all your drying efforts.

Flowers and leaves do not like to touch when drying. They change colour and look unappealing for medicine.

Cut roots into baby fingernail sized pieces while they are still fresh. Once hard, the roots become much harder to break. If you do not cut the root, put the whole roots in a couple of layers of paper bags, lie them on concrete and smash the roots with a hammer. It seems a bit violent to behave in such a way with medicine, but whole roots are difficult to make medicine with.

Characteristics of well -dried herbs

The leaves and flowers crumble but do not turn to powder.

Roots either snap easily or are really, really hard.

Flowers, leaves, roots and bark retain their colour. If they turn brown, black, grey or colourless, throw them in the compost.

All dried herbs smell like the medicine they will make.

Note: Dehydrators can be too hot for drying herbs. If using a dehydrator to dry your plant material, be sure your dehydrator is set on low.

www.ingramcontent.com/pod-product-compliance
Lightning Source LLC
Chambersburg PA
CBHW050449270326
41927CB00009B/1666